# Recent Advances in Prostate Cancer Research

# Recent Advances in Prostate Cancer Research

Edited by **Karl Meloni**

hayle
medical

New York

Published by Hayle Medical,
30 West, 37th Street, Suite 612,
New York, NY 10018, USA
www.haylemedical.com

**Recent Advances in Prostate Cancer Research**
Edited by Karl Meloni

International Standard Book Number: 978-1-63241-333-8 (Hardback)

Printed in the United States of America.

# Contents

# Preface

This book has been a concerted effort by a group of academicians, researchers and scientists, who have contributed their research works for the realization of the book. This book has materialized in the wake of emerging advancements and innovations in this field. Therefore, the need of the hour was to compile all the required researches and disseminate the knowledge to a broad spectrum of people comprising of students, researchers and specialists of the field.

Prostate cancer is one of the most widespread types of cancer in men and its cure was limited to surgery for confined state and androgen ablation for advanced disease until new alternatives became accessible. This book talks about a broad spectrum of novel facets of the epidemiology of prostate cancer, the diagnosis, cure and patient care, radiation therapy and various other available medical treatments.

At the end of the preface, I would like to thank the authors for their brilliant chapters and the publisher for guiding us all-through the making of the book till its final stage. Also, I would like to thank my family for providing the support and encouragement throughout my academic career and research projects.

**Editor**

# Epidemiology and Etiology

# Epidemiology of Prostate Cancer

Martin Dörr, Anne Schlesinger-Raab and Jutta Engel

Additional information is available at the end of the chapter

## 1. Introduction

This chapter presents the current state of prostate cancer epidemiology and compares data from different regions. The data are taken from several sources:

Globocan 2008 [1] gives a glance on the worldwide situation in cancer epidemiology and permits the comparison of more and less developed regions in every continent.

The "Surveillance, Epidemiology and End Results" Program (SEER) [2] in the USA and the Robert Koch Institute (RKI) [3] in Germany present epidemiologic data of highly industrialized nations with maximally developed medical systems.

The Munich Cancer Registry (MCR) [4], a population-based clinical cancer registry of Upper Bavaria, an area of 4.5 million inhabitants in the South of Germany, presents detailed analyses of clinical data, distributions of prognostic factors and therapy, and survival analyses. Data of the MCR have also contributed to the publication "Cancer Incidence in Five Continents, Volume IX" [5].

## 2. Incidence and mortality

In Table 1 absolute numbers and age-standardized rates of incidence and mortality are presented for selected regions and countries [1]. In 2008 it was estimated that nearly every seventh case of male malignoma was prostate cancer (899 thousand new cases, 13.6% of the total). Therefore, in men prostate cancer was the second most diagnosed cancer after lung cancer. Approximately three quarters of these cases were diagnosed in more developed countries. The highest incidence rates were measured in Australia, New Zealand, Northern and Western Europe and Northern America. Moderate incidence rates were found in South

America and Eastern Europe. The lowest incidence rates were reported from South-Central Asia.

| Region | Incidence absolute | Incidence ASR (W) | Mortality absolute | Mortality ASR (W) |
|---|---|---|---|---|
| World | 899 | 27.9 | 258 | 7.4 |
| More developed regions | 644 | 61.7 | 136 | 10.5 |
| Less developed regions | 255 | 11.9 | 121 | 5.6 |
| Asia | 133.2 | 7.2 | 59.6 | 3.2 |
| North America | 213.7 | 85.7 | 32.6 | 9.9 |
| Central America | 20.5 | 34.8 | 8.1 | 12.6 |
| South America | 84.1 | 50.2 | 29.2 | 16.2 |
| Australia and New Zealand | 21.0 | 104.2 | 4.0 | 15.4 |
| Central and Eastern Europe | 58.4 | 29.1 | 23.1 | 10.9 |
| Northern Europe | 64.9 | 73.1 | 17.4 | 15.4 |
| Southern Europe | 79.5 | 50.0 | 20.4 | 10.4 |
| Western Europe | 167.9 | 93.1 | 28.7 | 12.4 |
| Germany | 70.8 | 82.7 | 12.2 | 11.7 |
| Japan | 38.7 | 22.7 | 10.0 | 5.0 |
| USA | 186.3 | 83.8 | 28.6 | 9.7 |
| Brazil | 41.6 | 50.3 | 14.4 | 16.3 |
| China | 33.8 | 4.3 | 14.3 | 1.8 |
| India | 14.6 | 3.7 | 10.4 | 2.5 |
| Russian Federation | 22.1 | 26.1 | 9.5 | 10.8 |
| SouthAfricanRepublic | 7.5 | 59.7 | 2.5 | 20.8 |

Absolute numbers in thousands; ASR (W): age standardised rate per 100,000 by world standard

**Table 1.** Absolute numbers and age-standardised rates of incidence and mortality for selected regions and countries [1]

Despite its high proportion of cancer diagnoses, prostate cancer is the cause of cancer specific death in only every 16th case (258 thousand deaths, 6.1% of the total). This places prostate cancer on the sixth position of cancer-specific causes of death, topped by lung, liver, stomach, colorectal and oesophageal cancer. These deaths occur almost equally in both, more developed and less developed regions, thus leading to a twofold higher mortality rate in the more developed regions.

## 2.1. Incidence and mortality trends

Table 2 shows the current incidence and mortality of the USA [2], Germany [7, 8] and the Munich Cancer Registry [4]. These rates have changed considerably over time. Time series of more developed countries show that the incidence rates experience a drastic rise from 1985 to 1995 and remain at this high level. In the USA incidence (by world standard per 100,000) increases slowly from 1975 until 1985 (from 50 to 65). Then it rises rapidly reaching a peak of 135 in 1992. Then it decreased, since 1995 more slowly, but it remains on a higher level than before the peak (around 110). In Germany incidence is rising continuously since 1988 (from 30 to 75). The main explanation for these trends is the broad use of prostate specific antigen (PSA) testing as a screening method and performing biopsies, which started in the mid-1980s in the USA and in the early 1990s in Germany.

|  | USA (SEER, NCHS) [2, 6] | Germany (RKI) [7, 8] | MCR [4] |
|---|---|---|---|
| Absolute incidence | 241.7 | 70.8 | 2.9 |
| Crude incidence |  | 157.7 | 145.1 |
| Incidence ASR (W) | 106.1 | 82.7 | 76.4 |
| Mortality ASR (W) | 10.2 | 11.7 | 13.3* |
| Lifetime risk(%) | 16.2 | 13.0 |  |
| Median age at diagnosis(years) | 67.0 | 69.5 | 67.2 |
| Median age at death(years) | 80.0 |  | 76.7 |
| 5-year overall survival(%) , |  | 77.0 | 79.2 |
| 5-year relative survival(%) | 99.2 | 92.0 | 93.4 |
| 10-year overall survival(%) |  |  | 58.2 |
| 10-year relative survival(%) | 98.3 |  | 87.8 |

Absolute numbers in thousands

ASR (W): age standardised rate per 100,000 by world standard

Incidence and mortality from cohorts of 2008 (all regions)

Absolute incidence numbers of the USA are estimates of SEER data from 2012

* Mortality ASR (W) for singular prostate cancers is 9.9

median ages from cohorts of 2005-2009 (all regions)

5-year survival from cohorts of 2002-2008 (SEER and MCR)

10-year survival from cohorts of 1998-2008 (SEER and MCR)

**Table 2.** Epidemiologic basic numbers

In the USA, mortality initially increases slightly from 1975 and since 1992 it is decreasing more rapidly (from 14 over 17 to 10). In Germany the mortality rate (by world standard per 100,000) stays stable at 13.

## 2.2. Age distribution and age-specific incidence and mortality rate

Nearly all patients (≈ 99%) who are diagnosed with prostate cancer have reached an age of fifty or higher. The age distribution at diagnosis describes a positively skewed unimodal distribution with its modus at the age group 65-69. This age group contributes to nearly 25% of all prostate cancer cases. The risk of getting prostate cancer increases nearly exponentially with increasing age. This makes prostate cancer one of the most distinctive cancers in aging populations (Figure 1) with a ASIR of 800-1000 per 100,000 in the elderly of 70 years and older.

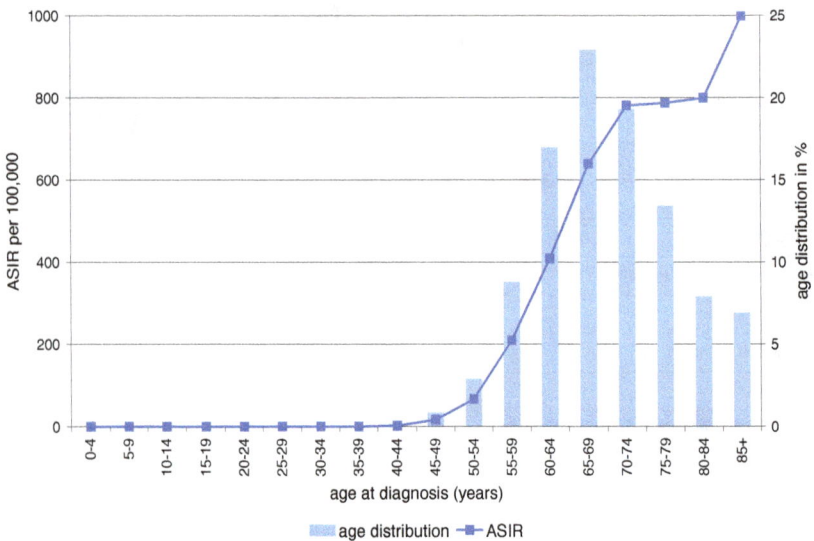

**Figure 1.** Age distribution at diagnosis and age-specific incidence rate (ASIR) of prostate cancer (1998-2008) [4]

Nearly all patients who died of prostate cancer (singular initial malignoma) have reached an age of fifty-five or higher. The distribution of age at death describes a negatively skewed unimodal distribution with its modus at the highest age group 85+. Here the age-specific mortality rates (ASMR) can perfectly be described by an exponential function. The risk of dying by prostate cancer increases accelerated with increasing age (Figure 2). The ASMR reaches 450 per 100,000 for men with an age of 80-84 and already 600 per 100,000 for men older than 84.

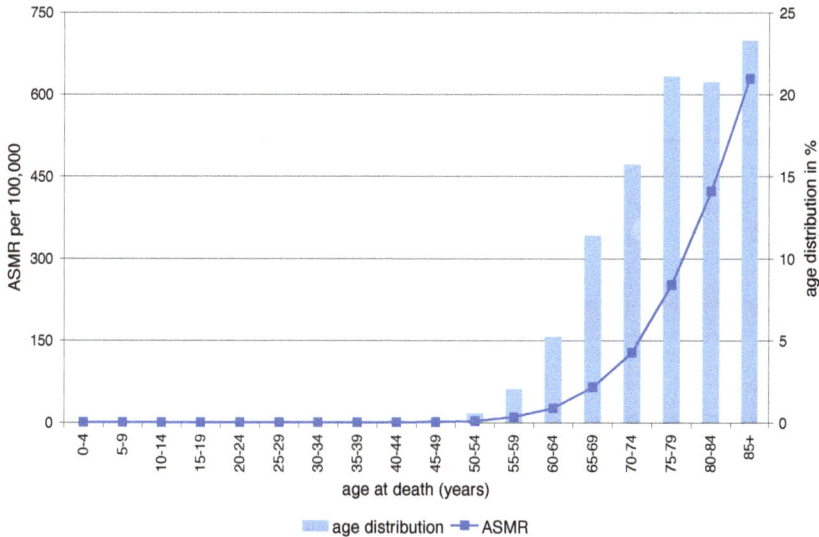

**Figure 2.** Age distribution at death and age-specific mortality rate (ASMR) of prostate cancer (1998-2009) [4]

## 3. Prognostic factors

According to Table 3 the conditional age distributions of the combined T categories 2 until 4 have the same shape and the modus at the age group of 65 until 69. These distributions are shifted slightly towards higher ages with the increasing T category. This simply reflects that it takes time to develop an advanced tumour. However, in those patients diagnosed with T1 category (clinically) the age distribution appears to be totally different. Here 80% of the men are older than 64 (about 60% within the other T categories) and every third man is older than 74.

Lymph node category (N), distant primary metastases (M), Gleason Score, initial PSA value and Gleason Score are positively correlated with the combined T category: the higher the T category, the higher the PSA value, the higher the Gleason Score and the higher the porportion of regional or distant metastases.

A positive lymph node status is mostly diagnosed when the tumour has spread through the prostatic capsule. Nearly 20% of those men with T3 and almost 50% with T4 tumours therefore are diagnosed with lymph node metastasis.

| | T category | | | | |
|---|---|---|---|---|---|
| | T1 % (n=1826 13.3%) | T2 % (n=8219 59.9%) | T3 % (n=3164 23.0%) | T4 % (n=503 3.7%) | All % (n=13712 100%) |
| Age (years) | | | | | |
| <50 | 0.5 | 2.3 | 1.4 | 1.8 | 1.8 |
| 50 - 54 | 1.5 | 4.5 | 3.5 | 3.0 | 3.8 |
| 55 - 59 | 3.0 | 11.0 | 10.2 | 11.1 | 9.8 |
| 60 - 64 | 9.7 | 20.2 | 18.2 | 15.1 | 18.2 |
| 65 - 69 | 20.9 | 31.4 | 32.8 | 26.4 | 30.1 |
| 70 - 74 | 26.1 | 20.2 | 23.1 | 19.7 | 21.7 |
| ≥75 | 38.3 | 10.4 | 10.8 | 22.9 | 14.7 |
| Lymph node status | | | | | |
| N+ | 2.5 | 1.6 | 18.4 | 45.1 | 7.3 |
| N0 | 40.6 | 85.2 | 73.5 | 33.6 | 76.2 |
| NX | 56.9 | 13.2 | 8.1 | 21.2 | 16.5 |
| Metastasis status | | | | | |
| M0 | 97.4 | 98.8 | 95.4 | 72.6 | 96.9 |
| M1 | 2.6 | 1.2 | 4.6 | 27.4 | 3.1 |
| PSA value (ng/ml) | | | | | |
| < 4 | 25.8 | 13.2 | 7.8 | 3.7 | 13.2 |
| 4 - <10 | 42.0 | 60.7 | 41.5 | 18.9 | 52.4 |
| 10 - <20 | 17.5 | 18.3 | 24.9 | 15.7 | 19.7 |
| ≥20 | 14.7 | 7.8 | 25.7 | 61.8 | 14.8 |
| Gleason Score | | | | | |
| 2 - 4 | 14.3 | 1.6 | 0.2 | 0.2 | 2.9 |
| 5 - 6 | 54.8 | 48.1 | 12.3 | 4.2 | 39.1 |
| 7 | 19.1 | 40.5 | 49.4 | 26.6 | 39.3 |
| 8 - 10 | 11.8 | 9.8 | 38.2 | 68.9 | 18.7 |

Presented numbers are column-wise percentages.

T category is a combination of cT and pT.

The disease cohort is limited to 2005-2009 to provide best current estimators.

**Table 3.** Prognostic factors by T category [4]

Although, only 2.4% of all prostate cancer cases have primary distant metastases, already 25% of the T4 patients are diagnosed with metastases.

About 50% of the men with prostate cancer have a PSA value of 4 to 10 ng/ml at initial diagnosis.

According to Figure 3aa shift from capsule exceeding tumours to capsule limited tumours took place in the 1990s. In the late 1980s about 15% of the diagnosed tumours were staged T4, some 45% T3 and nearly 25% T2. In the 2000s only some 5% of the diagnosed tumours were staged T4, good 20% T3 and about 60% T2. The T1 category was unaffected and oscillated around 12% during the whole time period. It seems that PSA-Screening has considerably lowered the proportion of locally advanced tumours.

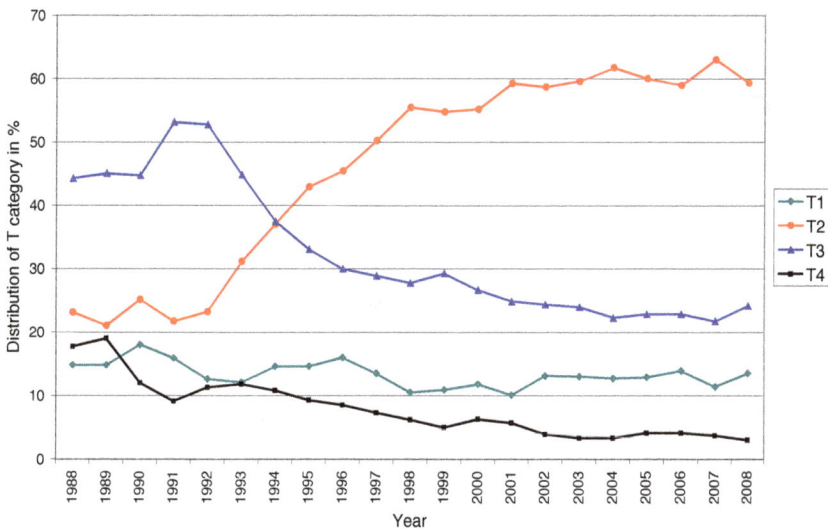

**Figure 3.** Distribution of T category over time (n = 35544) [4]. T category is a combination of cT and pT.

## 4. Therapy

Table 4 presents in detail the effects of combined T category on the choice of therapy. Guidelines [9] note that radical prostatectomy, radiation therapy and hormone therapy in combination with radiation therapy are the main primary treatment options when the tumour remains within the prostate capsule (T2) or does not invade nearby structures other than the seminal vesicles or the bladder neck (T3). A spreading prostate cancer should be treated with a hormone therapy. Active surveillance (AS) and watchful waiting (WW) are only noteworthy initial therapy strategies for tumours detected in an early stage. Although these are accepted treatment options in localised prostate cancer, they are seldom chosen compared to radical prostatectomy and hormone therapy. Transurethral resection of the prostate is not an appropriate surgical treatment option in prostate cancer but its proportion in T1 category (46.7%) indicates a greater proportion of incidentally found prostate cancers during a treatment of benign hyperplasia. Without further surgical or hormone therapy, one could classify these cases into the AS or WW groups.

| | T category | | | | |
|---|---|---|---|---|---|
| | T1 % (n=1826 13.3%) | T2 % (n=8219 59.9%) | T3 % (n=3164 23.0%) | T4 % (n=503 3.7%) | All % (n=13712 100%) |
| Initial therapy | | | | | |
| RPE | | 74.9 | 65.9 | 31.3 | 61.8 |
| TUR | 47.2 | 3.2 | 2.5 | 11.4 | 9.0 |
| HIFU | 4.5 | 3.4 | 0.8 | 0.2 | 2.8 |
| XRT | 16.6 | 6.1 | 9.8 | 12.7 | 8.5 |
| Hormone | 23.7 | 11.6 | 20.3 | 44.2 | 16.4 |
| AS and WW | 8.0 | 0.8 | 0.7 | 0.2 | 1.6 |

Presented numbers are column-wise percentages.

T category is a combination of cT and pT.

The disease cohort is limited to 2005-2009 to provide best current estimators.

RPE: radical prostatectomy, TUR: transurethral resection of the prostate, HIFU: high-intensity focused ultrasound, XRT: radiation therapy, Hormone: hormone therapy, AS: active surveillance, WW: watchful waiting

**Table 4.** Initial therapy by T category [4]

As Figure 4 shows impressively, initial therapy strategies have changed noticeably over the last 20 years. In the late 1980's radical prostatectomy was the initial therapy in about 25% of all treatments. Its rate increased continuously and finally reaches almost 60%, making this the most selected initial therapy per year since 1995. The curve of hormone therapy developed oppositely. To be more precise: hormone therapy was the most selected treatment till 1994. From 65% in 1989 it continuously decreased to now 20%. Radiation therapy (XRT) slightly increased to 10% as initial therapy. Finally, within the whole time span transurethral resection of the prostate (TUR) remains stable at a proportion of nearly 10%.

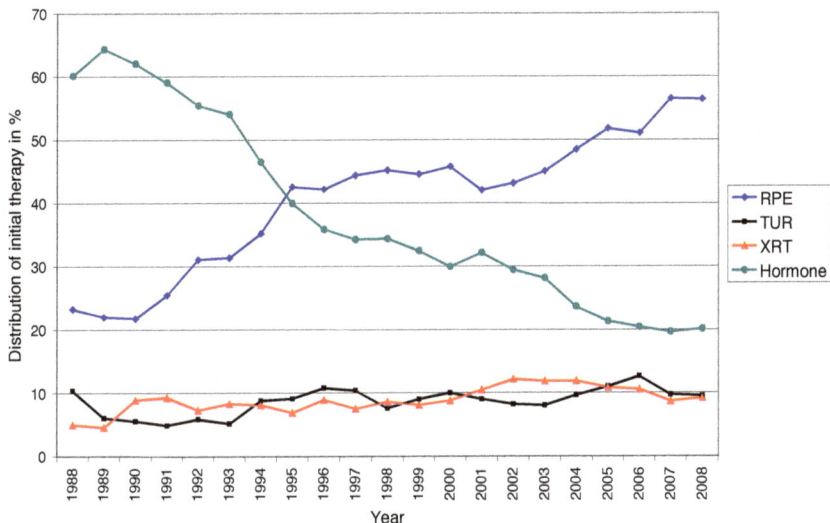

**Figure 4.** Distribution of initial therapy strategies over time (n = 35544) [4]. RPE: radical prostatectomy, XRT: radiation therapy, Hormone: hormone therapy, TUR: transurethral resection of the prostate

## 5. Survival

The following figures mainly present the relative survival (RS) curves, an estimator for the cancer specific survival. This is calculated by dividing the overall survival (OS) of the observed cohort by the expected survival of a normal population with the same distribution regarding birth-date and sex.

When looking at the influence of the year of diagnosis on the overall survival (Figure 5) or relative survival (Figure 6) only the curve of patients with a diagnosis in the years 1998 until 1992 noticeably differs from the other ones. Here the 5- and 10-year relative survival was 85.0% and 74.3%, respectively. In the group of patients diagnosed between 1993 and 1997 the 5- and 10-year relative survival was 94.9% and 88.6% in the group of 1998-2002 the 5- and 10-year relative survival was 94.0% and 84.1% and in the recent group of 2003-2008 the 5-year relative survival was 92.1%. Therefore, the following survival analyses are presented for patients with a diagnosis between 1998 - 2008.

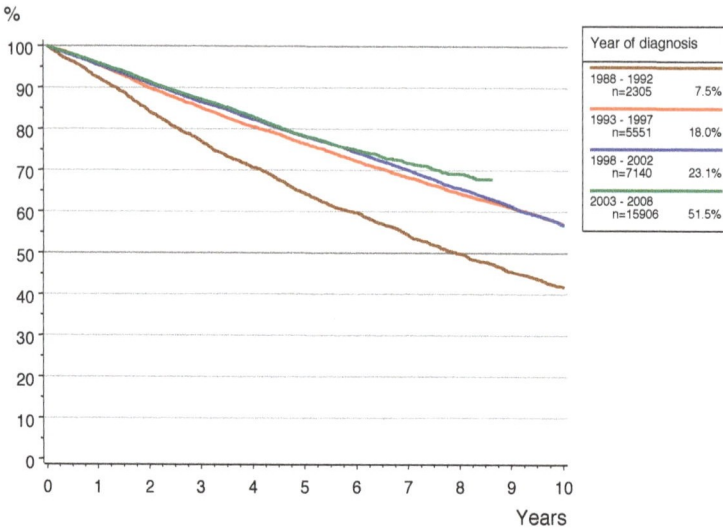

**Figure 5.** Overall survival by year of diagnosis (n=30902) [4]

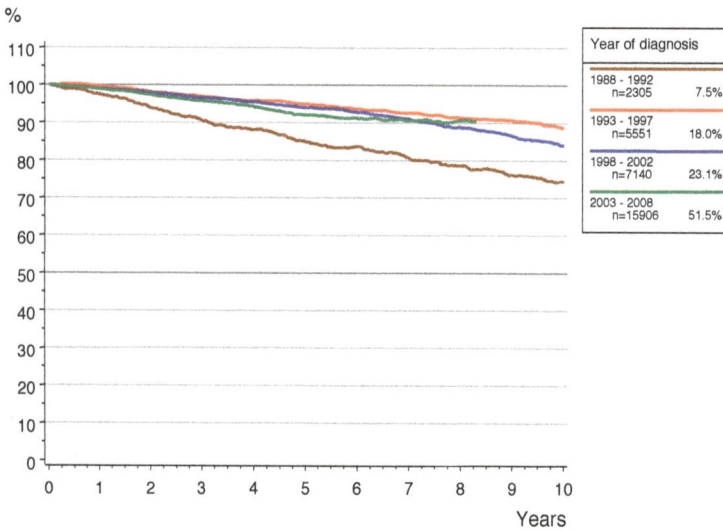

**Figure 6.** Relative survival by year of diagnosis (n=30902) [4]. Relative survival is the quotient of overall survival and expected survival and thus an estimator for the cancer specific survival.

The complete cohort of prostate cancer patients with a diagnosis between 1998 and 2008 (Figure 7) shows a 5-year overall survival of 78.8% and a 10-year overall survival of 57.7%. The relative survival is 93.6% and 84.1%, respectively. For comparison: SEER data show a 5-year relative survival of 99.2% for patients diagnosed between 2002 and 2008 and a 10-year relative survival of 98.3% for the cohort of 1998 – 2008.

Figure 8 presents the relative survival by the combined T category. As expected, patients with a T2-staging perform better than patients with a T1-Staging. The 5- and 10-year relative survival is 102.0% and 94.0% in T1, 104.9% and 108.8% in T2, 97.6% and 89.5% in T3 and 61.4% and 43.8% in T4, respectively. Relative survival can exceed 100%, because prostate cancer patients benefit from the better treatment of comorbidities during aftercare.

Lymph node status (N category) is an important prognostic factor. As Figure 9 shows, a positive lymph node status (N+) reduces the relative survival drastically (77.7% for 5-year and 61.9% for 10-year survival) compared to a 5- and 10-year survival of 105.5% and 107.5% in N0. Nonetheless, prostate cancer patients benefit from radical prostatectomy in the situation with lymph node metastases [10].

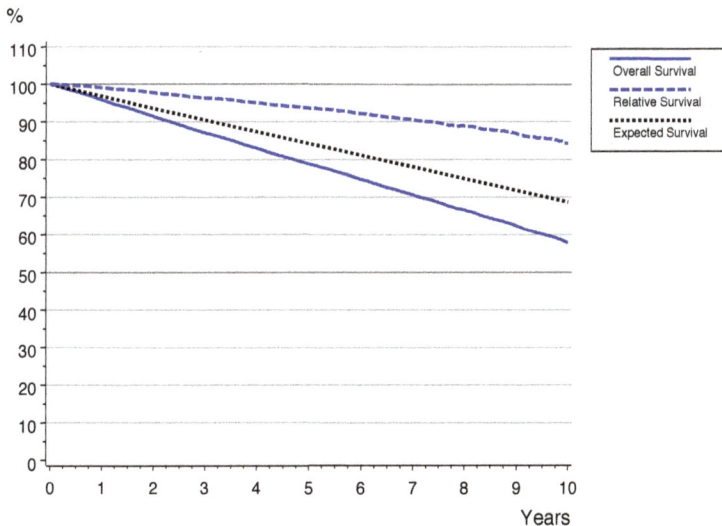

**Figure 7.** Overall, relative and expected survival of the complete collective (1998-2008, n = 25773) [4]. Relative survival is the quotient of overall survival and expected survival and thus an estimator for the cancer specific survival.

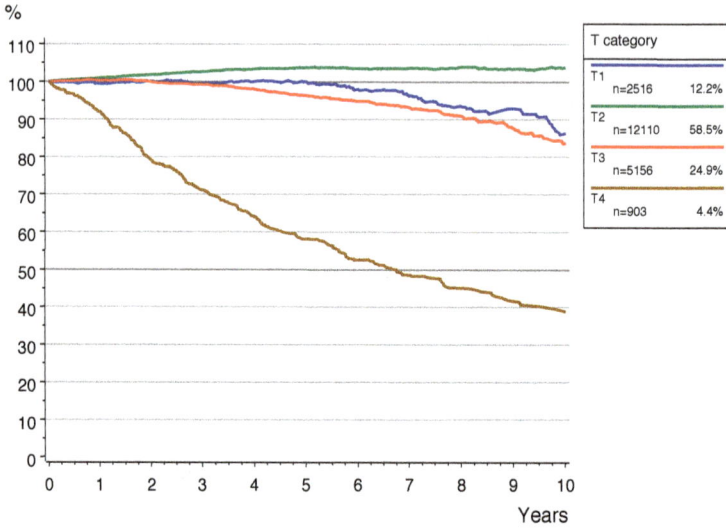

**Figure 8.** Relative Survival by T category (1998-2008, n = 20685) [4]. T category is a combination of cT and pT.

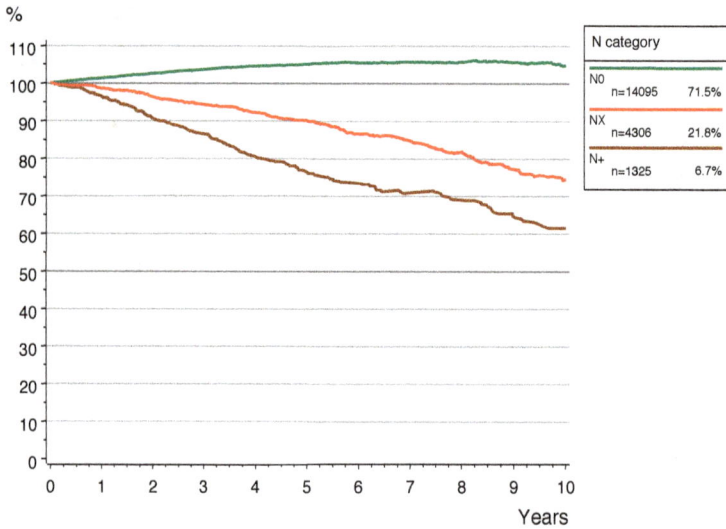

**Figure 9.** Relative Survival by N category (1998-2008, n = 19726) [4]. N category is a combination of cN and pN.

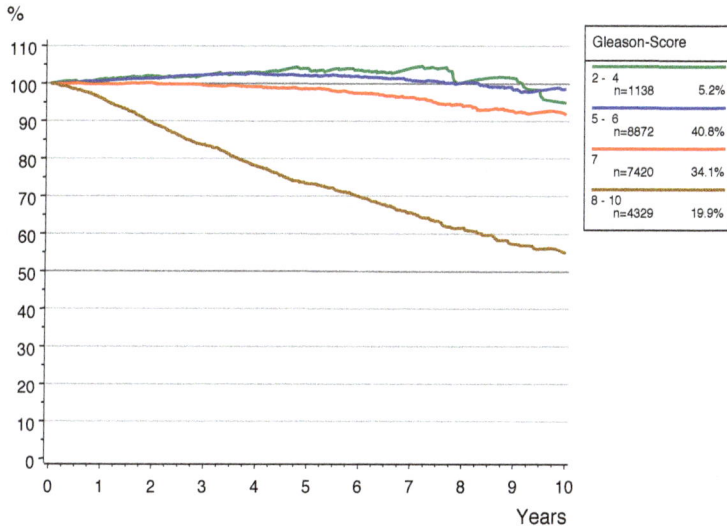

**Figure 10.** Relative survival by Gleason Score (1998-2008, n = 21759) [4]

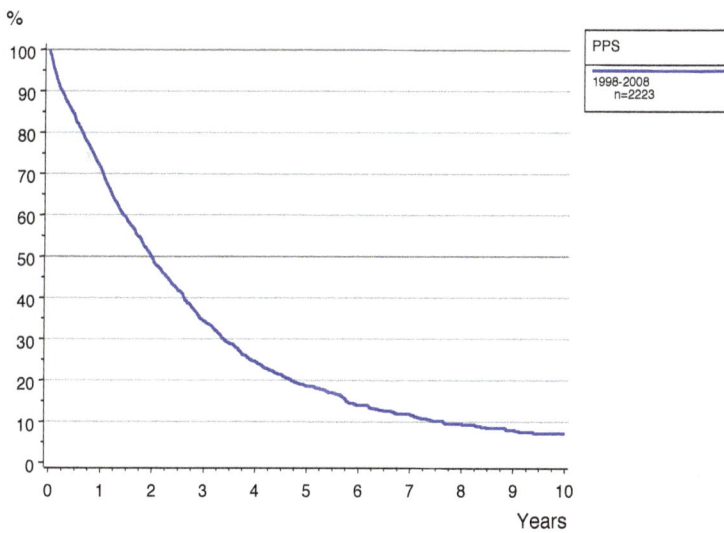

**Figure 11.** Post Progression Survival (1998-2008, n = 2223) [4]. Starting point of progression is from date of locoregional relapse or distant metastasis (primary M1 or metastases in further course of disease).

According to Figure 10 patients with the worst Gleason Score category (8 – 10) have a much poorer survival (73.4% for five year and 55.0% for ten year survival) than patients with a scoring of 7 and better, which does not discriminate very much (104.1% and 94.8% for Gleason Score 2 - 4, 102.2% and 98.6% for Gleason Score 5 – 6 and 98.6% and 91.8% for Gleason Score 7).

If the tumour has metastasised or locoregional recurrence has occurred, only 18.2% of the patients survive 5 years and 7.2% of the patients survive 10 years. The median survival is about two years (Figure 11).

## Nomenclature

WHO→World Health Organization

SEER→"Surveillance, Epidemiology and End Results" Program of the National Cancer Institute of the USA

NCHS→National Center for Health Statistics

RKI→Robert Koch Institut

MCR→Munich Cancer Registry

PSA→Prostate specific antigen

RPE→Radical prostatectomy

XRT→Radiation therapy

HIFU→High-intensity focused ultrasound

Hormone→Hormon therapy

TUR→Transurethral resection of the prostate

AS→Active surveillance

WW→Watchful waiting

ASR (W)→Age-standardised rate, using the proposed world standard population of Segi (1960)

ASIR→Age-specific incidence rate

ASMR→Age-specific mortality rate

## Author details

Martin Dörr, Anne Schlesinger-Raab and Jutta Engel

Munich Cancer Registry (MCR), Clinic Großhadern / IBE, Ludwig-Maximilians-University (LMU), Germany

# References

[1] Ferlay, Shin, Bray et al., Globocan 2008: Cancer Incidence and Mortality Worldwide; 2011. http://globocan.iarc.fr.

[2] National Cancer Institute: "Surveillance, Epidemiology and End Results" (SEER) Program. http://www.seer.cancer.gov.

[3] Robert Koch Institut (RKI). http://www.rki.de.

[4] Munich Cancer Registry (MCR). http://www.tumorregister-muenchen.de.

[5] IARC Scientific Publications, Cancer Incidence in Five Continents, Volume IX, 2009. http://ci5.iarc.fr/.

[6] Siegel, Naishadham and Jemal, Cancer statistics, 2012. CA: A Cancer Journal for Clinicians 2012; 62(1):10–29.

[7] Cancer in Germany 2005/2006. Incidence and Trends. Seventh edition Robert Koch Institut (ed) and Association of Population-based Cancer Registries in Germany (ed). Berlin, 2010.

[8] Cancer in Germany 2007/2008. Eighth edition. Robert Koch Institut (ed) and Association of Population-based Cancer Registries in Germany (ed). Berlin, 2012.

[9] National Institute for Health and Clinical Excellence. www.nice.org.uk.

[10] Engel, Bastian et al., Survival benefit of radical prostatectomy in lymph node-positive patients with prostate cancer. Eur Urol 2010; 57(5):754-61.

# Chapter 2

# Is There an Infectious Agent Behind Prostate Cancer?

Ugo Rovigatti

Additional information is available at the end of the chapter

## 1. Introduction

This CHAPTER deals with a more defined and specified issue: whether we can already identify, point our fingers toward a specific infectious agent or infectivity pathway most likely targeting and lurking behind prostate cancer (PCa). This issue became quite evident in the past 5-6 years, in view of the heated debate on the possible role of a what was considered a novel retrovirus: Xenotropic Murine Related Virus, or XMRV, in the aetiology of PCa and subsequently also of Chronic Fatigue Syndrome (CFS). Over two years ago, the same issue was discussed by the author at the International Congress on Muscle Fatigue held in Pisa in July 2010. That presentation has been now transformed in a paper, which is in press in the journal Neuro Muscolar Disease (NMD, Springer Verlag) [1]. The reader is therefore referred to that article -most likely already published by the time of this book printing- for aetiological considerations on CFS [1]. In this section, I will more extensively discuss the association of XMRV with PCa. Such an association was the first one to be discovered and this finding was the basis for also searching XMRV in CFS. In CFS, the potential association with an infective agent doesn't appear to be trivial, since "fatigue" has been widely associated with several types of cancer in the so called Cancer Related Fatigue (CRF), also discussed more extensively in the NMD paper [1] [2].

## 2. Discovery and falsification of XMRV

### 2.1. Linkage RNASEL – HPC-1

XMRV isolation was not a sudden or isolated finding, but it rather stemmed out of approximately twenty years of research by several groups, with a leading role by the group of R. Silverman [3] [4]. This work, as well, has even older roots, since it was initiated by deciphering the antiviral response triggered by Interferon (IFN). Robert Silverman's work was pioneering and seminal in this effort: together with Ian Kerr, he clarified the Interferon (IFN) response to viral infection, initially by characterizing the 5'-triphosporylated, 2',5'-linked oligoadenylates or 2-5A, a second messenger in the IFN response and its synthesizing enzyme (oligo-2',5'-A synthethase, or OAS) and finally discovering that 2-5A is the activator of an endogenous RNase activity, called RNase L [5] [3]. This is ubiquitously distributed but inactive inside cells, but it becomes strongly activated by binding 2-5A. By using radiolabelled 2-5A as probe, Silverman was able to identify and clone the gene *RNASEL* and to map later its location on chromosome 1q25 [5]. After approximately ten years, these studies intersected a totally different discovery path. Linkage studies on families with increased hereditary risk of prostate cancer, identified in 2002 the prostate carcinoma susceptibility gene (*Hereditary Prostate Carcinoma 1, HPC-1*) on chromosome 1q25, the same of *RNASEL* location [6]. Different alleles on this locus were associated with higher risk of PCa, such as the R462Q variant, which appeared to provide a 50% risk increase, while homozygosity doubled the risk [7]. This association between a locus behaving as a Tumor Suppressor Gene (*TSG*) and an Anti-Viral Response (*AVR*) gene is strongly suggestive of viral involvement in PCa. In the July 2010 presentation at the International Meeting on Muscle Fatigue -which was very critical of the XMRV identification- the sound evidence for viral involvement was emphasized. A logical-inference analysis showed that –most likely- a wrong viral candidate was chosen [1], Fig.1. Subsequent work has vindicated our first prediction (XMRV falsification), but additional work is required to strength the association with another candidate Virus that we propose: MFV (see later) [1]. Several studies have confirmed the RNASEL-HPC1 association [7] [8] [9] [4], but not all [10] [4] of them.

## 2.2. XMRV discovery

For another five years at the turn of the century, these discoveries on HPC-1 remained just suggestive of a viral involvement in PCA, for a locus –RNASEL- which behaves as a Tumor Suppressor Gene (TSG) –as already indicated by an interesting Editorial by Lengyel, in 1993 [11] and as suggested by others [12] [13]. Then Silverman with colleagues DeRisi and Ganem utilized a micro-array approach (*viro-chip*) [14], in order to try identifying the responsible virus [3, 15]. The first papers on XMRV appeared at the end of 2006/ beginning of 2007: they showed that XMRV was present at high frequency in patients homozygous for the R462Q allele (i.e., 8/20 or 40%) and that it is a xenotropic retrovirus with similarities with murine leukaemia viruses (MuLV) [16] [15]. Xenotropic retroviruses are endogenous viruses, which cannot infect cells of the original species, while ecotropic viruses do. Typically, endogenous murine retroviruses have been divided into two large families: ecotropic and non-ecotropic retroviruses [17] [18]. Ecotropic retroviruses -being still capable of active infection in the same species, i.e. mouse, cells- are present in only one or just a few copies (0-6) per genome. Their genetics is rather well clarified by several years of research [19]. The structure/genetics of the non-ecotropic retroviruses is more complex, also in view of the fact that they are present in a considerable (40-60) number of copies/genome. In recent years, particularly thanks to the work of J. Coffin and J. Stoye [20], non-ecotropic retroviruses have been clarified and subdivided into three subfamilies: xenotropic (XMP), not capable of replicating inside cells of the same species, polytropic (PMV), which are capable of replicating inside cells of several species including the original (mouse) and modified-polytropic (MPMV), which display altered properties in terms structure/function of the *env* gene [21] [17] [18]. The experiments, which distinguish among different subfamilies of non-ecotropic mouse retroviruses are: 1. infectivity/replication assays; 2. characterization of their structure by restriction enzyme and/or Southern blotting analysis; 3. complete sequencing [20, 21]. For a more detailed overview of this fascinating but rather complex scientific area, the reader is referred to two excellent review articles by J. Coffin and J. Stoye [17] [18].

### 2.3. Positive evidence

XMRV was also found integrated inside mesenchimal/stromal cells -rather than in tumour cell genomes- in proximity of genes of cell cycle or hormonal control, which could provide a reasonable link to carcinogenesis [16] [4]. Indeed, such mechanisms variably defined as "promoter insertion" or "insertional mutagenesis" appear to be the most likely involved in chronically (or non-acutely) transforming Retroviruses [22] [23]. This initial report by the discoverer group was followed up a few months later by another PNAS paper, by Schlaberg et al., in which XMRV was associated to approximately 23% of cases by immuno-histochemistry (IHC), while detection of viral DNA by PCR was quite lower (6%) [24]. Beside this rather surprising finding (since the opposite would be typically expected), this report also slightly contradicted the previous ones, since 1. XMRV was directly identified in the carcinoma cells and not in surrounding mesenchimal/stromal cells, 2. there was no evidence of an association between XMRV positive cases in PCa and RNAse-L involvement by mutation/lower function, as previously described in the Urisman et al. paper [15, 24]. In that report, 40% of cases which were homozygous for the R462Q variant in RNAse-L were XMRV+ [15]. In the following months of 2010, another group from Emory University in Atalanta (GA) also reported an association between XMRV and PCa, by employing three different and complementary technologies [25]: a) a very sensitive "nested" PCR assay, b) chromosomal fluorescence hybridisation (FISH) and c) very sensitive technology for detection of neutralizing antibodies (the same group and others had previously developed this technique for detecting anti-HIV antibodies) [26] [27] [25]. Also in this report, the serologic assay was the most sensitive, detecting XMRV antibodies in 27.5 % of cases (11/40), while positivity increased in carriers of the R462Q allele (8/20 –also in this study- or 40% of cases, which were RNASEL R462Q homozygous) [25]. Finally, this report confirmed, as in the original paper by Urisman et al., the presence of XMRV in stromal/mesenchimal and not in carcinoma cells [25]. In the same year, another group from Baylor College in Houston (TX) also detected an association between XMRV and PCa in 22% of cases [28]. However, virus was strangely detected in both tumour and normal cells of affected patients and there was no correlation –as in Schlaberg et. al - with RNaseL status [28].

### 2.4. Negative findings

Together with the appearance of such positive reports, however, a series of studies presenting negative findings started to appear in the literature. Many of these negative reports came from European laboratories, although an initial negative study –often ignored- was from Johns Hopkins University (JHU) in the US [29]: see below. While the issue of XMRV detection in PCa was getting more controversial, another "XMRV-front" opened with the publication in October 2009 of a paper in Science, where Lombardi et al. reported detection of XMRV in 67% (68/101) of Chronic Fatigue Syndrome (CFS) cases [30]. While controls showed much lower detection rates, i.e. 3.7% (8/218), such value (as well as previous ones) was alarming, since it suggested that a few million people may be infected in the general "healthy" population in the US and probably elsewhere [31]. The initial Lombardi et al. paper was followed by larger numbers of negative reports, appearing in the months immediately after its publication: they will not be reviewed extensively in this chapter and the reader is referred instead to the NMD paper [1], with only one exception. In September 2010, Lo et al. published a PNAS paper describing rather frequent association between CFS and a retrovirus different from XMRV: indeed this virus appeared to be polytropic (P-MLV) instead of xenotropic (X-MLV) [32]. While some scientists applauded this novel discovery [33], the PNAS paper was accompanied by an editorial by Andrew Mason's group, in which perplexities about these very findings were expressed [34]. Indeed, despite the relationship between the two viruses, it was extremely difficult to reconcile these findings or even to explain the discovery of XMRV as due to presence of P-MLV instead. In fact, the two viruses are clearly distinguishable by sequencing. Therefore, the idea presented at that time [33]: that the real culprit in CFS would be P-MLV and that the previous detection of XMRV should *de facto* be considered P-MLV detection, or that either virus could cause the same disease, was simply wrong.

The very first negative report for XMRV in PCa was from Hamburg, DE and was authored (1st) by one of the first co-authors of the original paper by Urisman: Nicole Fischer [35]. This suggests that very similar detection methods were employed in Germany: XMRV was detected only in one non-familiar PCa (of 87) and one control (of 70) sample. Neither one of these cases was homozygous for the R462Q allele [35]. An even more striking negative result was obtained by Hohn and collaborators in Berlin [36], who did not detect a single positive case among 589 PCa patients tested: this study employed a sensitive nested PCR detection, RT-PCR for *gag* sequences as well as serology for XMRV-specific antibodies [36]. A number of patients (76) were studied for the RNASEL allele and 12.9% scored positive [36]. Similar negative results were published in additional studies from Ireland (139 cases) [37], Holland (74 sporadic cases) [38], Mexico (55 cases) [39], USA (over 800 patients from a collaborative effort between Baylor, Johns Hopkins etc.) [40] and UK (437 patients from UK, Korea and Thailand) [41]. In the last study, a few patients scored positive: for example 2 out of 6 of Thailand's patients were positive, potentially reaching a score of 33%. However, evidence of contamination started emerging in this British International study: some of the amplified DNA did not contain a 24 bp deletion which is a hallmark of XMRV and other evidence suggested instead presence of P-MLV (as in the previous paper by Lo et al. on CFS) [41] [32]. A few assays, specific for contamination by mouse DNA, were therefore run to confirm identity of specimens. A very sensitive assay for Intracisternal A-type particles (IAPs) and mouse mitocondrial DNA was completely concordant with XMRV presence, clearly indicating presence of contamination [41]. Therefore, this 2010 paper by Robinson should have already signalled a red-flag warning for XMRV research [41].

### 2.5. Strength of RNASEL – HPC-1 paradigm

At the International Congress on Muscle Fatigue in 2010, I strongly criticized the association between *PCa* and *XMRV*, on the basis of such negative findings, most of which had been already published in the literature (July 2010). My analysis at the congress extended to the technology employed, thus suggesting that the *viro-chip* assay was –most likely- the source of error [1]. Still, data on the *RNase-L* association with *HPC-1* were indicative of viral involvement. Contrary to the situation in *PCa*, in which a few independent reports confirmed XMRV presence, while they were contradicted by a limited number of studies, CFS association with this virus was essentially based upon the unique paper by Lombardi et al. in 2009, somehow overwhelmed by a plethora of negative reports [1]. However, also in CFS, the case for the likely presence of an infectious agent, most probably a virus, can be made. This is particularly clear, in view of the presence of "micro-epidemics", often associated with CFS onset [1]. The rather strong evidence for a previous virus infection accompanied by the dramatic personal histories of CFS onset in thousands of patients could explain, but certainly NOT justify, the attachment of some patient-groups to the XMRV hypothesis, sometimes referred in the media as mass-hysteria [224]. We will later discuss whether the viral hypothesis should be completely dismissed in view of XMRV falsification or whether additional viral candidates should be investigated (see section 3).

### 2.6. XMRV controversy: looking back through 3 major Editorials

After 2010, the majority of XMRV reports documented negative results either in PCa or in CFS cases. Yet, the heated debate could have continued much longer, with some extreme defence of the XMRV hypothesis (J. Mikovits) and with a more balanced overview of the criticisms by R. Silverman (see for example, his excellent review in Nature Reviews of Urology, extensively discussing criticisms) [4]. Examples of debates on possible infectious agents present in human cancers are abundant in the literature: for PCa, HPVs are still extensively discussed as potential etiological agents or onset-cofactors see discussion in Sections 4.3 (3) and 4.3.1 (c). What or who was capable of rescinding the "Gordian Knot" of XMRV cancer/CFS association ? If we want to name a single scientist this is certainly John Coffin, although he extensively collaborated with other groups, especially with the group of S. Pathak. And yet, Coffin himself had written with J. Stoye in *Science*, accompanying one of the first papers on XMRV discovery -that of Lombardi et al. on the CFS association [30]- a positive editorial comment, which emphasized the future potential of such discovery [31].

i.      It may be instructive in this respect to re-analyse –so to speak: *after the facts*- the three major editorials, which accompanied the three major discovery-articles associated with XMRV. The first is the article by Dong et al. in PNAS at the beginning of 2007 [16], therefore immediately after publication of the Urisman et al. paper (December 2006). This article really gave credibility to the XMRV hypothesis, by showing that the virus was: 1. capable of replication in human cells, once a complete copy of the provirus was cloned and reconstructed; 2. responsive to the IFN pathway, as it had been predicted in view of the RNase L mutations; 3. uses a specific receptor, XPR-1 (therefore capable of mediating entrance for both xenotropic and polytropic retroviruses) for infecting human cells; 4. in three cases analysed, XMRV was integrated in tumour cells in regions surrounding potentially interesting/important genes, in two cases next to transcription factor genes (CREB and NFAT) and in the third, next to a hormone response gene, causing inhibition of androgen receptor trans-activation (APPB2/PAT1/ARA67). The accompanying editorial, by retro-virologist Hung Fan, is certainly the most cautious and critical of the three editorials [43]. Although underlying the potential importance of these findings, Fan clearly indicated that they were generating more questions than answers and that only by answering such questions could the XMRV hypothesis be strengthened or proven [43]. In one sentence, his cautionary criticism was particularly evident: *"However, another possibility is that XMRV is not causal to PC, but reflective of the reduced antiviral status of RNase L QQ individuals; another novel virus whose sequences were not detectd by the ViroChip might be the relevant agent"* (bold characters are my additions) [43].

ii.    The second fundamental paper for the XMRV hypothesis was the one by Lombardi et al. (2009), in which an astonishing 67% XMRV presence was documented in Chronic Fatigue Syndrome samples [30]. The paper was already briefly described, as well as the strong critical reaction it has generated, although this section is covered in more depth in the NMD review (see [1]) [30]. Surprisingly, the accompanying editorial written by John Coffin and Jonathan Stoye, appears to emphasize the positive aspects of these findings, rather than caution the readers about potential pitfalls, such as contaminations/artefacts [31]. It is apparent that the two Editorialists, among the major experts in mouse retro-virology, believed in 2009 that XMRV had strong connection to CFS, although it should be reminded that other viral infections have been previously associated with CFS (EBV, HHSV-6, HTLV etc., see [1]) [31]. And yet Coffin's with Pathak's groups eventually *"put the nails into the XMRV coffin one by one"* [44]. Far from being a "changing party" episode, reassessment of scientific data and even of personal believes is an essential and intrinsic process of scientific endeavour. One of the greatest epistemologists of past century, Karl Popper, has identified in the process of empirical *falsification* one of the essential logical characters of science in western world. In his *"All Life is Problem Solving"* Popper suggests that our scientific theories develop as an evolutionary (almost *Darwinian*) process, in which it is however *falsification* rather than *verification* the discriminating instrument (*Occam's razor*). Therefore, it is just natural and physiological that today in science, hypotheses and theories are continuously re-evaluated and reassessed, although in this process strong intellectual honesty and courage are also needed. Most likely, in 2009 Coffin/Stoye positively reacted and were convinced by 1. the fact that XMRV demonstrated a clear homology to MLV endogenous sequences, but different enough and with constant/homologous difference (approximately 10% throughout the viral genome) to let us believe that this was a totally new isolate. 2. The fact that all XMRV isolates detected showed strong homology among each other (less than 30 nucleotide variations in a genome of over 8000 bp.s), could be again evidence of an exogenous infecting agent (but also a contaminating virus). 3. Somehow, the general homology of XMRV with endogenous MLVs of approx. 90% may have been misleading still in 2009, since it might have suggested a mechanism of constant mutation accrual, as in phylogenetic analysis, of which the two editorialists are great experts [31]. In XMRV, however, recombination plays a major and determining role, as it was initially suggested in a PNAS editorial one year later, by Andrew Mason and colleagues (accompanying the third XMRV/MLV paper by Lo et al.) [34] [32].

iii.      Lo's paper initially appeared (or it was presented as) confirmatory of the infection hypothesis in CFS, since a murine retroviral sequence was detected in 86.5% of cases and only 7% of controls [32] [34]. The viral sequences however were not identical or very similar to XMRV, as previously reported, and appeared to be related to endogenous Polytropic retroviruses (PMLV). This generated some scepticism, as in previous work the viral sequences had little difference from the prototype retrovirus -XMRV. In his editorial, Mason underlines some discrepancies and yet does not clearly indicate that the finding of one xenotropic and one polytropic retroviruses are incompatible [34]. In other words, a general misconception could be –and apparently was- generated: there is an endogenous-like mouse retrovirus infecting cells in prostate carcinoma and CFS. In this scenario, *apparently* it didn't really matter whether it was marked with a P or with a X (for Polytropic and Xenotropic): the relevant and important point was that some type of murine endogenous-like retrovirus was infecting *Homo sapiens* in such disorders [34]. The paper by Ila Singh was also in line with such (mis-)interpretation [33]. On the other hand, as also pointed out in the previous editorial by Coffin and Stoye, the strength of the original XMRV hypothesis laid in the fact that all the isolates were similar to each other, although the prototype of XMRV appeared to be unique, different from any retrovirus known at that time [31]. Furthermore, Mason group's editorial suggested that, while the issue of which retrovirus exactly is present in PCa and/or CFS was being solved, a realistic and effective strategy could have been to test already potential therapeutic approaches with antiretroviral agents [34]. Again, such attitude is logically biased by the *caveat* that there was no firm evidence at that time for the real involvement of a retrovirus in both human conditions: this has been completely confirmed now by XMRV falsification. In fact, the paper by Lo et al. was rather good evidence *against* involvement of a retrovirus in both human conditions, since it suggested that contamination could be the cause [32]. Contamination, although denied in Lo's paper by a series of counter evidences, could explain the association with an endogenous murine polytropic retrovirus and, by extension, also with XMRV [32]. Andrew Mason group's editorial also emphasized the fact XMRV sequences appeared to be the result of recombinatory events [34]. They observed that in XMRV, while the 5' portion of its genome shares great homology to polytropic murine retroviruses, the 3' end is most similar to endogenous xenotropic MLV [34].

## 2.7. XMRV falsification

This observation, that inescapably leads to presence of recombination, was further developed approximately one year later in a seminal article by the groups of J. Coffin and S. Pathak [45]. In this Science paper in May 2011, Paprotka et al. convincingly showed that XMRV was generated by recombination during passage of the original tumor cells in nude mice [45]. The creation of human cell line 22 Rv1 was reported in 1999 after several passages by xenotransplantation, starting from 1993. The late passages /established cell line display presence of several copies of integrated XMRV provirus as well as high titers of virus production ($10^{10}$-$10^{11}$ PFU/ml). However, Paprotka et al. established a few essential and undermining criticisms: 1. First of all, fully infectious XMRV could not be detected in the original tumor explant (less than 1 copy/200 cells). 2. Second, two regions of strong homology with endogenous viruses could be detected: the 5′-end (called preXMRV-2) displays strong homology to PMLV endogenous sequences, while the 3′-end region (called PreXMRV-1) is most similar to an endogenous xenotropic retrovirus (XMLV). 3. Third, highly infectious "recombinant" XMRV started to appear in xenografts passaged in nude mice since 1996, i.e., three years after initial establishment of this tumour xenografts. This strongly suggests that infectious XMRV was created or has infected these cells between 1993 and 1996. 4. Fourth, the original nude mice strains utilized in xenotransplantation experiments did contain as endogenous viruses both the endogenous xenotropic virus (pre-XMRV-1, present in 6 out of 48 tested and typical of European mouse strains) as well as the endogenous PMLV (preXMRV-2, present in 25 out of 48 tested and typical of Asian mouse strains). 5. Fifth, the overall structure of the infectious XMRV could be explained by six recombinatory events between the two viruses: preXMRV-2 and preXMRV-1. Indeed, recombination is known to frequently occur during retrovirus replication, due to a polymerase (i.e., reverse transcriptase) switching between two different templates, therefore a mechanism of *"copy-choice"* as compared to the classical mechanism of *"cut-and-paste"* typical of general recombination [45] [46]. 6. Finally, the presence of a unique XMRV structure after so many recombinatory events strongly indicates that this *"creation"* occurred only once, most likely during xenograft passaging into nude mice [45]. The paper by Poprotka et al. therefore concluded the "XMRV Odyssey" with a most logical and well proven explanation and XMRV-falsification [45].

Additional evidence against XMRV as an exogenous virus infecting the human species were also obtained by the group of Jay Levy, who analysed some of the same CFS samples initially studies by Lombardi et al. Since these patients, initially reported as XMRV-positive, were found devoid of this retrovirus, this finding once more strengthened the evidence for contamination in positive samples [47]. A series of subsequent papers then reported evidence for contamination [45] [44] [48] [49] [50] in: 1. PCR reagents (even Taq polymerase) employed for XMRV detection; 2. microtomes or blades for tumours sections (even one year after the initial experiment); 3. contamination of several cell lines, beside the original 22Rv1. Prostate carcinoma cells lack the APOBEK-GA3 activity and are therefore susceptible to XMRV infection, while other human cells –for example human lymphocytes- appear to be highly resistant in view of the strong mutagenic activity of APOBEK-GA3.

# 3. MFV as potential candidate in PCa

Together with criticism of XMRV as potential candidate for CFS, we presented data in July 2010 [1] related to a novel viral candidate for both PCa and CFS: Micro-Foci inducing Virus or MFV. While the more specific aspects related to CFS association are presented elsewhere [1], MFV properties which link this virus to PCa will be here described.

## 3.1. Cancer Cluster Genetic Data

Micro-Foci inducing Virus was initially discovered in a paediatric tumor diagnoses-association generally defined as *"Cancer-Cluster"* (CC). A CC of neuroblastoma (NB) cases was diagnosed in Southern Louisiana in 1987-88 in the small town of Morgan City, while also the surrounding area appeared to be affected. A 12 fold increased NB incidence was recorded for a period of 18 months, while diagnoses then decreased to none [51]. This is a typical epidemiological behaviour of CCs, as it has been also recorded in other instances, such as paediatric leukaemia/lymphoma clusters [52]. Most of the tumours of this CC were conveyed to the Ochsner Foundation Research Center for further genetic analysis. The majority of them (66%) displayed elevated MYCN amplification, a well-known marker of aggressive NB. In one tumour with extremely elevated MYCN amplification (1000X the diploid value of controls), we started witnessing an elevated genetic instability in cultured tumor cells (see Fig. 1) [51]. This was accompanied by appearance of very small foci (Micro-Foci, MF) of rounded and refractile cells growing on top of the mesenchimal cells which typically grew up slowly and as monolayer in the initial tumor cultures (1ary cultures) [51] [53]. Furthermore, the initial dramatic amplification of MYCN seemed to disappear in growing primary cultures, apparently diluted out by the growth of mesenchimal flat cells (Fig. 1).

## 3.2. Isolation of MFV/MFRVs, partial cloning/sequencing

In order to find an explanation for this phenomenon, it was also noticed that the number of MFs was extremely variable, with some cultures having hundreds while others being devoid of them. An assay was therefore established by utilizing supernatants from cultures with hundreds MFs, with which we infected cells devoid of them. Since MF formation could be reproducibly transmitted even after ultra-filtration of such supernatants (through 100 μm filters), presence of a virus was hypothesized and confirmed by Electron Microscopy (EM). Transmission EM detected cytoplasmic particles of 65-73 nm for MFV (Fig. 2), while similar particles of larger size (85-92 nm) were identified in samples of paediatric lymphoma cases (MFV related Virus or MFRV), studied a few years later in Switzerland [51] [53] (Fig. 3).

Molecular cloning and partial sequencing of MFV/MFRV genome convincingly demonstrated that they share strong homology with members of the Reoviridae family, particularly Reovirus-3 (Dearing Strain) (Fig. 4).

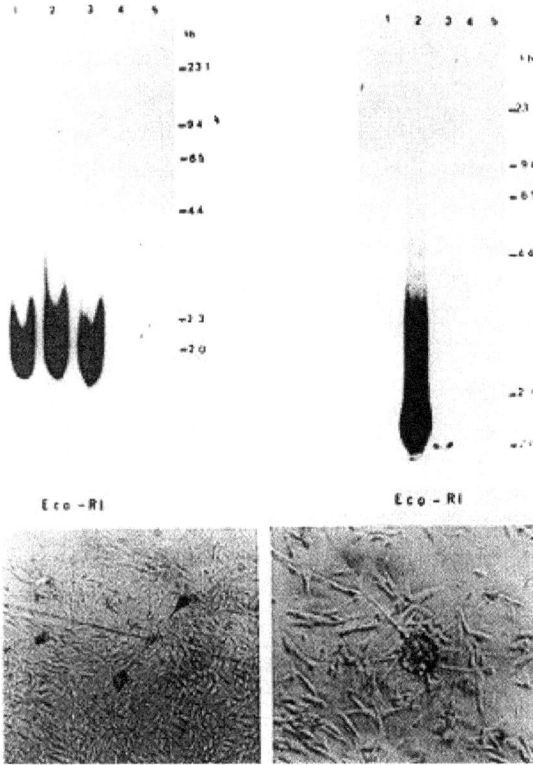

**Figure 1.** Top-left: Southern-blotting analysis shows high level of MYCN amplification in the original NB tumour from a Cancer-Cluster in Southern Louisiana. Lanes 1-3 contain DNA extracted from the original NB tumour, while lanes 4-5 two control DNAs (patient and normal blood donor peripheral leukocytes). Amplification was evaluated as 1000X fold by dilution experiments (not shown). Top-right: Southern-blotting analysis of DNA from the original tumour (lane 2) and from tumour cells passaged in culture for 2 weeks (lane 3) and 4 weeks (lanes 4-5). Bottom left: two microfoci, composed by small, rounded neuronal cells growing on top of a monolayer of large flat mesenchimal cells with Schwann cell markers. Lower magnification (40 X). Microfocus shown at higher magnification (100X).

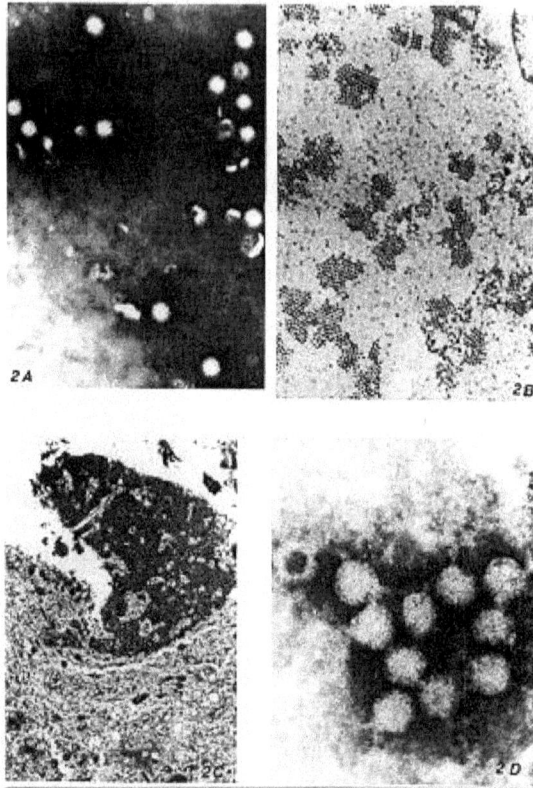

**Figure 2.** Electron Microscopy of MFV particles. 2A: negative staining of MFV particles (magnification = 100.000X). 2B and 2C: MFV viral "factories" in the cytoplasms of infected and transforming cells (magnifications: 15.000 and 10.000 respectively). 2D: Negative staining of MFV highest magnification (350.000X).

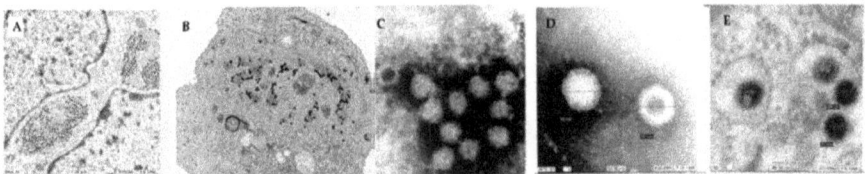

**Figure 3.** Electron Microscopy of MFV and MFRV particles. In 3A: MFV particles display a more localized pattern (15K X magnification), while in 3B, MFRV are spread through cell cytoplasm (5K X magnification). Fig.s 3C displays MFV at 350K X magnification (as in 2D) and Fig.s 3D-E MFRVs at 300K X and 175K magnification, respectively).

**Figure 4.** Comparison of sequences for Micron-NS –μNS- gene from MFV, a classical Reoviridae (Reovirus-3) and one isolate from Burkitt's Lymphoma (BL). Divergence from Reo-3 is approximately 20%.

### 3.3. MFV-transformed cells growth *in vitro* and *in vivo*

Furthermore, extensive work *in vitro* and *in vivo* has convincingly shown that MFV causes malignant transformation in vitro and tumours in animals (see Fig.s 5-8) [51] [53].

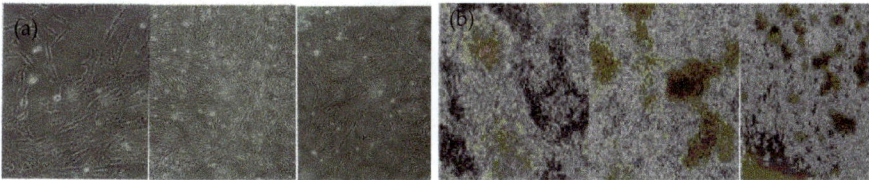

**Figure 5.** As shown in Fig. 5A normal, quasi-diploid SK-N-SH cells grow as mesenchimal cell (or Schwann-Cells) mono-layers, but after MFV infection they transform (Fig. 5B) into aggressively growing NB cells. Transformed cells extensive-ly grow in these *in vitro* conditions in the presence of low serum (2%), forming masses of rounded, small and packed cells (similar to MFs), which are loosely attached to the mesenchimal cell monolayer, othen floating in the medium supernatant.

Fig. 5 shows the different patterns of growth of uninfected neuroblastic SK-N-SH cells (a) and MFV-infected/transformed SK-N-SH (b). While the original SK-N-SH cells grow slowly in low serum conditions (Fig. 6), MFV-transformed cells are undistinguishable in their growth properties from cells obtained from aggressive NB tumours -for example, SK-N-BE cells (Fig. 6).

### 3.4. Carcinogenesis Mechanism(s)

The molecular mechanism of carcinogenesis induced by MFV has been partially clarified when it became evident that normal non-tumorigenic diploid neuroblasts are rapidly de-stroyed by MFV infection: most monolayers are "wiped-out" in 36-72 hrs [54] [53] [55]. The only cells, which appear to sustain MFV infection without extensive apoptosis, have amplified the *MYCN* locus [54]. In Fig. 7, in the left panel, Southern blotting analysis (employing a *MYCN* specific probe) of the cell line *SK-N-AS* shows that the *MYCN* is diploid in mock-infected cells (-), but becomes highly amplified (approx. 100X) upon MFV infection and relative transformation (line 2: *SK-N-AS* +). A similar result was obtained with cell line *VA-N-BR* (3rd lane) [51]. Similar results were also obtained with cell line *SK-N-SH* (which is also initially diploid and non-tumorigenic in nude mice) by Q-PCR analysis. Upon MFV infection, these cells acquire a *MYCN* DNA level intermediate between the mock-infected cells (yellow, green lines) and cell line *IMR-32* (MYCN amplification approx. 20X: black line): SH-10 cells (i.e., MFV-infected *SK-N-SH)* display an amplification level –by comparison- of approximately 10X (blue line).

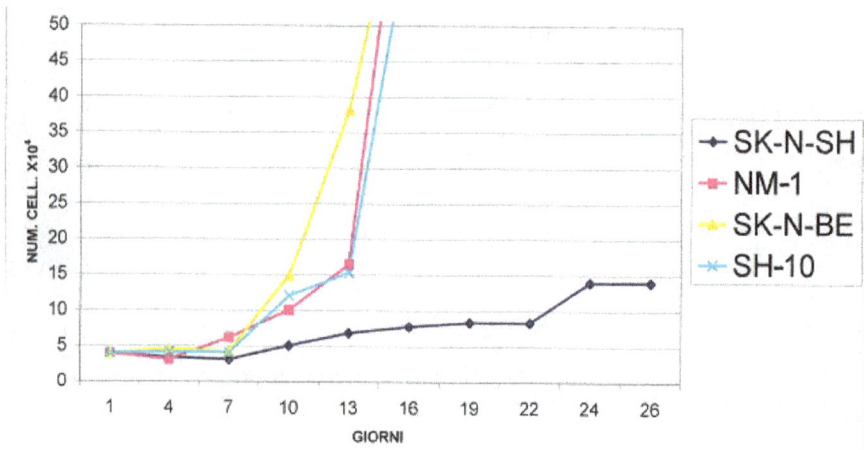

**Figure 6.** All cells were grown in Dulbecco's Modified MEM with the addition of 2 % Foetal Bovine Serum (FBS). NM-1 and SH-10 are two different clones of MFV- transformed SK-N-SH cells, while SK-N-BE is a a Neuroblastoma cell line established from an aggressive tumour with MYCN amplification.

The same MFV-infected/transformed *SK-N-SH* cells -, shown in previous page [53]- were also employed in *in vivo* experiments of nude mice inoculation and relative tumour growth. Inoculation of MFV-transformed SK-N-SH cells into the left flank of a nude mouse causes the appearance of large tumoral masses of NB cells (uninfected SK-N-SH cells were injected in the contra-lateral flank as control, Fig. 8).

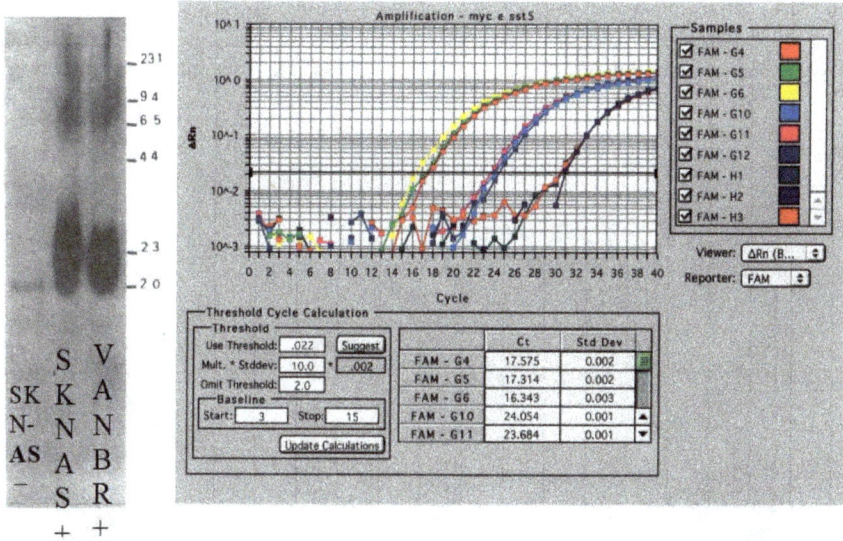

**Figure 7.** Southern Blotting and Q-PCR analysis of genomic DNA from cells infected/transformed by MFV. Left panel: Southern blotting analysis of cell line SK-N-AS before (lane 1) and after (lane 2) MFV infection; in lane 3, cell line SK-N-VR after infection/transformation with MFV (see also text description). Right panel: Q-PCR analysis of SK-N-SH cell DNA, DNA from SH-10 (the same line infected/transformed by MFV) and DNA from IMR-32 a cell line from aggressive neuroblastoma with MYCN amplification (approximately 20X). The relative level of MYCN amplification in SH-10 cells is estimated –by comparison- in the order of 10X.

# 4. Evidence for the association between MFV/MFRVs and prostate cancer

## 4.1. The Interferon (IFN) pathway

Evidence presented so far indicate that 1. in prostate carcinoma, an interferon-sensitive pathway appears to be affected. Attempts to identify an infectious agent (also on the basis of these observations), had led to identification of XMRV, a candidate virus, which has been eventually falsified by several groups (see part 1). However, as it has been emphasized in this chapter, evidence for viral involvement in PCa are rather strong and independent from the particular isolate XMRV. Indeed, as previously underlined, XMRV isolation is based upon usage of *viro-chip* technology and logical inference analysis predicts that this step is most error-prone [1]. In order to list and underline numerous elements indicating MFV as a strong candidate, the general IFN pathway is here considered and RNase-L as next point.

Although RNase-L is also an essential part of IFN pathway, it will be discussed separately, since it is prominent in view of numerous evidence and studies performed in PCa and other pathologies. Furthermore, the fact that transgenic animals *knockouts* for *RNASEL* gene do not develop tumours at higher frequency, suggests that additional elements in the IFN pathway may also be relevant [56] [57]. Since several years ago, the IFN pathways has been extensively dissected: beside RNase-L, two additional pathways are prominent: a) the PKR signal transduction and b) the Adenosine-Deaminase of RNA (ADAR) mechanism.

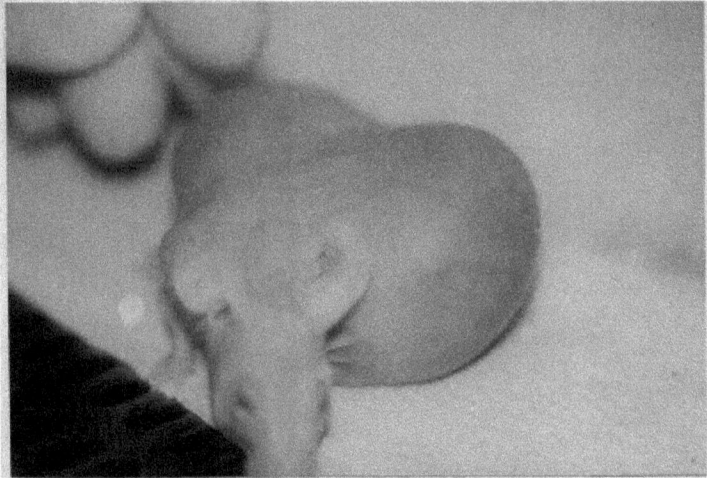

**Figure 8.** Tumorigenesis in nude-mice of SK-N-SH cells infected/transformed by MFV. Injection of $10^7$ SK-N-SH cells (right flank) or SH-10 clone (left flank) with the same number of MFV-transformed SK-N-SH cells shows the outgrowth 3 weeks later of large tumoral masses in the case of MFV-infected/transformed cells (SH-10). Histological analysis confirmed the presence of human neuroblastoma cells after xenotransplantation [53].

*4.1.1. PKR*

PKR was one of the best characterized pathways in the IFN signal transduction, starting from pioneering work of Isaacs and Lindenman, who initially characterized the IFN activity [58] [59]. One of the first enzymatic activities induced by IFN and its inducers (i.e., dsRNAs) is the dsRNA dependent Protein Kinase or PKR. PKR conveys the IFN message in several ways but especially by phosphorylation of: 1. PKR itself (autocatalysis); 2. the $\alpha$ subunit of eIF-2a ; 3. the inhibitor of transcription factor NFkB, IkB, thus releasing such inhibition; 4. the TAT transcription factor, essential activator of HIV; 5. the NFAT protein and 6. the phosphoprotein MPP4, which binds dsRNA and is activated during the M phase of cell cycle [58] [59] [60]. Among the different activities elicited by PKR activation, the best studied and known is certainly the inhibitory effect on protein synthesis (eIF-2a) [61]. Ser-51 Phosphorylation in this case blocks initiation of protein synthesis, by inhibiting the exchange of guanine nucleotide [61] [62] [63]. There are some discussions and discrepancies on the regulation of PKR from different portions of the gene/structure: two knockout transgenic mice were generated by the groups of Karomillas/Bell [64] and Ch. Weissmann [65] [66].

The first one has been targeted in the carboxy-terminal of PKR, where is present the kinase activity, and doesn't show impairment of antiviral response or TNF-α responses, thus indicating the redundant role of PK activity [60, 64]. To the contrary, Weissmann's lab ko mouse and its MEFs are strongly inhibited in view of the deletion of the NH2- portion of the protein, where the dsRNA-binding domain of PKR resides [65] [66] [60]. Effectors of PKR are several types of dsRNA molecules, both artificial and natural [67]. In this respect, the genome of MFV is a strong/ideal inducer of PKR in acutely infected cells, as we have documented in both mouse and human cells. Most likely, PKR induction also contributes to the strong apoptotic effects we have documented 36-72 hours post-infection [53]. In particular, MFV-infected cells completely block protein synthesis and strongly impair rRNA production (see later) and these effects seem to be mediated by PKR and RNase-L respectively. In prostate cancer, the same pathway of PKR appears to be downstream of another essential regulator and also Tumor Suppressor function of prostate cells: PTEN [68]. Therefore, typically the deletion of PTEN (which is extremely common in prostate cancer [69]) will lead to ablation of the TSG function of PKR by phosphorylation of eIF-2a and block of protein synthesis [68] [69]. In view of the MFV/MFRV connection hypothesis, it is speculated that infection by this family of viruses will eventually cause/select for PTEN deletion, as this will inhibit cellular apoptosis, which would otherwise be inescapable [53] [55] [69].

### 4.1.2. ADAR

The additional and last form of IFN response here considered is the RNA-specific Adenosine Deaminase or ADAR, which is strongly induced after viral infection [70] [71]. Although such RNA editing was initially considered a rare phenomenon, almost a curiosity of RNA regulation and fine tuning, extensive genomic sequencing by NGS and high-throughput technologies have allowed to discern considerable editing in several DNA genomic sequences by a related Deaminase activity which targets DNA, called APOBEC, as well as ADAR activity on expressed mRNAs [72] [73] [74]. It is still not clear how efficient such mechanism may be at the RNA level, since ADAR activity may protect cells but also favour virus aggression or persistence inside infected cells [70]. DNA deaminase activity as well is still poorly understood, but new phenomena discovered in human cancer cells through Next Generation Sequencing (NGS) technology suggest that genome modulation and plasticity by APOBEC could also play a major role in carcinogenesis [73] [75].

Could the ADAR activity induced by Interferon (ADAR-1) be responsible for important antiviral effects in human and other cells ? Although the question is still open and there are also examples of opposite regulation as previously mentioned –for example in Hepatitis Delta Virus (HDV) [70]-, important inhibitory effects were documented, with Measles Virus [76] [77] and with Influenza Virus in mouse cells [78]. Furthermore, a specific gene of the Adenovirus genome is responsible for counteracting the RNA-editing activity of ADAR: the VAI gene [79]. In the case of Reoviridae, little is still known but there is at least one animal model in which ADAR was induced by both artificial dsRNA and reoviridae genome (which obviously is dsRNA), although the response modality of ADAR appeared quite different [80] [81].

Among human cancer as well very little is known, particularly in the case of prostate carcinoma [82] [73]. More data have been obtained in the case of brain tumours, since ADAR is known to effect important editing in brain neurons. In at least two tumour examples, hypoediting seems to characterize cancer cells. In *glioblastoma multiforme*, rectification of a mutated permeable glutamate receptor to Ca++-impermeable receptor suppressed proliferation [83] [84], while in hypo-editing astrocytoma cells, re-balancing editing expression induced regression [85]. Additional work on ADAR/APOBEC in prostatic cancer and reoviridae is certainly warranted.

### 4.2. RNase-L, an essential pathway

The clearest evidence for viral involvement in prostate carcinoma and in human cancer in general was obtained through studies of the IFN response leading to RNase-L activation. The general scheme of IFN genes activation has been clarified through years of intense studies with several models, cell lines, laboratory and transgenic animals, in vitro assays and molecular/biochemical systems [60] [86]. Without getting into too many details –and referring instead the readers to some excellent review articles on this subject [60] [86] [87] [88] - two general types of IFN molecules are known: viral IFN and immune IFN. Both IFN-α and IFN- β (as well as IFN-omega) belong to the viral form, induced by viral infection [60], while the immune form is essentially composed by IFN-γ and is induced by immune stimulation. Focusing on viral genes, this is a rather large family in humans, since 13 genes for IFN-α, 1 for IFN-β and one for IFN-omega were mapped on the short arm of human chromosome 9 [89] [90]. None of these genes contains introns, while the only IFN gene with introns is the IFN-γ form with 3, on the long arm of chromosome 12. Two types of IFN receptors, IFNAR-1 and IFNAR-2 are known on human chromosome 21: they must heterodimerize for activation by IFN-α/β [91] [92] [93]. The following signalling is today understood mostly in the JAK-STAT transduction pathway, thanks to the work of several molecular biologists, first and foremost the group of Jim Darnell at Rockefeller University [94] [95] [96]. STATs are "signal transducers and activator of transcription" molecules: at least seven of them are known, i.e. Stat-1, Stat-2, Stat-3, Stat-4, Stat-5a, Stat-5b and Sta-6. STATs are activated by members of the Janus family of Tyrosine kinases (JAKs), of which 4 members are known, i.e. Jak-1, Jak-2, Jak-3 and Tyk-2. Various combinations of Jak's and Stat's elements are active in transducing both viral and immune IFN signalling [87] [88]. Additional important elements are the IRFs, (IFN Regulatory Factor) family [97], which cooperate in the activation of IFN-responsive genes. These are characterized by presence of regulatory elements: ISRE or IFN-stimulated Response elements [98], usually for viral IFNs and the GAS (gamma IFN activation sites) [99]. In conjunction with Stat's, IRFs constitute the so called ISGF (IFN stimulated gene factor's) [100]. Having clarified this terminology, ds-RNA activation of IFN pathway does not always or only use Jak-Stat elements. The transcription factor IRF-3 (IFN response Factor 3) acts as subunit of a complex called ds-RNA activated transcription factor complex (DRAF) by sereine/threonine phosphorylation, translocation to the nucleus, association with p300/CBP and gene activation [101]. Among the activated genes, the Oligo Adenylate Synthetase gene family, or OAS, is one of the most important, because it conveys the anti-viral signal to the next and final effector: RNase-L. In humans, three OAS genes of different sizes (proteins of 40-46 kDa -OAS1-, of 69 kDa –OAS2- and of 100 kDa -OAS3-) have been mapped on the long arm of chromosome 12 (12q24.2), thus suggesting genome duplications in *H. sapiens* [102]. Similarly to the effectors previously considered –PKR and ADAR-, OAS proteins do contain regions for binding dsRNA, the signalling and activating effector [103] [104] [105]. However, all three effectors contain separate regions with peculiar enzymatic activities: kinase, deaminase, synthethase [60]. The exact nature of dsRNA activators is not always completely clear, but hypothesized to be formed by or to contain dsRNA elements. In the case of interest, i.e. MFV/MFRVs infection, since these belong to Reoviridae family, it is clearly fragments or segments of viral genome (dsRNA) [53] [55]. Great variation has been documented in the extent/level of OAS activation and 2-5 A production [80].

Last element, RNase-L, is activated by 2-5 A signal molecules, typically oligomers with >2 elements for optimal induction, while RNase-L must dimerize for activation [106] [107]. This endoribonuclease is typically present as monomer in a latent form, essentially in every cell (tested so far), but -after 2-5 A interaction- it homodimerizes and is activated [107], although heterodimers with RLI (RNase-L inhibitor) have been also described. As previously mentioned, RNase-L gene, called RNS4, has been mapped on the long arm of chromosome 1 (1q25), on a location corresponding to the chromosomal site for the Human Prostate Carcinoma susceptibility (HPC-1) [108], as mapped with linkage studies by Jeff Trent and others [108] [6].

In view of the coincident chromosomal location of RNASEL and HPC-1 [6] [108] and the initial speculations by Lengyel and others that this gene may behave as a bona fide Tumor Suppressor [109] [12] [13], Silverman with DeRisi and Ganem undertook the described *viro-chip* high-throughput search for potential viral candidates, leading to XMRV isolation [15]. As previously described and discussed in Section 1, XMRV identification has been clearly falsified as a recombination artefact arising during xenograft transplantation in nude mice [45].

In view of the coincidental chromosomal localization of HPC-1 and RNASEL, what are the evidence for RNase-L involvement after MFV/MFRV infection ? The acute phase of infection by these viruses is accompanied by a very high activation of RNase-L [53]. An assay, detecting ribosomal RNA (rRNA) degradation in infected and transforming cells was developed (U. Rovigatti, unpublished), thus confirming the extremely high levels of RNase-L induction, often leading to block of cell proliferation and apoptosis [53] [55]. In the past several years, groups in USA, France and Belgium have also documented a strong deregulation of this endoribonuclease in patients affectd by Chronic Fatigue Syndrome. Pioneering work by Suhadolnick et al at Temple Univ. initially disclosed that 2-5 A activated RNase-L is upregulated in CFS patients [110] [111] [112]. This finding was followed up by description of a lower molecular weight form (37 kDa) of the same enzyme in CFS patients by the same group [113]. The French-Belgian group of De Meirleir et al. then showed that the 37 kDa fragment is proteolytically cleaved from the original enzyme of 87 kDa, by human elastase and/or calpain [114]. The same authors also speculated that the levels of 2–5 A molecules with structures larger than dimers (trimers/tetramers) protect the 83 kD moiety from degradation [115] [116]. Presence of the 37 kD RNase-L could also explain the higher enzymatic activity (associated with the low MW form) and the ratio between the two forms was proposed as potential marker for CFS [117] [111] [118].

In conclusion, the extremely elevated levels of RNase-L in every cell type infected by MFV indicate that this could be an important parameter to be evaluated. Analysis is being performed for addressing the question of whether cells with impaired/mutated alleles of RNase-L (such as the R462Q allele) may be more resistant to the apoptogenic effect(s) of MFV/MFRV and could become better targets for carcinogenesis [53] [55] [1].

## 4.3. Inflammation - ubiquitous in PCa

Inflammation has been estimated as being somehow responsible for 20% of human cancers: these are typically linked to infectious agents, causing chronic infections as well as by other environmental factors [119] [120] [121]. While it appears to be an essential component of carcinogenesis –being defined as "the seventh hallmark of cancer" [122]– inflammatory processes are particularly prominent in PCa [121] [119]. Furthermore, inflammation in PCa adds an enigmatic component, which could be or become one of the best clue for deciphering its aetiology [55]. This enigmatic nature is however rather complex, as it can be distinguished by several elements:

1.  The **paradox of a rather common disease** (most common cancer among men), afflicting this year over 300.000 people and killing more than 33.000 patients, only in the US [123]. For comparison, it has been observed that there is just a handful of cases described in the literature for Primary Seminal Vesicle Carcinoma, essentially in the same anatomical location [124]. This shows a peculiar and striking difference between two very close histological sites: PCa is diagnosed only in the prostate peripheral zone, rarely in the transition zone and almost never in the central zone [125]. This pattern is accompanied by typical phenomena of inflammation which is almost never of acute type (at time of diagnosis) and is characterized in the described zones by: a. chronic inflammation, b. benign prostatic hyperplasia (BPH), d. focal atrophy, e. a new type of inflammatory response defined as prostatic inflammatory atrophy (PIA) and finally developing into f. prostatic intraepithelial neoplasia (PIN) and/or g. prostatic carcinoma (PCa) [125] [126] [127] [128]. This pattern associates with an extremely common disease, the most common form of cancer in men, again suggesting a rather "common" causality [55]. As we will also consider other clues (see 2,3,4), the best explicatory mechanism is that of a common infection, in particular an infectious agent which is "endogenous" or "persitent" in *H. sapiens* and apparently much more frequent in certain human populations or races [129] [130] (see below)

2.  **Variation in epidemiological data** for Chinese, Japanese or Arab men in comparison with the male population in Western Countries: for example, men born in South East Asia who then migrated to the US acquire a higher incidence within the first two gener-

ations [130] [131] [132]. In Shri-Lanka men, the incidence was recently assessed as 5.7 per 100.000 males, while such incidence rose up by twenty folds in immigrants to the Western Countries (for example, UK) [133]. This is again indicative of "life-style" rather than genetic factors being responsible for prostate carcinogenesis. Similar data are also present in Japanese men who migrate to the US [134]. Using similar epidemiological approaches, Hsing has recently divided different nations into three risk groups for incidence and mortality of PCa. The high risk group includes USA and several European Countries; to medium risk group belong European Nations such as UK, Italy and Spain, while Asian Countries are mostly included in the third, low risk group [130]. There is a general trend of increasing incidence, which the authors attribute to westernisation of life-style in the low-risk nations, but to TUR (trans-uretral resection) and PSA-testing in the high risk Nations [130, 134]. Interestingly, the incidence in US black males is 50-60 fold higher that that in Shanghai, China [130] [135]. The data by Julian Peto and others have confirmed these trends and the rapid changes in incidence/mortality in migrant populations (often within the first generation), thus emphasizing the concept that factors different from genetics (i.e. environmental, such as infectious agents) may be responsible [129].

3.   The fact that inflammation, BPH and PCa **typically occur in the prostate peripheral area**, with almost no tumours in the central zone. This led initially LM Franks to hypothesize that in prostate cancer, the inflammatory effects are always accompanied by hyperproliferation and/or atrophy/necrosis [126]. Later, McNeal et al. have elaborated the same concept, by noticing in 1988 that in the whole gland, there is a clear-cut zonal distribution [125]. Out of 88 tumours studied, the majority (68%) arose in the peripheral gland, while 24% in the transitional zone and only 8% in the central gland zone. As mentioned, this suggests that infection through ascending urethra could be a responsible/associated factor [125] [136] [119]. Although bacteria have been initially suspected as responsible for inflammatory phenomena and as causes of carcinogenesis (*Neisseria Gonorrhoeae, Clamydia Trachomatis, Trichomonas Vaginalis,* and *Treponema Pallidum*), such intepretation has been reconsidered in post-antibiotics era, since prostatic persistant bacterial infections have dramatically dropped [137]. Still, bacteria can be often grown even from expressed fluids of asymptomatic men [138]. The possible causality by viruses is still an open question, as extensively discussed in the first section on XMRV discovery and refusal. Among viruses, several have been extensively investigated throughout the years and particularly: **i.** *Cytomegalovirus (CMV)* has been investigated in view of its association with malignant transformation in vitro. Seven studies on tissues and 2 on serology do not support an association with PCa. [139] [140, 141] **ii.***Epsten Barr Virus (EBV)* levels were shown to be not significantly different in PCa/BPH by Ab's, PCR and IHC; [142] **iii.** *HHV-8* was initially detected by Chang and Moore in *Kaposi Sarcoma (KS)* by subtractive hybridisation [143]. Initial positive results in PCa by Monini et al. [144] were later explained by infiltration with lymphocytes, most likely in *HIV-1* positive (and therefore *HHV-8+*) patients [145, 146]. Also, the strongly positive findings by Hoffman in men from Trinidad and Tobago can be probably explained by bias of selected controls [147] [148]. **iv.** *Polyoma* **Viruses** have been also associated with PCa: an ini-

tial report by Monini et al. [149] was followed by an interesting paper by Das et al., since they found *BKV* DNA positivity more frequently in malignant tissue [150]. However, also these studies were not confirmed [151] [152]. **v.** *Human Papilloma Viruses (HPVs)* : Extensive work has focused on these viruses throughout the years. Their relevance was also surmised from studies on women cervical/uterine cancer –pioneered by Harald zur Hausen (Nobel Prize for Medicine in 2008)- where *HPVs* are clearly involved in >90% of cases [153]. However: i) even Zur Hausen in reviewing this subject in his Nobel lecture dismisses the role of HPVs in PCa: in this sense, men would be some kind of "healthy carriers" of the viral carcinogen [154]; ii) Several studies have been published, some of which with positive results (for example, in an Argentinean study, 42% PCa were positive versus 0% BPH samples) [155]. However, in 24 studies from other Countries, there is no evidence of different *HPV* involvement between cancer specimens and controls [156]. Furthermore, the most recent meta-analysis didn't show significant OR for PCa associated with *HPV-16* (OR = 1.09) or with *HPV-18* (OR = 1.08) infections [157]. Similar results were obtained by a recent review article (in press) [156]. iii) Another element which does not fit *HPVs* as potential carcinogens in PCa is the observation –initially made by Woodsworth [158] - that *HPV* infections do not elicit high inflammation or inflammation at all ([158], see also later discussion). As already mentioned, inflammation –most likely associated with a prostatic infection- is one of the Hallmarks of Cancer, particularly in this tumor type, PCa [122] [121].

4.   Several reports (Platz; Mahmoud; Chan; Jacobs) have documented that **assumption of aspirin or Non-Steroidal Anti-Inflammatory Drugs (NSAIDs)** for different periods could considerably lower PCa risk [159] [160] [161] [162]. These studies have been expanded in recent years, particularly by the work of Mahmud with several Meta-Analyses [163] [164, 165] [166] [167]. A positive correlation has been detected for aspirin usage (protection) with OR in the range of 0.81- 0.83 and this is confirming what was already known from animal studies, which typically display stronger and clear-cut protective effects (also with NSAID). In the case of NSAID, the effect is less apparent, or maybe diluted out [166]. In most recent nested case-control studies, Mahmud has confirmed a modest but significant effect with all propionates, ie. Ibuprofen, Naproxen etc., but not with other NSAIDs [167]. The question is somehow connected also to the relationship between BPH and PCa, since the former has been often considered a precursor and initial inflammatory response leading to the latter [168] [169] [170]. Additional findings hower do not lend support to this hypothesis [171] [172]. Finally, a very recent study by Sutcliffe and others also does not show any effect for NSAID treatment in BPH as well as LUTS (Low Urinary Tract Symptoms) [173]. In either cases and also in view of the Mahmud meta-analyses, there may be a positive (protective) effect, but too small and/or diluted out [173].

*4.3.1. How can this Inflammation-Scenario fit the proposed role of MFV/MFRVs*

a.   First of all, this family of viruses infects the human population in the first years of life. By age 5, >95% of human population displays antibodies against Reoviridae and this type of viruses have been shown to be capable of persisting in infected patients and animals for several months/years [174]. Furthermore and as discussed in the next section, MFV/MFRVs display all the features of a "Stem Cell Virus" (SCV), with features of interaction in early childhood with a developing immune system [53, 175]. That a prostate cancer stem cell may be present in PCa and targeted in the first phase of carcinogenesis has been longly hypothesized and recently confirmed [176] [177] [178]. Further studies are certainly warranted in order to assess presence of MFV/MFRVs in early childhood and during ontogeny [55].

b. Different levels/types of MFV/MFRVs appear to be present in different human populations worldwide. However, a clear picture of the specific subtypes involved is still missing, particularly for what concerns MFV/MFRVs. This should be clarified experimentally (by viral nucleic acid and specific protein detection, presence of antibodies etc.) [174]. Furthermore, essential aspects of these viruses features are still missing as we do not have full knowledge of these viruses genome sequence/structure [53]. Patterns of infections and micro/mini-epidemics in different populations could be deduced and mirrored by what is happening with Rotaviruses (another member of Reoviridae) in the paediatric population, where dominance of one particular genotype was shown to dramatically change from year to year, at least in Central and Eastern Europe [179].

c. The question of inflammation in PCa leads to the search of a causing agent in both affected patients and experimental systems. This chapter has dwelled trough different aspects of this essential question. The presented appraisal of potential responsible agents clearly indicates today a lack of credible candidates among bacterial infections. Even for viral candidates, the previous discussion showed that Herpes Viruses (CMV, EBV, and HHV-8), Polyoma Viruses and Papilloma Viruses lack some of the essential features as triggering agents [157] [156]. For all these viruses, extensive detection studies were performed for years without reaching any consensus nor obtaining evidence for their presence but in a limited percentage of cases [157] [156]. Same negative result was finally obtained for a Retrovirus, XMRV, after much controversy and discussion [4] [45] [44] [48] [49] [180], while a previously retroviral candidate (HTLV-II) had been previously falsified in the case of CFS [181] [1]. It must be stressed that the essential feature discussed here is inflammation and the two most likely candidates in the previous list, i.e. Retroviruses and Papillomaviruses do not appear to induce inflammation as expected from analysis of PCa: I) Retroviruses are known to be capable of replicating inside cells, even without causing cytopathic effects or transformation for that matter [182]; II) for HPVs, the quoted work by Woodworth has clarified this point. He wrote [158]: "*A hallmark of HPV infection is absence of an inflammatory response. Basal cells express low levels of HPV early proteins, they don't undergo lysis, and they are not rapidly recognized and destroyed by resident leukocytes such as NK cells and tissue macrophages.....HPV infections can persist and remain latent for long periods and may induce tolerance to HPV antigens.."*

To the contrary and as described in Section II, MFV/MFRVs are strongly apoptogenic and capable of inducing strong/very strong inflammatory responses in several experimental systems [53] [1]. In preliminary experiments, we have established primary cultures from approximately 20 cases of PCa. In the majority of cases, cultured cells displayed extensive cytopathic effects and did not survive for extensive passages, with three exceptions. While these results confirm previous descriptions by Frank, McNeal and by De Marzo's group [125] [126] [127] [128], they also suggest that whatever factor elicited strong inflammatory mechanisms in the prostate, with cycles of hyperplasia and of necrosis, the same factor may increase its effects during in vitro culturing [55]. We are presently testing this set of PCa tumors and relative cultures (different passages) for presence of MFV/FMRVs.

**d.** Although never specifically tested, sialycilic acid and similar salts have been shown to be effective for the containment/ replication-inhibition of this family of viruses (reoviridae) [183] [184]. Any strategy or molecule capable of reducing their inflammatory responses would probably elicit similar results.

### 4.4. Stemness in PCa: MFV as a "Stem Cell Virus"

*4.4.1. Prostate Cancer stem Cell or Cells ?*

Essential aspects of PCa have been here discussed with emphasis on viral models [55] [1]. In this last section of the chapter and also in dealing with peculiar aspects of PCa carcinogenesis in connection with an infecting virus (with MFV/MFRVs as potential candidates), the issue of Cancer Stem Cells (*CSC*) or *stemness* will be discussed. The concept of Cancer Stem Cell dates back to much ground work in the past two centuries, with several pioneers such as Julius Cohnheim and Rudolf Virkow already in the 19th century: they predicted the existence of *"embryonic rests"* at the origin of tumor formation [185] [186]. At the beginning of XXth century, Pappenheim hypothesized the existence of embryonic stem cells, but it was only in the second half of '900 that experimental evidence was provided for them [187]. In Toronto, in the '60s and '70s, the research of Ernest McCulloch and James Till demonstrated that only a minute fraction of myeloma cells grew in *in vitro* assays in order to form colonies in semisolid media [188, 189]. The Toronto school settled the basis for further work by John Dick (see later). In the same years, similar work was carried on by Robert Bruce, showing that only 1-4% of lymphoma cells did transplant into recipients [190], and by Jim Griffin, who demonstrated low clonogenic potential for Acute Myelogenous Leukaemia cells growing in methylcellulose [191]. Three additional lines of research paved the way for the final development of CSC hypothesis. 1. Mutations or translocations were discovered in cells at birth, which became markers of leukaemia-precursor cells (i.e., TEL-AML1, MLL-AF4, AML-ETO, OTT-MAL): these cells behave as leukaemia stem cells, since they could differentiate into several lineages/compartments, while additional mutations were required for achievment of full-leukemogenesis [192] [193] [194] [52], 2. the work of Peter Fialkow clearly indicated clonal expansions of leukaemia stem cells in specific diseases such as CML, AML and Myelodisplastic Syndromes (MDS) [195] [196]. Most of this work was carried on using genetic markers such as G6PD, present on the X chromosomes: in females, one of the X is silenced by the so-called lyonization phenomenon (from Mary Lyon's work) [197], thus allowing to distinguish the expansion of individual clones in cases of heterozygosity (for ex., A/B alleles for G6PD) [198] [199]; 3. The work of A. Hamburger and S. Salmon in Tucson,

AZ, who also showed low frequency ($1/10^{-3}$ to $1/10^{-4}$) of colony formation from solid tumours [200, 201]. These experiments were, however only partly convincing or reproducible (for example, in S. Salmon's work) and further ethical questions and concern were raised by experiments of C. Sautham and A. Brunschwig who injected harvested cancer cells into the same cancer patients, again discovering that only large numbers (i.e., $10^6$) were capable of tumor iniriation [42]. Only at the end of the 80's and with the advent of authomated high-speed Flurescence Activated Cell Sorting (FACS) [202], the group of John Dick in Toronto was capable of convincingly and reproducibly demonstrating the existence of Leukemic Stem Cells (LSCs). This was accomplished by xenotransplantation assays, in which LSCs from AML were transplanted into Severe Combined Immunodeficient (SCID) mice, often crossed with Non-Obese Diabetic (NOD) mice, in which also the natural immune response (NK cells) is defective [203] [204]. In order to demonstrate stemness, these experiments had to prove the three essential features of stem cells, i.e. a. their capability of remaining dormant, b. their pluripotency, being capable of reproducing the full spectrum of cancer (i.e. leukaemia) phenotype; c. their capability of self-renewal by asymmetric division, thus, giving rise to both bulk tumour cells and their immature precursors [205] [206]. The paper by Bonnet and Dick in 1997 is considered the first clear-cut demonstration of the LSC concept by xenotransplantation [207]. Subsequently, the same concept (Cancer Stem Cell or CSC) was also proven in solid tumours, initially in breast cancer by Al-Hajj et al. in 2003, where the CSC was shown to be CD44+CD24-/low lineage [208]. However, additional markers were subsequently identified in breast cancer, one of the most interesting ones being Aldehyde Dehydrogenase (ALDH), which appears to affect the phenotype of cancer cells, being associated to capacity of detoxification and a more aggressive behaviour also in other types of CSC [209] [210]. ALDH however doesn't seem to be an universal marker, as it is not, for example, associated with a more aggressive phenotype in melanoma cells [211]. Another controversial issue in recent years has concerned the frequency of Cancer Stem Cells (CSC) in different tumours. For example, a recent paper by Quintana et al. calculated that with an assay employing NOD/SCID IL2Rg mice, up to 25% of melanoma cells were tumorigenic [212]. Similar controversies are also present for the identification of prostate CSC [176] [177] [178]. In fact, two different populations of SC and prospective CSC were isolated in PCa [213] [214]. An initial paper in Nature described regeneration of the whole prostate from a single basal cell, which in addition to classical markers of prostate cell differentiation (Sca-1+, CD133+, CD44+) also displayed presence of c-KIT receptor (CD117+) [215]. However, a subsequent paper by the group of Michael Shen convincingly showed that among luminal cells, rare precursors exist which display presence of the homeobox gene NKx3-1 in absence of androgens and are therefore called castration-resistant Nkx3-1 expressing cells (CARNs) [216]. These cells can reconstitute prostate ducts after transplantation and, upon deletion of the suppressor gene PTEN, rapidly form carcinomas *in vivo* [216]. Finally, the group of Owen Witte has recently shown that it is also a basal cell which can initiate tumorigenesis in nude mice through cooperation of AKT, ERG and androgen receptor [217]. It is therefore possible that more than one precursor stem cell is the target of malignant transformation in prostate cancer. Furthermore, this could also fit with the described PCa carcinogenesis, in which a rather diffuse "field effect" has been known for some time [218] [219].

*4.4.2. Evidence for MFV as Stem Cell Virus, possibly involved in PCa Carcinogenesis.*

a.  In initial preliminary experiments, we have shown that dilutions of MFV/MFRVs for several log.s (from $10^{-2}$ to $10^{-8}$ FFU/ml) will cause a similar number of transformants, thus indicating that the limiting factor was not the virus itself, but rather its target. Since an equal number of precursor stem cells are believed to be present in such cultures, it is hypothesized that the target is indeed a SC [1].

b.  The Micro-Foci induced by MFV have several features of deranged stem cells, in which genetic aberrations took place, such as MYCN amplification in neuroblasts and t(8;14) / t(2;8) in paediatric lymphomas (BL-type). Even the so-called organoids or tumorspheres of PCa (prostaspheres) have similar fetures of MFs: we are now performing experiments in order to convert normal prostate tissue/cell lines into prostaspheres by MFV infection [53].

c.  As mentioned, PCa is characterized by an initial oligoclonality, which underlines carcinogenesis through a "field-effect" (FE). Evidence of oligoclonality were also obtained by molecular biology studies (see next point). However a molecular explanation for FEs is still lacking [218] [219]: MFV/MFRVs could explain FE alterations in view of the slowly progressing infection, mostly through cell-to-cell contacts [53] [55].

d.  In approximately 50% of PCa, peculiar translocations TMPRSS2-ERG have been detected, which join together an androgen regulated gene: the transmembrane protease serine 2 gene, TMPRSS2, with at least 26 different genes for transcription factors [220] [221, 222]. Although data on association of translocations with PCa aggressiveness are controversial, the translocation is an excellent marker of clonality (individual breakpoints): they have shown initial existence of oligoclonal disease, further evolving into monoclonality during metastatic disease [223].

e.  We have shown in several experiments –and previously discussed in section 2- that MFV/MFRVs infection is associated or causing peculiar genetic aberrations such as MYCN amplification (I.E., Fig. 7) or t(8;14) / t(2;8) translocations in paediatric lymphoma [53]. Similarly, we hypothesize that the associated translocations induced by MFV/MFRVs in prostate cells are TMPRSS2-ERG translocations, which would confer resistance to virus-induced apoptosis [55]. Experiments are being carried out in several PCa biopsies already characterized for presence of translocations (in 25% of cases).

## 5. Summary and conclusion

In this chapter, a review of general literature, as well as data previously published or unpublished by the author, was presented with the specific aim of fostering an ongoing debate on prostate cancer aetiology. This debate was particularly spurred in the past six years by the controversy arising after isolation of a new retrovirus, highly homologous to endogenous xenotropic and polytropic murine retroviruses, called XMRV [55] [1].

The first part of the chapter has focused on XMRV, its isolation and eventual falsification, also as a "parable" of scientific trajectories and behaviours in science. The most heated episodes are probably missing (but the reader could easily find them in some well-written editorials, for example the one in Science: *False Positive*, [224]), but the scientific rationale should be easily followed from isolation to falsification. In this first section, I underlined the difference between RNASEL – HPC-1 association and XMRV identification. While the first is rather logically strong and corroborated by several evidence and years of research, the second was essentially based on just one high-throughput technology –kind of *shot-in-the-dark*- experiment. It is easily biased and prone to artefacts, as it happened in this instance. However, the idea of an infecting agent in PCa is strengthened by several other elements, of which RNASEL involvement is only one (also: IFN, PKR, etc are affected; presence of inflammation, involvement of peripheral prostate, field cancerization effects, etc.).

In the second part, the candidate MFV virus was presented, in view of its affinity with PCa (IFN involvement, RNase-L strong induction, generation of inflammatory mechanisms). For RNase-L, evidence was also coming from CFS studies, again pointing toward similarities between the two conditions (and cancer related fatigue –CRF ? [2] [1]). Furthermore, MFV was isolated from a cancer-cluster (NOT through PCR enrichment) in view of its strong/powerful biological activity. This is exemplified by its very strong apoptogenic mechanisms (entire cultures wiped-out in 36-72 hours) or its capability of inducing strong genetic instability, leading to genomic aberrations, such as MYCN amplification and t(8;14) or t(2;14) [53].

Finally, in the third section, the elements of PCa carcinogenesis, where MFV/MFRVs could show more clearly its effects, were underlined: they included IFN pathways, RNASEL, inflammation and MFV capability of infecting/transforming stem-like cells [53] [55].

What are then the MFV/MFRVs properties which should be emphasized or taken home as messages? Or how we should rationalize them in this ongoing debate on PCa carcinogenesis ? As mentioned, the RNASEL – HPC-1 paradigm is logically strong and also in CFS numerous evidence point toward infections (micro-epidemics, virus-infection symptoms, IFN pathway etc.) [3] [1].

One essential property of MFV/MFRVs is its biological power, which could lead to strong and persistent infections and long-lasting inflammations in affected hosts. This could easily explain cycles of necrosis/regeneration, which we witness in BPH, PIA, PCa [53] [119].

A second important question -not addressed by this review for limited space- regards the nature of these viruses and whether they have been isolated before. In view of the persistent/ long-lasting infections they can initiate, an easy comparison/association is with EBV, which infects *H. sapiens* in early childhood/youth (depending from geographic areas), then remaining latent, and has been also associated with lymphomagenesis and other human cancers. Indeed, in the *hospital-safari's* expeditions of Dennis Burkitt, there was a second type and non-Herpes virus (not EBV) constantly isolated [225] [226] [227] [228] [229] [230] [231] [232] (also: Jay Levy/ Thomas Bell, personal communications). All the data available today point toward a virus similar to MFV/MFRVs: in this sense and in view of our MFRVs data, these viruses could be the missing link to malignancy in BL (EBV does not cause malignancy, it just immortalizes lymphoblasts) [53] [233].

A final question, in view of the close relationship of these viruses in terms of persistence in the human population, is what justifies this proximity, which –at least for its *"cousin* EBV"- resembles parasitism. Several authors and M. Greaves among them, have introduced elements of *"Darwinian-medicine"* analysis in our interpretation of carcinogenesis [234] [235] [52] [175] [236] [237] [53] [55] [1]. The *take-and-give* of MFV/MFRVs with *H. sapiens* infections could certainly be associated to some of their properties. For example, to their strong apoptogenic effects, leading to inflammatory reactions in BPH/PIA/PCa, but also possibly to useful tissue modelling/reshaping in other instances. The described strong relationship of these viruses with stem-like cells further suggests a closer partnership of MFV/MFRVs with *H. sapiens* in *Darwinian-medicine* terms. With all possible consequences.

## Author details

Ugo Rovigatti

Address all correspondence to: profrovigatti@gmail.com

University of Pisa Medical School, Pisa, Italy

## References

[1] Rovigatti, U., Chronic Fatigue Syndrome (CFS) and Cancer Related Fatigue (CRF): two "fatigue" syndromes with overlapping symptoms and possibly related aetiologies. Neuro-Muscolar Disorders, 2012. In the Press.

[2] MEEUS, M., et al., Immunological Similarities between Cancer and Chronic Fatigue Syndrome: The Common Link to Fatigue? . Anticancer Research November 2009 29 (11 ): p. 4717-4726

[3] Silverman, R., A scientific journey through the 2-5A/RNase L system. Cytokine Growth Factor Rev, 2007. 18: p. 381 - 388.

[4] Silverman, R.H., et al., The human retrovirus XMRV in prostate cancer and chronic fatigue syndrome. Nature Reviews of Urology, 2010. 7(7): p. 392-402.

[5] Silverman, R.H., Viral encounters with OAS and RNase L during the IFN antiviral response. 2007. J. Virol., 81: p. 12720-12729.

[6] Carpten, J., et al., Germline mutations in the ribonuclease L gene in families showing linkage with HPC1. Nature Genetics, 2002. 30(2): p. 181-184.

[7]  Casey, G., et al., RNASEL Arg462Gln variant is implicated in up to 13% of prostate cancer cases. Nature Genetics, 2002. 32(4): p. 581-583.

[8]  Roekman, A., et al., Germline Alterations of the RNASEL Gene, a Candidate HPC1 Gene at 1q25, in Patients and Families with Prostate Cancer. The American Journal of Human Genetics, 2002. 70(5): p. 1299-1304.

[9]  Noonan-Wheeler, F.C., et al., Association of hereditary prostate cancer gene polymorphic variants with sporadic aggressive prostate carcinoma. The Prostate, 2006. 66(1): p. 49-56.

[10] Wiklund, F., et al., Genetic Analysis of the RNASEL Gene in Hereditary, Familial, and Sporadic Prostate Cancer ClinCanRes 2004 10 (21 ): p. 7150-56

[11] Lengyel, P., Tumor-suppressor genes: news about the interferon connection Proceedings of the National Academy of Sciences 1993 90 (13 ): p. 5893-5895

[12] Hassel, B.A., et al., A dominant negative mutant of 2-5A-dependent RNase suppresses antiproliferative and antiviral effects of interferon. EMBO J., 1993. 12: p. 3297-3304.

[13] Zhou, A., Interferon action and apoptosis are defective in mice devoid of 2-5 A- oligoadenylate-dependent RNase L. EMBO J., 1997. 16: p. 6355-6363.

[14] Wang, D., et al., Microarray-based detection and genotyping of viral pathogens Proceedings of the National Academy of Sciences 2002 99 (24 ): p. 15687-15692

[15] Urisman, A., et al., Identification of a novel Gammaretrovirus in prostate tumors of patients homozygous for R462Q RNASEL variant. PLoS Pathog, 2006. 2: p. e25.

[16] Dong, B., et al., An infectious retrovirus susceptible to an IFN antiviral pathway from human prostate tumors. Proc Natl Acad Sci USA, 2007. 104: p. 1655 - 1660.

[17] Stoye, J.P. and J.M. Coffin, The four classes of endogenous murine leukemia virus: structural relationships and potential for recombination. . Journal of Virology 1987 61 (9 ): p. 2659-2669

[18] COFFIN, J.M., J.P. STOYE, and W.N. FRANKEL, Genetics of Endogenous Murine Leukemia Virusesa. Annals of the New York Academy of Sciences, 1989. 567(1): p. 39-49.

[19] Jenkins, N.A., et al., Organization, distribution, and stability of endogenous ecotropic murine leukemia virus DNA sequences in chromosomes of Mus musculus. . Journal of Virology 1982 43 (1 ): p. 26-36

[20] Stoye, J.P. and J.M. Coffin, Polymorphism of murine endogenous proviruses revealed by using virus class-specific oligonucleotide probes. . Journal of Virology 1988 62 (1 ): p. 168-175

[21] Dorner, A.J., J.P. Stoye, and J.M. Coffin, Molecular basis of host range variation in avian retroviruses. . Journal of Virology 1985 53 (1 ): p. 32-39

[22] Hayward, W.S., B.G. Neel, and S.M. Astrin, Activation of a cellular onc gene by promoter insertion in ALV-induced lymphoid leukosis. NATURE, 1981. 290(5806): p. 475-480.

[23] Varmus, H.E., Retroviruses and Oncogenes I (Nobel Lecture). Angewandte Chemie International Edition in English, 1990. 29(7): p. 707-715.

[24] Schlaberg, R., et al., XMRV is present in malignant prostatic epithelium and is associated with prostate cancer, especially high-grade tumors. Proc Natl Acad Sci USA, 2009. 106: p. 16351-16356.

[25] Arnold, R.S., et al., XMRV Infection in Patients With Prostate Cancer: Novel Serologic Assay and Correlation With PCR and FISH. Urology, 2010. 75(4): p. 755-761.

[26] Montefiori, D.C., et al., Demographic Factors That Influence the Neutralizing Antibody Response in Recipients of Recombinant HIV-1 gp120 Vaccines Journal of Infectious Diseases 2004 190 (11 ): p. 1962-1969

[27] Li, B., et al., Evidence for Potent Autologous Neutralizing Antibody Titers and Compact Envelopes in Early Infection with Subtype C Human Immunodefic. Virus Type 1 Journal of Virology, 2006. 80(11): p. 5211-5218.

[28] Danielson, B.P., G.E. Ayala, and J.T. Kimata, Detection of Xenotropic Murine Leukemia Virus-Related Virus in Normal and Tumor Tissue of Patients from the Southern United States with Prostate Cancer Is Dependent on Specific Polymerase Chain Reaction Conditions Journal of Infectious Diseases 2010 202 (10 ): p. 1470-1477

[29] Sfanos, K., et al., A molecular analysis of prokaryotic and viral DNA seq.s in prost. tissue from patients with prostate cancer indicates the presence of multiple and diverse microorganisms. Prostate, 2008. 68: p. 306 - 320.

[30] Lombardi, V.C., Detection of an infectious retrovirus, XMRV, in blood cells of patients with chronic fatigue syndrome. SCIENCE, 2009. 326: p. 585-589.

[31] Coffin, J.M. and J.P. Stoye, A New Virus for Old Diseases? Science 2009 326 (5952 ): p. 530-531

[32] Lo, S.-C., Detection of MLV-related virus gene sequences in blood of patients with chronic fatigue syndrome and healthy blood donors Proceedings of the National Academy of Sciences 2010 107 (36 ): p. 15874-15879

[33] Singh, I.R., Detecting Retroviral Sequences in Chronic Fatigue Syndrome. Viruses, 2010. 2(11): p. 2404-2408.

[34] Courgnaud, V., et al., Mouse retroviruses and chronic fatigue syndrome: Does X (or P) mark the spot? Proceedings of the National Academy of Sciences 2010 107 (36 ): p. 15666-15667

[35] Fischer, N., et al., Prevalence of human gammaretrovirus XMRV in sporadic prostate cancer. J Clin Virol, 2008. 43: p. 277 - 283.

[36] Hohn, O., et al., Lack of evidence for xenotropic murine leukemia virus-related virus(XMRV) in German prostate cancer patients. Retrovirology, 2009. 6(1): p. 92.

[37] D'Arcy, F., et al., No evidence of XMRV in Irish prostate cancer patients with the R462Q mutation. European Urology Supplements, 2008. 7: p. 271.

[38] Verhaegh, G.W., et al., Prevalence of human xenotropic murine leukemia virus-related gammaretrovirus (XMRV) in dutch prostate cancer patients. The Prostate, 2011. 71(4): p. 415-420.

[39] Martinez-Fierro, M., et al., Identification of viral infections in the prostate and evaluation of their association with cancer. BMC Cancer, 2010. 10(1): p. 326.

[40] Aloia, A.L., et al., XMRV: A New Virus in Prostate Cancer? Cancer Research 2010 70 (24 ): p. 10028-10033

[41] Robinson, M., et al., Mouse DNA contamination in human tissue tested for XMRV. Retrovirology, 2010. 7(1): p. 108.

[42] Brunschwig, A., C. M. Southam, et al. (1965). "Host resistance to cancer. Clinical experiments by homotransplants, autotransplants and admixture of autologous leucocytes." Ann Surg 162(3): 416-25.

[43] Fan, H., A new human retrovirus associated with prostate cancer Proceedings of the National Academy of Sciences 2007 104 (5 ): p. 1449-1450

[44] Groom, H.C.T. and K.N. Bishop, The tale of xenotropic murine leukemia virus-related virus Journal of General Virology 2012

[45] Paprotka, T., et al., Recombinant Origin of the Retrovirus XMRV Science 2011 333 (6038 ): p. 97-101

[46] Coffin, J.M., S.H. Hughes, and H.E. Varmus, Retroviruses. 1997.

[47] Knox, K., et No Evidence of Murine-Like Gammaretroviruses in CFS Patients Previously Identified as XMRV-Infected Science 2011 333 (6038 ): p. 94-97

[48] Cingoz, O. and J.M. Coffin, Endogenous Murine Leukemia Viruses: Relationship to XMRV and Related Sequences Detected in Human DNA Samples. Adv Virol. 2011: p. 940210.

[49] Kang, D.E., et al., XMRV Discovery and Prostate Cancer-Related Research. Adv Virol, 2011. 2011: p. 432837.

[50] Sfanos, K.S., et al., XMRV and prostate cancer[mdash]a 'final' perspective. Nature Reviews Urology, 2012. 9(2): p. 111-118.

[51] Rovigatti, U., Isolation and initial characterization of a new virus: Micro-Foci inducing virus or MFV. C R Acad Sci III, 1992. 315(5): p. 195-202.

[52] Greaves, M., Infection, immune responses and the aetiology of childhood leukaemia. Nature Reviews of Cancer, 2006. 6(3): p. 193-203.

[53]  U. Rovigatti, A.T., A. Piccin, R. Colognato amd B. Sordat. Preliminary Characteriza-
      tion of a New Type of Viruses Isolated from Paediatric Neuroblastoma and Non-
      Hodgkin's Lymphoma: potential Implications for Aetiology. in Intn. Conference
      Childhood Leukaemia. Section P1-18 pp I-IV, September 2004. 2004. London, United
      Kingdom: Editor: CwL.

[54]  Rovigatti, G.B.a.B.S.M. MFV Virus unduces MYCN DNA amplification and trans-
      forms benign neuroblastsinto cells tumorigenic in nude mice. in 18th International
      Congress of Biochemistry and Molecular Biology "Beyond the Genome". 2000. Lon-
      don, UK.

[55]  Rovigatti, U., C. Selli, and R. Bartoletti, Of Mice and Men - Viruses and Prostate Can-
      cer: What Is the Next Step? European Urology, 2010. 58(5): p. 684-686.

[56]  Liu, W., et al., Tumour suppressor function of RNase L in a mouse model. European
      Journal of Cancer, 2007. 43(1): p. 202-209.

[57]  Zhou, A., et al., Interferon action and apoptosis are defective in mice devoid of
      2[prime],5[prime]-oligoadenylate-dependent RNase L. EMBO Journal, 1997. 16(21):
      p. 6355-6363.

[58]  Garcia, M.A., E.F. Meurs, and M. Esteban, The dsRNA protein kinase PKR: Virus and
      cell control. Biochimie Interferons 1957-2007: from discovery to mechanism of action
      and clinical applications, 2007. 89(6â€"7): p. 799-811.

[59]  Garcia, M.A., et al., Impact of Protein Kinase PKR in Cell Biology: from Antiviral to
      Antiproliferative Action. Microbiology and Molecular Biology Reviews, December
      2006. 70(4): p. 1032-1060.

[60]  Samuel, C.E., Antiviral Actions of Interferons Clinical Microbiology Reviews 2001 14
      (4 ): p. 778-809

[61]  Williams, B.R., PKR; a sentinel kinase for cellular stress. Oncogene., 1999. 18(45): p.
      6112-20.

[62]  Pathak, V.K., D. Schindler, and J.W. Hershey, Generation of a mutant form of protein
      synthesis initiation factor eIF-2 lacking the site of phosphorylation by eIF-2 kinases.
      Molecular and Cellular Biology 1988 8 (2 ): p. 993-995

[63]  Samuel, C.E., Mechanism of interferon action: Phosphorylation of protein synthesis
      initiation factor eIF-2 in interferon-treated human cells by a ribosome-associated kin-
      ase processing site specificity similar to hemin-regulated rabbit reticulocyte kinase
      Proceedings of the National Academy of Sciences 1979 76 (2 ): p. 600-604

[64]  Abraham, N., et al., Characterization of Transgenic Mice with Targeted Disruption of
      the Catalytic Domain of the Double-stranded RNA-dependent Protein Kinase, PKR
      Journal of Biological Chemistry 1999 274 (9 ): p. 5953-5962

[65]  Yang, Y.L., et al., Deficient signaling in mice devoid of double-stranded RNA-de-
      pendent protein kinase. Embo J., 1995. 14(24): p. 6095-106.

[66] Balachandran, S., et al., Essential Role for the dsRNA-Dependent Protein Kinase PKR in Innate Immunity to Viral Infection. Immunity, 2000. 13(1): p. 129-141.

[67] Li, X.-L., et al., A central role for RNA in the induction and biological activities of type 1 interferons. Wiley Interdisciplinary Reviews: RNA, 2011. 2(1): p. 58-78.

[68] Mounir, Z., et al., Tumor Suppression by PTEN Requires the Activation of the PKR-eIF2{alpha} Phosphorylation Pathway SciSig., 2009. 2(102): p. ra85-.

[69] Squire, J.A., et al., Prostate Cancer as a Model System for Genetic Diversity in Tumors Advances in Cancer Research, D. Gisselsson, Editor. 2011, Ac. Press. p. 183-216.

[70] Samuel, C.E., Adenosine deaminases acting on RNA (ADARs) are both antiviral and proviral. VirologySpecial Reviews 2011, 2011. 411(2): p. 180-193.

[71] George, C.X., et al., Adenosine deaminases acting on RNA, RNA editing, and interferon action. J Interferon Cytokine Res. 31(1): p. 99-117.

[72] Galeano, F., et al., A-to-I RNA editing: The "ADAR" side of human cancer. Developmental Cell Behavior, 2012. 23(3): p. 244-250.

[73] Dominissini, D., et al., Adenosine-to-inosine RNA editing meets cancer Carcinogenesis 2011 32 (11 ): p. 1569-1577

[74] Li, J.B., et al., Genome-Wide Identification of Human RNA Editing Sites by Parallel DNA Capturing and Sequencing Science 2009 324 (5931 ): p. 1210-1213

[75] Zaranek, A.W., et al., A Survey of Genomic Traces Reveals a Common Sequencing Error, RNA Editing, and DNA Editing. PLoS Genet, 2010. 6(5): p. e1000954 EP -.

[76] Cattaneo, R., et al., Accumulated measles virus mutations in a case of subacute sclerosing panencephalitis: Interrupted matrix protein reading frame and transcription alteration. Virology, 1986. 154(1): p. 97-107.

[77] Cattaneo, R., et al., Biased hypermutation and other genetic changes in defective measles viruses in human brain infections. Cell, 1988. 55(2): p. 255-265.

[78] tenOever, B.R., et al., Multiple Functions of the IKK-Related Kinase IKKÎµ in Interferon-Mediated Antiviral Immunity Science 2007 315 (5816 ): p. 1274-1278

[79] Lei, M., Y. Liu, and C.E. Samuel, Adenovirus VAI RNA Antagonizes the RNA-Editing Activity of the ADAR Adenosine Deaminase. Virology, 1998. 245(2): p. 188-196.

[80] Samuel, C.E., Reoviruses and the interferon system. Curr Top Microbiol Immunol., 1998. 233(Pt 2): p. 125-45.

[81] Yang, C., et al., Identification and expression profiles of ADAR1 gene, responsible for RNA editing, in responses to dsRNA and GCRV challenge in grass carp (Ctenopharyngodon idella). Fish & Shellfish Immunology, 2012. 33(4): p. 1042-1049.

[82] Paz, N., et al., Altered adenosine-to-inosine RNA editing in human cancer Genome Research 2007 17 (11 ): p. 000

[83]  Ishiuchi, S., et al., Blockage of Ca2+-permeable AMPA receptors suppresses migra-tion and induces apoptosis in human glioblastoma cells. Nature Medicine, 2002. 8(9): p. 971-978.

[84]  Ishiuchi, S., et al., Ca2+-Permeable AMPA Receptors Regulate Growth of Human Glioblastoma via Akt Activation The Journal of Neuroscience 2007 27 (30 ): p. 7987-8001

[85]  Cenci, C., et al., Down-regulation of RNA Editing in Pediatric Astrocytomas Journal of Biological Chemistry 2008 283 (11 ): p. 7251-7260

[86]  Stark, G.R., et al., How Cells Respond To Interferons. Annual Review of Biochemis-try, 1998. 67(1): p. 227-264.

[87]  Darnell, J.E., Jr., Interferon research: impact on understanding transcriptional control. Curr Top Microbiol Immunol., 2007. 316: p. 155-63.

[88]  Stark, G.R. and J.E. Darnell Jr., The JAK-STAT Pathway at Twenty. Immunity, 2012. 36(4): p. 503-514.

[89]  Roberts, R.M., et al., The evolution of the type I interferons. Journal of Interferon and Cytokine Research, 1998. 18(10): p. 805-816.

[90]  Deonarain, R., et al., Impaired Antiviral Response and Alpha/Beta Interferon Induc-tion in Mice Lacking Beta Interferon Journal of Virology 2000 74 (7 ): p. 3404-3409

[91]  Bach, E.A., M. Aguet, and R.D. Schreiber, THE IFNÎ³ RECEPTOR:A Paradigm for Cy-tokine Receptor Signaling. Annual Review of Immunology, 1997. 15(1): p. 563-591.

[92]  Prejean, C. and O.R. Colamonici, Role of the cytoplasmic domains of the type I inter-feron receptor subunits in signaling. Seminars in Cancer Biology, 2000. 10(2): p. 83-92.

[93]  Malmgaard, L., Induction and regulation of IFNs during viral infections. J Interferon Cytokine Res., 2004. 24(8): p. 439-54.

[94]  Darnell, J., I. Kerr, and G. Stark, Jak-STAT pathways and transcriptional activation in response to IFNs and other extracellular signaling proteins Science 1994 264 (5164 ): p. 1415-1421

[95]  Schindler, C. and J.E. Darnell, Transcriptional Responses to Polypeptide Ligands: The JAK-STAT Pathway. Annual Review of Biochemistry, 1995. 64(1): p. 621-652.

[96]  Darnell, J.E., Jr., Studies of IFN-induced transcriptional activation uncover the Jak-Stat pathway. J Interferon Cytokine Res., 1998. 18(8): p. 549-54.

[97]  Nguyen, H., J. Hiscott, and P.M. Pitha, The growing family of interferon regulatory factors. Cytokine & Growth Factor Reviews, 1997. 8(4): p. 293-312.

[98]  BraganÃ§a, J. and A. Civas, Type I interferon gene expression: Differential expres-sion of IFN-A genes induced by viruses and double-stranded RNA. Biochimie, 1998. 80(8â€"9): p. 673-687.

[99] Decker, T., P. Kovarik, and A. Meinke, GAS elements: a few nucleotides with a major impact on cytokine-induced gene expression. J Interferon Cytokine Res., 1997. 17(3): p. 121-34.

[100] Copeland, K.F., Modulation of HIV-1 transcription by cytokines and chemokines. Mini Rev Med Chem., 2005. 5(12): p. 1093-101.

[101] Daly, C. and N.C. Reich, Characterization of Specific DNA-binding Factors Activated by Double-stranded RNA as Positive Regulators of Interferon /-stimulated Genes Journal of Biological Chemistry 1995 270 (40 ): p. 23739-23746

[102] Rebouillat, D., et al., Characterization of the Gene Encoding the 100-kDa Form of Human 2â€²,5â€²Oligoadenylate Synthetase. Genomics, 2000. 70(2): p. 232-240.

[103] Clemens, M.J. and B.R. Williams, Inhibition of cell-free protein synthesis by pppA2[prime]p5[prime]A2[prime]p5[prime]A: a novel oligonucleotide synthesized by interferon-treated L cell extracts. Cell, 1978. 13: p. 565-572.

[104] Floyd-Smith, G., E. Slattery, and P. Lengyel, Interferon action: RNA cleavage pattern of a (2[prime]-5[prime])oligoadenylate-dependent endonuclease. Science, 1981. 212: p. 1030-1032.

[105] Zhou, A., B.A. Hassel, and R.H. Silverman, Expression cloning of 2-5A-dependent RNAase: a uniquely regulated mediator of interferon action. Cell, 1993. 72: p. 753-765.

[106] Dong, B., et al., Intrinsic molecular activities of the interferon-induced 2-5A-dependent RNase. . Journal of Biological Chemistry 1994 269 (19 ): p. 14153-14158

[107] Dong, B. and R.H. Silverman, 2-5A-dependent RNase Molecules Dimerize during Activation by 2-5A Journal of Biological Chemistry 1995 270 (8 ): p. 4133-4137

[108] Smith, J., et al., Major susceptibility locus for prostate cancer on chromosome 1 suggested by a genome-wide search. Science, 1996. 274: p. 1371 - 1374.

[109] Lengyel, P., Tumor-suppressor genes: news about the interferon connection. Proc. Natl Acad. Sci. USA, 1993. 90: p. 5893-5895.

[110] Suhadolnik, R.J., et al., Upregulation of the 2-5A Synthetase/RNase L Antiviral Pathway Associated with Chronic Fatigue Syndrome Clinical Infectious Diseases 1994 18 (Supplement 1 ): p. S96-S104

[111] Shetzline, S.E., et al., Structural and functional features of the 37-kDa 2-5A-dependent RNase L in chronic fatigue syndrome. J Interferon Cytokine Res, 2002. 22(4): p. 443-56.

[112] De Meirleir, K., et al., Antiviral Pathway Activation in Chronic Fatigue Syndrome and Acute Infection Clinical Infectious Diseases 2002 34 (10 ): p. 1420-1421

[113] Suhadolnik, R.J., et al., Biochemical evidence for a novel low molecular weight 2-5A-dependent RNase L in chronic fatigue syndrome. J Interferon Cytokine Res, 1997. 17(7): p. 377-85.

[114] Demettre, E., et al., Ribonuclease L Proteolysis in Peripheral Blood Mononuclear Cells of Chronic Fatigue Syndrome Patients Journal of Biological Chemistry 2002 277 (38 ): p. 35746-35751

[115] Nijs, J., et al., Chronic fatigue syndrome: intracellular immune deregulations as a possible etiology for abnormal exercise response. Medical Hypotheses, 2004. 62(5): p. 759-765.

[116] Frémont, M., et al., 2-5 A Oligoadenylate size is critical to protect RNase L against proteolytic cleavage in chronic fatigue syndrome. Experimental and Molecular Pathology, 2005. 78(3): p. 239-246.

[117] NIJS, J. and K. DE MEIRLEIR, Impairments of the 2-5A Synthetase/RNase L Pathway in Chronic Fatigue Syndrome In Vivo November-December 2005 19 (6 ): p. 1013-1021

[118] MEEUS, M., et al., Unravelling Intracellular Immune Dysfunctions in Chronic Fatigue Syndrome: Interactions between Protein Kinase R Activity, RNase L Cleavage and Elastase Activity, and their Clinical Relevance In Vivo January-February 2008 22 (1 ): p. 115-121

[119] De Marzo, A., et al., Inflammation in prostate carcinogenesis. Nat Rev Cancer, 2007. 7(4): p. 256 - 269.

[120] Nelson, W., et al., The role of inflammation in the pathogenesis of prostate cancer. J Urol, 2004. 172(5 Pt 2): p. S6 - 11.

[121] Nelson, W., A. De Marzo, and W. Isaacs, Prostate cancer. N Engl J Med, 2003. 349: p. 366 - 381.

[122] Colotta, F., et al., Cancer-related inflammation, the seventh hallmark of cancer: links to genetic instability Carcinogenesis 2009 30 (7 ): p. 1073-1081

[123] Siegel, R., et al., Cancer statistics, 2011. CA: A Cancer Journal for Clinicians, 2011. 61(4): p. 212-236.

[124] Bostwick, D.G., Urologic Surgical Pathology. 1997. p. 423-456.

[125] McNeal, J.E., et al., Zonal distribution of prostatic adenocarcinoma. Correlation with histologic pattern and direction of spread. Am. J. Surg. Pathol., 1988. 12: p. 897-906.

[126] Franks, L.M., Atrophy and hyperplasia in the prostate proper. J. Pathol. Bacteriol., 1954. 68: p. 617-621.

[127] De Marzo, A., et al., Proliferative inflammatory atrophy of the prostate: implications for prostatic carcinogenesis. Am J Pathol, 1999. 155: p. 1985 - 1992.

[128] Putzi, M.J. and A.M. De Marzo, Morphologic transitions between proliferative inflammatory atrophy and high-grade prostatic intraepithelial neoplasia. Urology, 2000. 56: p. 828-832.

[129] Peto, J., Cancer epidemiology in the last century and the next decade. Nature, 2001. 411: p. 390-395.

[130] Hsing, A.W., L. Tsao, and S.S. Devesa, International trends and patterns of prostate cancer incidence and mortality. Int J Cancer, 2000. 85: p. 60-67.

[131] Cook, L.S., Et Al., Incidence Of Adenocarcinoma Of The Prostate In Asian Immigrants To The United States And Their Descendants. The Journal of urology, 1999. 161(1): p. 152-155.

[132] Sion-Vardy, N., et al., Ethnicity and its significance in the pathobiology of prostatic carcinoma in Southern Israel. Urologic oncology, 2008. 26(1): p. 31-36.

[133] Ranasinghe, W.K.B., et al., Incidence of prostate cancer in Sri Lanka using cancer registry data and comparisons with the incidence in South Asian men in England. BJU International, 2011. 108(8b): p. E184-E189.

[134] Shiraishi, T., et al., The frequency of latent prostatic carcinoma in young males: the Japanese experience. In Vivo, 1994. 8(3): p. 445-7.

[135] Zhu, Y.P., et al., Prevalence of incidental prostate cancer in patients undergoing radical cystoprostatectomy: data from China and other Asian countries. Asian J Androl, 2009. 11(1): p. 104-8.

[136] McNeal, J.E., Normal histology of the prostate. Histology for Pathologists (Ed. Sternberg), 1988. 12: p. 619-633.

[137] Pelouze, P.S., Gonorrhea in the male and female: a book for practitioners. 1935, W B Sounders Company: Philadelphia.

[138] Handsfield, H.H., et al., Asymptomatic gonorrhea in men. Diagnosis, natural course, prevalence and significance. New England Journal of Medicine, 1974. 290: p. 117-123.

[139] Boldogh, I., et al., Human cytomegalovirus and herpes simplex type 2 virus in normal and adenocarcinomatous prostate glands. Journal of the National Cancer Institute, 1983. 70(5): p. 819-826.

[140] Eizuru, Y., et al., Herpesvirus RNA in human urogenital tumors. Proceedings of the Society for Experimental Biology and Medicine, 1983. 174(2): p. 296-301.

[141] Bergh, J., et al., No link between viral findings in the prostate and subsequent cancer development. Br J Cancer, 2006. 96(1): p. 137-139.

[142] Berrington de Gonzalez, A., et al., Antibodies against six human herpesviruses in relation to seven cancers in black South Africans: A case control study. Infectious Agents and Cancer, 2006. 1(1): p. 2.

[143] Chang, Y., et al., Identification of herpesvirus-like DNA sequences in AIDS-associated Kaposi's sarcoma. Science, 1994. 266(5192): p. 1865-9.

[144] Monini, P., et al., Kaposi's Sarcomaâ€"Associated Herpesvirus DNA Sequences in Prostate Tissue and Human Semen. New England Journal of Medicine, 1996. 334(18): p. 1168-1172.

[145] Corbellino, M., et al., Absence of HHV-8 in prostate and semen [2]. New England Journal of Medicine, 1996. 335(16): p. 1237-1239.

[146] Diamond, C., et al., Human herpesvirus 8 in the prostate glands of men with Kaposi's sarcoma. Journal of Virology, 1998. 72(7): p. 6223-6227.

[147] Hoffman, L.J., et al., Elevated Seroprevalence of Human Herpesvirus 8 among Men with Prostate Cancer Journal of Infect. Diseases 2004 189 (1 ): p. 15-20

[148] Sutcliffe, S., et al., Plasma Antibodies against Chlamydia trachomatis, Human Papillomavirus, and Human Herpesvirus Type 8 in Relation to Prostate Cancer: A Prospective Study Cancer Epidemiology Biomarkers & Prevention 2007 16 (8 ): p. 1573-1580

[149] MONINI, P., et al., DNA Rearrangements Impairing BK Virus Productive Infection in Urinary Tract Tumors. Virology, 1995. 214(1): p. 273-279.

[150] Das, D., R.B. Shah, and M.J. Imperiale, Detection and expression of human BK virus sequences in neoplastic prostate tissues. Oncogene, 2004. 23(42): p. 7031-7046.

[151] Newton, R., et al., Antibody levels against BK virus and prostate, kidney and bladder cancers in the EPIC-Oxford cohort. Br J Cancer, 2005. 93(11): p. 1305-1306.

[152] Das, D., K. Wojno, and M. Imperiale, BK virus as a cofactor in the etiology of prostate cancer in its early stages. J Virol, 2008. 82: p. 2705 - 2714.

[153] zur Hausen, H., Papillomaviruses in the causation of human cancers - a brief historical account. Virology, 2009. 384: p. 260 - 265.

[154] zur Hausen, H., The search for infectious causes of human cancers: Where and why. Virology, 2009. 392(1): p. 1-10.

[155] Leiros, G., et al., Detection of human papillomavirus DNA and p53 codon 72 polymorphism in prostate carcinomas of patients from Argentina. BMC Urology, 2005. 5(1): p. 15.

[156] Hrbacek, J., et al., Thirty years of research on infection and prostate cancer: No conclusive evidence for a link. A systematic review. Urologic Oncology: Seminars and Original Investigations, In the Press (0).

[157] Hrbacek, J., et al., Serum antibodies against genitourinary infectious agents in prostate cancer and benign prostate hyperplasia patients: a case-control study. BMC Cancer, 2011. 11(1): p. 53.

[158] Woodworth, C.D., HPV innate immunity. Front Biosci, 2002. 7: p. d2058-71.

[159] Platz, E.A., Nonsteroidal anti-inflammatory drugs and risk of prostate cancer in the Baltimore Longitudinal Study of Aging. Cancer Epidemiology Biomarkers Prevention, 2005. 14: p. 390-396.

[160] Mahmud, S., E. Franco, and A. Aprikian, Prostate cancer and use of nonsteroidal anti-inflammatory drugs: systematic review and meta-analysis. Br. J. Cancer, 2004. 90: p. 93-99.

[161] Chan, J.M., et al., The epidemiology of prostate cancer [mdash] with a focus on nonsteroidal anti-inflammatory drugs. Hematl Oncol Clin. North Am., 2006. 20: p. 797-809.

[162] Jacobs, E.J., A large cohort study of aspirin and other nonsteroidal anti-inflammatory drugs and prostate cancer incidence. J. Natl. Cancer Inst., 2005. 97: p. 975-980.

[163] Mahmud, S., E. Franco, and A. Aprikian, Prostate cancer and use of nonsteroidal anti-inflammatory drugs: systematic review and meta-analysis. Br J Cancer, 2004. 90(1): p. 93-99.

[164] Mahmud, S.M., et al., Non-steroidal anti-inflammatory drug use and prostate cancer in a high-risk population. Eur J Cancer Prev, 2006. 15(2): p. 158-64.

[165] Dasgupta, K., et al., Association between nonsteroidal anti-inflammatory drugs and prostate cancer occurrence. Cancer J, 2006. 12(2): p. 130-5.

[166] Mahmud, S.M., E.L. Franco, and A.G. Aprikian, Use of nonsteroidal anti-inflammatory drugs and prostate cancer risk: A meta-analysis. International Journal of Cancer, 2010. 127(7): p. 1680-1691.

[167] Mahmud, S.M., et al., Use of Non-Steroidal Anti-Inflammatory Drugs and Prostate Cancer Risk: A Population-Based Nested Case-Control Study. PLoS ONE, 2011. 6(1): p. e16412 EP -.

[168] Chokkalingam, A.P., et al., Prostate carcinoma risk subsequent to diagnosis of benign prostatic hyperplasia. Cancer, 2003. 98(8): p. 1727-1734.

[169] Dennis, L.K., C.F. Lynch, and J.C. Torner, Epidemiologic association between prostatitis and prostate cancer. Urology, 2002. 60: p. 78-83.

[170] Sarma, A.V., Sexual behavior, sexually transmitted diseases and prostatitis: the risk of prostate cancer in black men. J. Urol., 2006. 176: p. 1108-1113.

[171] Sondergaard, G., M. Vetner, and P.O. Christensen, Prostatic calculi. Acta Pathol. Microbiol. Immunol. Scand., 1987. 95: p. 141-145.

[172] Sutcliffe, S., Gonorrhea, syphilis, clinical prostatitis, and the risk of prostate cancer. Cancer Epidemiol Biomarkers Prev, 2006. 15: p. 2160-2166.

[173] Sutcliffe, S., et al., Non-steroidal anti-inflammatory drug use and the risk of benign prostatic hyperplasia-related outcomes and nocturia in the Prostate, Lung, Colorectal, and Ovarian Cancer Screening Trial. BJU International, 2012. 110(7): p. 1050-1059.

[174]  Ogilvie, I., et al., Burden of community-acquired and nosocomial rotavirus gastroen-
       teritis in the pediatric population of Western Europe: a scoping review. BMC Infec-
       tious Diseases, 2012. 12(1): p. 62.

[175]  Greaves, M., Darwinian medicine: a case for cancer. Nature Reviews of Cancer, 2007.
       7(3): p. 213-221.

[176]  Wang, Z.A. and M.M. Shen, Revisiting the concept of cancer stem cells in prostate
       cancer. Oncogene, 2011. 30(11): p. 1261-1271.

[177]  Kasper, S., Identification, characterization, and biological relevance of prostate cancer
       stem cells from clinical specimens. Urologic oncology, 2009. 27(3): p. 301-303.

[178]  Li, H. and D.G. Tang, Prostate cancer stem cells and their potential roles in metasta-
       sis. Journal of Surgical Oncology, 2011. 103(6): p. 558-562.

[179]  Ogilvie , I., et al., Burden of rotavirus gastroenteritis in the pediatric population in
       Central and Eastern Europe: Serotype distribution and burden of illness. vaccines,
       2011. 7(5) 2164-5515): p. 523-533.

[180]  Sfanos, K.S., et al., XMRV and prostate cancer[mdash]a 'final' perspective. Nature Re-
       views of Cancer, 2012. 9(2): p. 111-118.

[181]  DeFreitas, E., et al., Retroviral sequences related to human T-lymphotropic virus type
       II in patients with chronic fatigue immune dysfunction syndrome Proceedings of the
       National Academy of Sciences 1991 88 (7 ): p. 2922-2926

[182]  John Coffin, S.H.H.a.H.V., Retroviruses. 1997: Cold Spring Harbor Laboratory Press.

[183]  Daniel, P. and R. Morin, [Effect of sodium salicylate on the "in vitro" development of
       RNA viruses (author's transl)]. Ann Microbiol (Paris), 1975. 126(3): p. 381-7.

[184]  Ward, R.L., D.S. Sander, and D.R. Knowlton, In vitro activities of bismuth salts
       against rotaviruses and other enteric viruses. Antimicrobial Agents and Chemothera-
       py 1985 27 (3 ): p. 306-308

[185]  Cohnheim, J., Ueber entzundung und eiterung. Path. Anath. Physiol. Klin., 1867. 40:
       p. 1-79.

[186]  Virchow, R.E., Editorial. Virchows. Path. Anath. Physiol. Klin., 1855. 3: p. 23.

[187]  Pappenheim, A., Prinzipen der neuren morphologischen haematozytologie nach zy-
       togenetischer grundlage. Folia Hematol., 1917. 21: p. 91-101.

[188]  McCulloch, E.A. and J.E. Till, Perspectives on the properties of stem cells. Nature
       Medicine, 2005. 11(10): p. 1026-1028.

[189]  BECKER, A.J., E.A. McCULLOCH, and J.E. TILL, Cytological Demonstration of the
       Clonal Nature of Spleen Colonies Derived from Transplanted Mouse Marrow Cells.
       Nature, 1963. 197(4866): p. 452-454.

[190] Bruce, W.R. and H. Van Der Gaag, A quantitative assay for the number of murine lymphoma cells capable of proliferation in vivo. nature, 1963. 199: p. 79-80.

[191] Sabbath, K.D., et al., Heterogeneity of clonogenic cells in acute myeloblastic leukemia. J. Clin. Invest., 1985. 75: p. 746-753.

[192] Greaves, M., Childhood leukaemia. Bmj, 2002. 324(7332): p. 283-7. 2.

[193] Greaves, M.F., et al., Leukemia in twins: lessons in natural history. Blood, 2003. 102: p. 2321-2333.

[194] Greaves, M.F. and J. Wiemels, Origins of chromosome translocations in childhood leukaemia. Nature Reviews Cancer, 2003. 3: p. 639-649.

[195] Fialkow, P.J., S.M. Gartler, and A. Yoshida, Clonal origin of chronic myelocytic leukemia in man. Proc Natl Acad Sci U S A, 1967. 58(4): p. 1468-71.

[196] Fialkow, P.J., et al., Leukaemic transformation of engrafted human marrow cells in vivo. Lancet, 1971. 1(7693): p. 251-5.

[197] Fialkow, P.J., Is lyonisation total in man? Lancet, 1970. 2(7667): p. 315.

[198] Fialkow, P.J., et al., 6-Phosphogluconate Dehydrogenase: Hemizygous Manifestation in a Patient with Leukemia Science 1969 163 (3863 ): p. 194-195

[199] Fialkow, P.J., Use of genetic markers to study cellular origin and development of tumors in human females. Adv Cancer Res, 1972. 15: p. 191-226.

[200] Hamburger, A. and S. Salmon, Primary bioassay of human myeloma stem cells. J Clin Invest, 1977. 60: p. 846 - 854.

[201] Hamburger, A. and S. Salmon, Primary bioassay of human tumor stem cells. Science, 1977. 197: p. 461 - 463.

[202] Herzenberg, L.A., et al., The history and future of the fluorescence activated cell sorter and flow cytometry: a view from Stanford. Clin. Chem., 2002. 48: p. 1819-1827.

[203] McCune, J.M., The SCID-hu mouse: murine model for the analysis of human hemato-lymphoid differentiation and function. Science, 1988. 241: p. 1632-1639.

[204] Kamel-Reid, S., A model of human acute lymphoblastic leukemia in immune-deficient SCID mice. Science, 1989. 246: p. 1597-1600.

[205] Sirard, C., et al., Normal and leukemic SCID-repopulating cells (SRC) coexist in the bone marrow and peripheral blood from CML patients in chronic phase, whereas leukemic SRC are detected in blast crisis. Blood, 1996. 87(4): p. 1539-48.

[206] Lapidot, T., et al., A cell initiating human acute myeloid leukaemia after transplantation into SCID mice. Nature, 1994. 367(6464): p. 645-8.

[207] Bonnet, D. and J.E. Dick, Human acute myeloid leukemia is organized as a hierarchy that originates from a primitive hematopoietic cell. Nat Med, 1997. 3(7): p. 730-7.

[208] Al-Hajj, M., et al., Prospective identification of tumorigenic breast cancer cells. Proc Nat Acad Sci, 2003. 100: p. 3983-3988.

[209] Moreb, J.S., Aldehyde dehydrogenase as a marker for stem cells. Curr Stem Cell Res Ther, 2008. 3(4): p. 237-46.

[210] Marcato, P., et al., Aldehyde dehydrogenase: Its role as a cancer stem cell marker comes down to the specific isoform. Cell Cycle, 2011. 10(91538-4101): p. 1378-1384.

[211] Prasmickaite, L., et al., Aldehyde Dehydrogenase (ALDH) Activity Does Not Select for Cells with Enhanced Aggressive Properties in Malignant Melanoma. PLoS ONE, 2010. 5(5): p. e10731 EP -.

[212] Quintana, E., et al., Efficient tumour formation by single human melanoma cells. Nature, 2008. 456: p. 593 - 598.

[213] La Porta, C.A., Thoughts about cancer stem cells in solid tumors. World J Stem Cells. 4(3): p. 17-20.

[214] Tu, S.-M. and S.-H. Lin, Prostate Cancer Stem Cells. Clinical Genitourinary Cancer, 2012. 10(2): p. 69-76.

[215] Leong, K.G., et al., Generation of a prostate from a single adult stem cell. Nature, 2008. 456(7223): p. 804-808.

[216] Wang, X., et al., A luminal epithelial stem cell that is a cell of origin for prostate cancer. Nature, 2009. 461(7263): p. 495-500.

[217] Goldstein, A.S., et al., Identification of a Cell of Origin for Human Prostate Cancer Science 2010 329 (5991 ): p. 568-571

[218] Mackinnon, A.C., et al., Molecular Biology Underlying the Clinical Heterogeneity of Prostate Cancer: An Update. Archives of Pathology & Laboratory Medicine, 2009. 133(7): p. 1033-1040.

[219] Nonn, L., V. Ananthanarayanan, and P.H. Gann, Evidence for field cancerization of the prostate. The Prostate, 2009. 69(13): p. 1470-1479.

[220] Tomlins, S.A., et al., Recurrent fusion of TMPRSS2 and ETS transcription factor genes in prostate cancer. Science, 2005. 310(5748): p. 644-648.

[221] Kumar-Sinha, C., S.A. Tomlins, and A.M. Chinnaiyan, Recurrent gene fusions in prostate cancer. Nature Reviews of Cancer, 2008. 8(7): p. 497-511.

[222] Tomlins, S.A., et al., ETS Gene Fusions in Prostate Cancer: From Discovery to Daily Clinical Practice. European Urology, 2009. 56(2): p. 275-286.

[223] Clark, J.P. and C.S. Cooper, ETS gene fusions in prostate cancer. Nat Rev Urol, 2009. 6(8): p. 429-39.

[224] Cohen, J. and M. Enserink, False Positive Science 2011 333 (6050 ): p. 1694-1701

[225]  Bell, T.M., et al., Isolation of a Reovirus from a Case of Burkitt's Lymphoma. Br Med J., 1964. 1(5392): p. 1212-3.

[226]  Bell, T.M., et al., Further isolations of reovirus type 3 from cases of Burkitt's lymphoma. Br Med J., 1966. 1(5502): p. 1514-7.

[227]  Bell, T.M. and M.G. Ross, Persistent latent infection of human embryonic cells with reovirus type 3. Nature., 1966. 212(5060): p. 412-4.

[228]  Bell, T.M., G.M. Munube, and D.H. Wright, Malignant lymphoma in a rabbit inoculated with reovirus. Lancet., 1968. 1(7549): p. 955-7.

[229]  McCrae, A.W., et al., Trans-stadial maintenance of reovirus type 3 in the mosquito Culex (C) pipiens fatigans Weidmann and its implications. East Afr Med J., 1968. 45(10): p. 677-86.

[230]  Munube, G.M., et al., Sero-epidemiology of reovirus type 3 infections in four areas of Uganda with varying incidence of Burkitt's tumour. East Afr Med J., 1972. 49(5): p. 369-75.

[231]  Levy, J.A., E. Tanabe, and E.C. Curnen, Occurrence of reovirus antibodies in health African children and in children with Burkitt's lymphoma. Cancer., 1968. 21(1): p. 53-7.

[232]  Levy, J.A., et al., Effect of reovirus type 3 on cultured Burkitt's tumour cells. Nature., 1968. 220(5167): p. 607-8.

[233]  Macsween, K.F. and D.H. Crawford, Epstein-Barr virus-recent advances. Lancet Infect Dis., 2003. 3(3): p. 131-40

[234]  Maley, C.C., Cancer: The Evolutionary Legacy. Heredity, 2002. 88(3): p. 219.

[235]  Greaves, M., Cancer causation: the Darwinian downside of past success? The Lancet Oncology, 2002. 3(4): p. 244-251.

[236]  Greaves, M., Darwin and evolutionary tales in leukemia ASH Education Program Book 2009 2009 (1 ): p. 3-12

[237]  Greaves, M. and C.C. Maley, Clonal evolution in cancer. Nature, 2012. 481(7381): p. 306-313.

# Supportive Care

# Chapter 3

# The Role of Physiotherapy in the Pre and Post Treatment Interventions in Prostate Cancer Patients

Mario Bernardo Filho and
Mauro Luis Barbosa Júnior

Additional information is available at the end of the chapter

## 1. Introduction

### 1.1. Cancer and physiotherapy

Cancer is the common term for all malignant tumours and its consequences are a concern for people worldwide. Advances in health and medical science procedures (early diagnosis, improved chemotherapy and radiotherapy) and surgical techniques, and their utilization in the field of oncology, have significantly improved survival and have thus strongly influenced the practice of physiotherapy [1, 2, 3, 4].

People are living longer with their cancers, which in many cases are treated as chronic disease, due to the early detection and advances in treatment options. Thus, physiotherapists require greater knowledge of the clinical conditions and improved skill in managing patients with cancer, before, during and after the specific medical procedures. They also have the responsibility of managing and treating patients during the pre and postoperative periods with the provision of the best particular physiotherapeutic intervention to each patient [5, 6].

Besides the knowledge about clinical interventions, the physiotherapist needs to be in contact with the recent advances in the scientific literature in general. Moreover, this professional must know about the risk factors to cancer and participate in actions to aid in the prevention of this disease [5, 6, 7].

In oncology, for example, there is increasing evidence, initially only from epidemiological studies but increasingly from individuals case studies, that risk of some cancers, such as prostate, may be reduced in people living in areas of high ambient solar radiation or with high sun exposure than in those where the converse is the case. Naturally, the information about the protection against the unnecessary exposition of the sunlight is also very important [8, 9].

Images are suitable tools to aid in the early diagnosis of several types of cancer. However, some modalities of images, as the positron emission tomography (PET) dependenting on the radiopharmaceutical, and in some clinical condition, false negative information can be obtained. As a profisssional of an interdisciplinar team, the physiotherapist must have enough knowledge to suggest a modality of image and to know about the limitations of each procedure [4, 10, 11]

Epidemiological researches have put in evidence the benefits of physical activity in relation to the risk of cancer. Moreover, the physical activity has been considered as a modifiable lifestyle risk factor that has the potential to reduce the risk of the majority of the types of diseases, as the cancer. The physiotherapist must be also involved in public and private actions to guide the Society to have correct style of the life also related to adequate exercise (kinesiotherapy) and physical activities in general. Naturally, these actions must consider the individual characteristic of each subject [5, 12].

Undesirable clinical conditions due to the use of some techniques to treat cancer can bring bothersome that can comprise the sexual health and the quality of life. It is important that the interprofessional team be prepared to discuss these questions [13, 14].

## 2. Role of physiotherapy

Physiotherapeutic procedures have an important role in the healthcare of people of all ages and with different types of clinical status. These procedures are relevant in the treatment, in the prevention of diseases or complications and in the management or treatment of undesirable pathological conditions to thus minimize the impact these may have in the quality of life of the patient [7].

Physiotherapy is a profession defined by great diversity in areas of clinical practice with the purpose of developing, maintaining and restoring the maximum movement and functional ability of each person, considering the specific limitations of the individual. The role of the physiotherapist within the interdisciplinary group (physician, nurse, nutritionist, occupational therapy, social worker, psychologist, speech therapist) is well defined in various clinical conditions, as with the patient with cancer [5, 7].

The pressing need arises for the existence of a differentiated care system with the purpose to cater for the particular needs of the patients and their families. It is desirable that the physiotherapist working in oncology has a broad knowledge of other clinical areas, such as neurology, the musculoskeletal and cardiopulmonary systems and in rehabilitation and kinesiotherapy in general, as well as in services along the entire spectrum of patient care. There is also a considerable role for the physiotherapists in the evaluation of the clinical conditions and management of the patients, as well as in assisting people's return to work and normal life following treatment [6, 14].

It is often the fatigue and weakness caused by the disease and/or its treatment that delay this return to normal functions and limit the quality of life of a specific individual. An important aspect related to cancer and its treatment is the typically induced muscle atrophy. Probably this clinical condition is due to perturbations in different pathways of the muscle protein metabolism, including decreased muscle protein synthesis, increased muscle protein degradation, or a combination of both [5, 12, 15].

The most prevalent symptom in cancer is fatigue, which has now overtaken pain as the most common distressing symptom of the disease. The intensity of the fatigue varies from patient to patient and it is a complex and subjective phenomenon. Non-pharmacological fatigue cares are desirable. There is much evidence to suggest that appropriately prescribed physical exercises (kinesiotherapy) play an important role in the decrease of cancer fatigue and the improvement of the quality of life of the patient. The reduction of fatigue is highly relevant and desirable for the patient to (i) have the ability to continue or return to work; (ii) develop daily activities at home; and (iii) participate in social activities, all of which are clear parts of the overall quality of life of the patient [2-4, 15, 16]

It is thus essential that physiotherapists working with cancer patients have a clear and comprehensive understanding of the individual cancers and their staging and development, as well as the techniques that are being used in the diagnosis and treatment of the patient. The physiotherapist must have knowledge of the consequences and complications of clinical procedures, such as surgery, chemotherapy and radiotherapy, and their potential side effects such as neuropathies and cardiomyopathies. Moreover, the physiotherapist must be informed about the specific procedures that were used in the patient during medical intervention. A discussion about these procedures and the possible complications and occurrences are relevant to the management of the patient before and after the surgery. In addition, the physiotherapist must also know how these medical procedures can affect the physiotherapeutic interventions and thus select the best and convenient procedure for each patient [5, 7, 14]

The physiotherapist also needs to know more about individual medications as patients can survive longer using new cancer treatments, but often with severe side effects, which leave them weaker and often feeling quite unwell during the process. Hormonal therapy, for example, has an important effect on the muscle mass. The decrease in muscle mass, leading to muscle weakness and general debility, can be minimized by specific kinesiotherapyprogrammes. These appropriated exercises are established and implemented by physiotherapists considering the anatomical area of the disease and specific capabilities and limitations of each patient [5, 6, 7, 14].

Whole body vibration exercises (WBV) performed in oscillating platform could be a good option to aid the patient with cancer. The vibrations generated in these platforms can be transmitted to body of the patient, and, it is suggested that, in appropriated conditions, these vibrations could improve walking function, muscle strength, bone mineral density, cardiovascular fitness and body balance. Moreover, the health-related quality of life is increased and the fall risk is decreased. The frequency and the amplitude of the vibration can be totally controlled by the physiotherapist that is supervising the clinical procedure. The duration of the work, as well as, the time to rest, the number of sets in a session and the number of sessions are also controlled. All these conditions depend on, mainly, the clinical and physical conditions of the patient. The mechanisms responsible for the WBV benefits are not fully understood, however it is hypothesized that these effects are probably related to direct and indirect actions. The direct effects would be related with the transmission of energy of the vibration, for example, to a muscle that would be stimulated. The indirect effects might to be associated with the neuroendocrine system. Whole body mechanical vibration on the muscle performance would be due to the induction of a myotatic reflex contraction referred as the tonic vibration reflex [17, 18, 19].

Normally, the person is standing on the platform, but other positions are possible, as it is shown in the Figure 1. It is possible to see in the Figure 1.c that the man has bent knees.

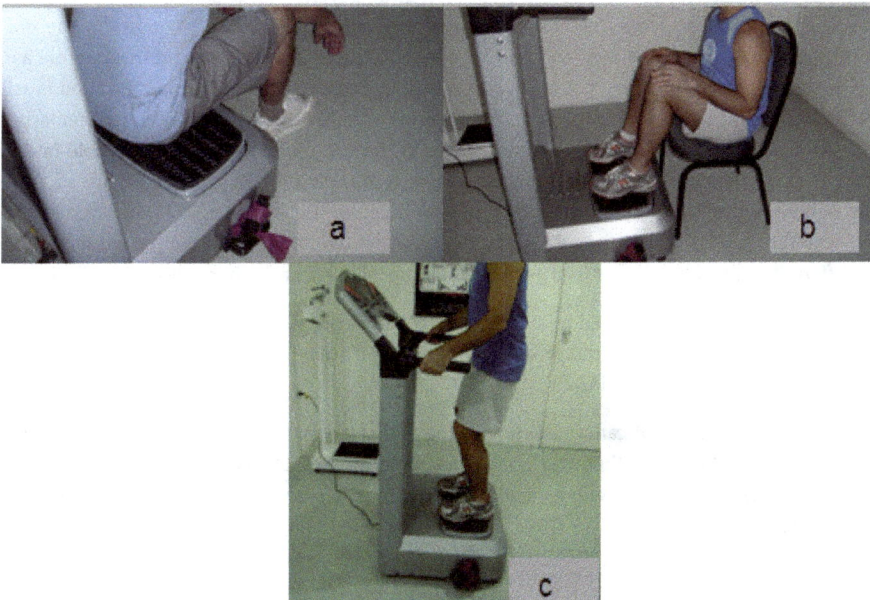

**Figure 1.** Some of the positions of the person in the oscillating platform. (a) sitting, (b) sitting in a chaise and the feet in the platform, (c) standing.

Physiotherapists utilize physical agents, such as therapeutic exercises (kinesiotherapy), electrotherapy and manipulative therapy to provide a holistic approach to the prevention, diagnosis and therapeutic management of clinical disorders, as well as possible future complications [5, 7]. Involving the movements of the body and the optimization of the functions of the tissues, they aim to enhance the health, welfare and quality of life and thus they can play an important role in the management and rehabilitation of patients with prostate cancer (PCa). In patients with PCa, the physiotherapist will also guide the patient in relation to the knowledge and understanding of the anatomic structures related directly with the pelvic floor, the correct breathing and the perception of the muscles of the pelvic floor, as other muscles of the pelvis. Specific attention is given to the comprehension of the functions of these muscles, especially to the levatorani muscle [20-26]

Sexual health is a state of physical, emotional, mental and social well-being in relation to sexuality; it is not merely the absence of disease, dysfunction or infirmity. Sexuality is considered as a personal and human dimension that is characterized as a strong aspect of the human personality and it is an aspect of the emotional and physical intimacy that men and women experience through their lives. Moreover, sexuality is experienced and expressed in thoughts, fantasies, desires, beliefs, attitudes, values, behaviours, practices, roles and relationships [27, 28, 29]

Sexuality is influenced by the interaction of biological, psychological, social, economic, political, cultural, ethical, legal, historical, religious and spiritual factors. Sexuality is present from the conception up to the dead and it consists of three interrelated and inseparable aspects, that are biological, psychological and social. In consequence, particular attention must be done to the relevance and hole of the organs related to the biological components involved in the sexuality [29, 30]. The importance of the comprehension of the possible undesirable consequences of the clinical procedures used to treat the PCa must be discussed with the patient and/or with the partner. The physiotherapist must have also knowledge about the sexuality to define specific exercises and techniques available to aid the patient with PCa in different steps of his life, as well as the limitations of these and other procedures. [6, 14]

Figure 2 shows some tools used to explain the patient about the anatomic structures directly and indirectly involved with the prostate and the structures that can be damaged in the surgery for the treatment of the PCa.

During the final stages of cancer treatment, the palliative care becomes paramount and the participation of the physiotherapist is also desirable in the interdisciplinary team. The care with the patient with cancer will contribute to minimize the progression of secondary symptoms [5, 6, 26].

The correct and appropriated mobilization of the scars to avoid adherence and important alterations in the posture of the patient is also highly relevant. This procedure contributes to the improvement of the quality of life of the patient immediatly and in the future [5].

Procedures of the physiotherapy in palliative care is also used for pain, lymphoedema, dyspnoea and other symptom assessment and treatment, as well as for the education on safe transfer and mobility management of the patient. Constipation, nausea, sleep disturbance (insomnia), anxiety, fatigue, dyspnoea, pain scores and appetite are all improved by physiotherapeutic intervention. Some of these clinical complications can be also prevented or minimized. Along the time, the lymphoedema management in the terminally diseases has developed more effectively, with evidence supporting the complex physiotherapy treatment and the integration with other professionals [5, 7, 16].

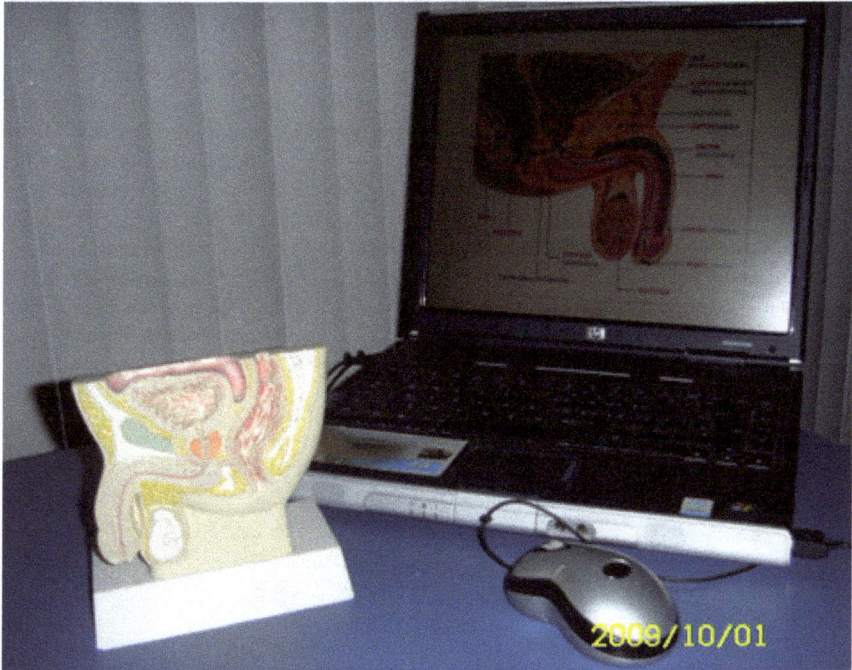

**Figure 2.** Tools used to explain to the patient about the anatomic structures of the pelvic floor

## 3. Prostate cancer in the world

Cancer is an important public problem and is considered a national health priority area in several countries due to the burden that it places on the individual, families and the community [1, 2, 31].

The World Health Organization (WHO) develops strategies towards the prevention, research, education and control of the cancer. Important medical developments and relevand scientific findings have permitted that people with cancer can survive with their disease and with the side effects of their disease and its treatment for longer [31].

The high relevance of the cancer in public health and research activity can also be demonstrated by the number of scientific research identified in the database system PubMed (a service of the National Library of Medicine and the National Institutes of Health) [32].

It is possible to see in the Table I, the number of publications in the PubMed related to cancer and cancer and some organs. It is possible to identify in the Table I approximately 2 700

000 full papers in this databank with the keyword cancer and 2.22% of these publications are related with PCa.

The mainly risk factors for PCa are (a) age (it is the strongest risk factor for PCa andthe probability of developing this disease is 1 in 12,833 for men aged birth to 39, 1 in 44 for men aged 40 to 59, and 1 in 7 for men aged 60 to 79 years), (b) family history (greater risk if father or brother had the disease and slightly higher for men whose mothers or sisters have had breast cancer ), (c) Race/Ethnicity (greater risk among African American men compared with white, Asian, and American Indian men), (d) prostate changes (abnormal cells described as high-grade prostatic intraepithelial neoplasia), and (e) diet ( food with high animal fat and low in fruits and vegetables).Moreover, between 5 to 10% of the PCa cases are believed to be due primarily to high-risk inherited genetic factors or PCa susceptibility genes. Genetic testing has been a reality and it has been well documented that genetic factors might increase the risk of cancer onset [33, 34].

| Keyword | Number of publications |
|---|---|
| Cancer | 2 656 222 |
| "Breast cancer" | 49 804 |
| "Prostate cancer" | 59 245 |
| "Colorectal cancer" | 47 010 |

**Table 1.** Number of publications in the PubMed with keywords related to cancer

PCa is the most common solid cancer in men worldwide and is the most common of all cancers in the North America. In an epidemiological study was reported that the estimated PCa incidence rates remain most elevated in North America, Oceania, and Western and Northern Europe. Mortality rates tend to be higher in less developed regions of the world including parts of South America, the Caribbean, and sub-Saharan Africa. Increasing PCa incidence rates were observed in 32 of the 40 countries examined, which clearly demonstrates the increasing problem related to this disease, that it would be not desirable. However, PCa mortality rates decreased in 27 of the 53 countries under study, whereas rates increased in 16 and remained stable in 10 countries [2, 15, 33, 34].

## 4. The importance of the early diagnosis of the prostate cancer

The early diagnosis of PCa has been facilitated by the determination of the prostate specific antigen (PSA), rectal touch and ultrasonography, which has subsequently led to a high cure rate in the early stages (stage I/II) of the disease. However, it is important to have in mind, that these current diagnostic techniques have not, in several cases, sufficient specificity and sensitivity to determine the stage and aggressiveness of the PCa and to identify appropriate treatment [2, 6, 35-37].

International guidelines support opportunistic PSA screening in well-informed patients and recommend a baseline PSA at 40 years of age. Although some relevant controversies contin-ue about the real benefit of the screening program, the undisputable finding is that an in-creasing percentage of young men have an early PCa diagnosis and this condition has the advantage to permit curative interventions [2, 35-37].

When a man has the PCa early diagnosed, he has a number of treatment options, which carry similar success rates. Surgery, brachytherapy or external beam radiotherapy in combination with several months of initial hormone treatment all carry the same chance of cure but they all have very different recovery times, or number of visits to the hospital to consider [4, 6].

Concerning to the recurrent PCa, a key treatment decision is based on whether the disease is only localized in the prostate fossa. If the sites of cancer in the early phase of recurrent dis-ease were known, patients would be treated properly, leading to fewer side effects, a better prognosis with curative approach, and reduced treatment cost. Nuclear medicine imaging has been considered a reliable technique to be used with this purpose and an important as-pect of the nuclear imaging that should be understood is that this type of imaging demon-strates physiology rather than anatomy [4, 6, 10, 11].

PET is a nuclear medicine technique for tumor imaging. The radiopharmaceutical 18F-FDG was firstly introduced to image brain tumors. Along the time, this radiopharmaceutical has been widely accepted and it was considered a highly effective and successfully way to im-age several types of cancers. In consequence, investigations using 18F-FDG were performed to evaluate the use of this radiopharmaceutical in the diagnosis of the PCa. Unfortunately, in general, the PCacan not be imaged with this radiopharmaceutical. This poor performance of 18F-FDG is mainly related to the low glucose metabolic rate in the PCa, as well as, a relevant excretion of the radiopharmaceutical into the adjacent urinary bladder. Moreover, it is well known that the ability of FDG-PET to detect cancer is based on an increased expression of cellular membrane glucose transporter and enhanced hexokinase II enzyme activity within the tumor cells, where the 18F-FDG undergoes enzymatic transformation to FDG-6 phos-phate [10, 11].

Due to the limitations to use the 18F-FDG to detect PCa, other molecules to be labeled with a radionuclide, to be utilized as PET-radiopharmaceuticals, have been investigated with this purpose. Choline is a substrate for phosphatidylcholine, which is incorporated into cell membrane phospholipids, and is not dependent on cell proliferation and this molecule can be labeled with 11C or 18F for detection. 11C-choline has been shown to be superior to 18F-FDG to detect PCa, in part due to its negligible urinary secretion. 11C-choline PET has been shown to be able to localize primary PCa to the fossa of the prostate gland in up to 86.5% of patients and localize lymph node spread in up to 81.8% of patients [10, 11].

Another molecule, acetate, as 18F or 11C-labeled acetate, which is involved in cytoplasmic lipid synthesis, has been investigated to detect PCa. The retention of radiolabeled acetate in PCa cell lines has been shown to be related to fatty acid metabolism and enhanced beta-oxidation pathway. As PET-labeled acetate has minimal urinary activity, it is considered very suitable for evaluation of local prostatic disease with a high sensitivity for PCa lesions. When compared with 18F-FDG-PET for detection of primary tumors, there is a markedly increased sensitivity of 11C-acetate PET compared with 18F-FDG-PET, and the uptake of 11C-acetate is higher if the PSA is >3 ng/mL [10, 11].

The considerations about the early detection of the PCa is necessary, due to, there is considerable variation in the likely side effects and risks of long-term consequences such as urinary incontinence (UI) and erectile dysfunction (ED) in patients with PCa. With the early diagnosis there is an expectation of curing cancer, minimizing the risk of UI and ED and increasing the quality of life of the patient [38-41].

In general, radical prostatectomy (RP) is a curative and appropriated therapy for any patient whose tumour is clinically confined to the prostate, has a life expectancy of 10 years or more, and has no serious co-morbid conditions that would contraindicate surgery. Other factors affecting treatment decisions include patient factors, such as (i) Current symptoms (International Prostate Symptom Score, urinary flow rate), (ii) Current age (preference under the age of 70 years), (iii) Concurrent illnesses may determine suitability or not for surgery, (iv) Patient preference (psychological factors including patients ideas, concerns and expectations). Tumor/cancer factors, such as (a) Grade of tumour (the "aggressiveness" determines the risk of relapse), (b) Stage of tumour (determines radical of palliative approach), (c) Chance of response to treatment, (d) Chance of recurrence, and (e) Possibility of second curative treatment modalities if the first treatment fails must be also considered [6, 34, 38-41].

It is also important to consider that the risk of death under the anaesthetic for a RP is about 1 in 250 patients. The procedures used in the surgery become technically more challenging when the patient is overweight or obese and the risks of surgery increase. Improved knowledge about the anatomy of the organs of the pelvis and the muscles of the pelvic floor and the functions related to them had resulted in major improvements in this surgical technique [38-41].

Radiation therapy (RT) is another option for treatment of PCa. RT uses high-energy X-rays or other types of ionizing radiation to try to kill the cancer cells in various organs/tissues. There are mainly two types of radiotherapy: (i) External radiotherapy that uses a source of ionizing radiation that is outside of the body and (ii) Internal radiotherapy that uses a radioactive substance sealed in needles, seeds, wires, or catheters that are placed directly into or near the cancer (brachytherapy). The external radiotherapy is a complex procedure and requires the patient to make a number of steps, as (i) positioning and immobilization of the patient, (ii) localization of the tumor, (iii) determination of the size of the tumor, (iv) delineation of the target (tumor) and critical tissues structures in the neighborhood, (v) dose prescription, (vi) type of ionizing radiation, (vii) treatment planning, (viii) simulation and verification of the treatment and (ix) evaluation.Concerning to the brachytherapy to the PCa, several radioactive seeds (in general with iodine-125] are implanted into the prostate gland with the aim to irradiate the tumor. These seeds are not removed and will be permanently in the prostate. As the iodine-125 emits low level energy electromagnetic radiation, the energy of the radiation is deposited in the prostate, treating locally the tumor [4].

Various severe complications following RT can occur and these complications depend on the type of the procedure used in the treatment. In addition, clinical complications, such as UI and ED have also been associated with the RT [6, 14, 40, 42].

In Figure 3 is shown some modalities of treatment for PCa and possible adverse effects associated with some of these treatments.

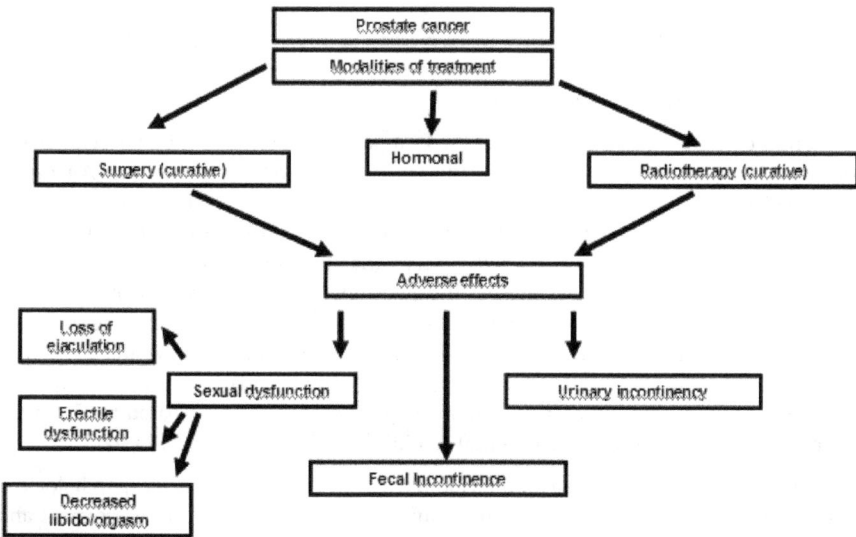

**Figure 3.** Modalities of treatment for the prostate cancer and possible adverse effects associated.

As presented before, UI and ED are undesirable side effects normally associated with the RP and RT due to the damage of the muscles of the pelvic floor. [26, 38, 39, 43]

UI has a prevalence ranging from 5 to 60 per cent. UI after RP is the most bothersome complication of this operation and has a major impact on the quality of life and it is therefore of the utmost importance to minimize its prevalence after this kind of surgery. In the clinical routine with the patient that was submitted to treatment to PCa, it is verified that the UI is an unpleasant condition [21, 24, 26].

The types and characteristics of UI secondary to PCa are (a) Stress UI, which is mainly associated with RP; (b) Urge incontinence, which is associated with RT and consists of a strong, unpleasant and sudden urge to urinate, with burning sensation or irritation in the bladder; and (c) Mixed incontinence, which affects mainly older patients on radiation and/or hormone therapy [21, 24]

In addition to the functional problem of the UI, this clinical condition causes a psychosocial disorder characterized by distress. Moreover, this is potentialised and augmented by the inability of the patient to perform habitual activities. Furthermore, the impossibility of controlling leakage and the resulting feeling of regression, and the inability to overcome the fatigue resulting from the interruption in the number of hours and the quality of sleep in the case of nocturia and anxiety increase dissatisfaction. In consequence, a restrictive social situation can be usually observed, characterized by shyness, shame from the leakage, and social stigmatization and isolation. Additionally, UI may trigger an undesirable, obsessive and strong psychological behavior related to the control of leakage of urine and of associated odors. These factors can increase the anxiety and to cause a reduction of the social life of the patient. Additionally, UI may trigger an obsessive and strong psychological behavior related to the control of leakage and odors. These factors can contribute to cause a reduction of the social life of the patient [6, 14, 20, 24, 42].

The impact of UI on the quality of life of the PCa patient is determined by the self-perception of the severity and the disruption of daily activities caused by the symptoms. An important consideration is that the cases of UI and ED (and other sexual dysfunctions, see Figure 3] recorded in clinics seem to be much higher than the number described in the publications. This discrepancy could be attributed to the great variability of definitions, measurement instruments, and manners of assessing UI. If a good interview with the patient before the treatment of the PCa is not performed, it is also difficult to determine whether the symptom is a result of the treatment of the disease or of the natural involution that would occur with age. Moreover, there is a fatalistic and resigned attitude that makes the patients hide or mask the symptom from the professional or the professional is not prepared to obtain the informations that are relevant to the clinical conditions of the patient [6, 20, 24, 42].

ED, in general, is usually due to a multifactorial etiology, comprising organic, psychological, or mixed aspects, and may often require a multidisciplinary approach for assessment and treatment. Organic causes encompass vascular, neurologic, hormonal, as a result of medications, pelvic surgery (mainly RP), RT, diabetes or mixed factors. In general, any condition that can cause damages to the nerves or impair blood flow in the penis may lead to ED. Pelvic surgery (especially RP and bladder surgery for cancer) might damage cavernous nerves and arteries near the penis, causing ED [23, 30, 39].

Penile erection is the consequence of a complex neurovascular process in which nerves, endothelium of sinusoids and blood vessels, and smooth muscle cells are involved. Several central nervous and peripheral transmitters and transmitter systems participate in the process and the nitric oxide (NO) is the main mediator of penile erection. It is produced by a group of enzymes called nitric oxide synthase (NOS) which utilizes the amino acid L-arginine and molecular oxygen as substrates to produce NO and L-citrulline. The endothelial NOS is constitutively expressed within the vascular system, it is tightly regulated and produces physiologically relevant levels of NO.The investigations about the NO, that can readily cross plasma membranes to enter target cells, and its functions as a mediator synthesized and released from the vascular endothelium and as a neurotransmitter in inhibitory nerves innervating the penis represented a breakthrough in the comprehension of the neurophysiological basis of erection. Moreover, the synthesis of NO and the consequences of NO binding to soluble guanylylcyclase is essential for the erectile process [44, 45, 46].

Impaired erectile function, or the total inability to maintain or achieve sufficient penile rigidity for satisfactory sexual intercourse performance, it was firstly used as a definition of impotence. On 1992, it was recommended that the term "erectile dysfunction" replace the term "impotence," but, sometimes, the two terms have been used interchangeably. The term ED is more precise and eliminates the confusion of multiple meanings and connotations associated with the word impotence. ED is defined as a "consistent or recurrent inability of a man to attain and/or maintain penile erection sufficient for sexual activity". The condition must be present for a minimum of 3 months to establish the diagnosis. The exception to this is when ED is preceded by trauma or pelvic surgery [47, 48, 49]

In addition, penile erection involves a complex interaction between the central nervous system and local factors. The penis is innervated and regulated by autonomic (sympathetic and parasympathetic) and somatic (sensory and motor) nerve fibers. Overall, erection is a neurovascular event modulated by psychological and hormonal factors. The economic burden of ED is not just limited to the cost of diagnosis and treatment. Subtle impacts on the society that are difficult to quantify are (i) lost time at work, (ii) decreased productivity of the patient due to distress, (iii) impact on the partner and family and (iv) alteration of the social interactions. The comprehensive knowledge and the understanding of these conditions have also reflected in the number of papers published in important scientific journals that have increased along of the years [27, 38, 39, 41, 46].

Reports of studies describing ED after RP have shown a range from 29% to 97.5% with less ED occurring in younger men. Men with ED may suffer from depression and low self-esteem, and experience difficulties establishing and maintaining relationships. Treatment regimens currently available for ED include psychotherapy, sex therapy, oral pharmacological agents, androgen replacement therapy, intraurethral therapy, intracavernosal injections, several procedures related to the physiotherapy and surgery [27, 38, 39, 41, 50].

The pelvic floor muscles, besides other functions, play an important role in sexual activity and contractions of the ischiocavernosus and bulbocavernosus muscles produce an increase in the intracavernous pressure and influence penile rigidity. The bulbocavernosus muscle compresses the deep dorsal vein of the penis to prevent the outflow of blood from an engorged penis. The procedures of the physiotherapy, associated with a interdisciplinar team, including exercises for the muscles of the pelvic floor muscle only or associated with manometric biofeedback, electrotherapy, vaccum pumps can be used successfully in various patients with ED [20-26]

In addition, it is highly desired to consider that beneficial effects of pre- and postoperative pelvic floor interventions (RT or RP) using physiotherapy procedures, since both the duration and degree of UI after RP decrease in these case [24, 51-53].

When a patient with PCa is referred to undertake physiotherapy procedures before the surgery or radiotherapy, it is possible to teach him about the perception of the muscles of the pelvic foor, facilitating the performance of exercises involving these muscles associated with an ideal breathing, just after the RP or RT [6, 22-24].

As it is possible to see in the Figure 3, besides the ED, another clinical conditions related to the sexual functions can appear in the patient submitted to a RP, as the loss of ejaculation and the decrease of the libido and orgasm [6, 27, 39, 41].

The interventions related to the physiotherapy will contribute to aid the patient to live your sexuality. Moreover, it is important to show to the patient that sexuality is not only genitality, but it goes beyond the limits of genital impulse and is characterized as a strong experience of human personality [6, 13, 27, 39, 41].

Several options of treatment are available to treat ED, as psychosexual counseling, medication, use of physiotherapy (exercises to the pelvic floor muscles, electrotherapy, acupuncture and external vacuum devices), intracavernous injection therapy, vascular surgery, and use of a penile prosthesis. The etiology of the ED, the acceptability for the patient, the available information about methods and the success rate have been used to determine the choice of intervention. The clinical interventions used in the physiotherapy provide noninvasive methods that are easy to perform, painless, and inexpensive [6, 39, 41, 50, 51].

## 5. Physiotherapy procedures in the management of the patient with prostate cancer

The physiotherapist, from his assessment, can also help the patient with PCa in the presurgical period in which the exercises for the pelvic floor and for the respiration that will be performed in the post-surgical period can be learned early by the patient. Moreover, the knowledge and the perception of the muscles of the pelvic floor by the patient will be very important. As these muscles are located inside the pelvis, they are considered a continence muscle group giving structural support for the pelvic organs and the pelvic sphincters (urethra and anus, for exemple in men). Based on urethral continence maintained by muscles of the pelvic floor, the procedures of the physiotherapy of this muscle group can retake the control of the urinary continence or maximize it, also by nerve stimulation, according to the consensus, which can inhibit the detrusor muscle, increasing the quality of life of patients with Pca [20-26].

Patient assessment by the physiotherapist is accomplished through the anamnesis, voiding diary, pad test, data collection of the urodynamic study and/or other complementary examinations, if any, physical examination and specific maneuvers to assess urine leakage [24].

In the interview, beyond identifying the main complaint and history of the patient, issues inherent in urination are of utmost importance to be addressed. The voiding diary is a useful tool because it allows the physiotherapist to objectively quantify the volume of urine loss, as well as the frequency of the urination. As the voiding diary is fully performed by the patient over a period of about two to three days, with notes of drinking water, the type of the drink, volume voided, urgency severity, quantification of loss and its association to carry out some activity at the time,he is leding to observe his behavior voiding, generating his self-knowledge [20-26].

The completion of the pad test lasts one hour, and after that the pad is weighed, depicting the severity of UI. When the weigth is less than 3g, the UI is considered light. The UI is moderated to 3 up to 10 g, and over 10g is considered severe incontinence [20-26].

Urodynamic investigations involve the evaluation of the dynamic function of the lower urinary tract. The urodynamic study, an examination of the gold standard, evaluates the morphology, pressure (urethral, vesical and abdominal under static and dynamic conditions), physiology and hydrodynamic transport urine of the voiding mechanism, thus detailing the stages of filling and emptying as well as the sphincter behavior. Common urodynamic findings in post-RP patients are (a) internal sphincter deficiency and (b) bladder dysfunction (detrusor instability and decreased compliance) [20-26].

On physical examination is evaluated the strength and the tone of the pelvic floor muscles through the anal sphincter, perineal sensation and bulb-cavernosum reflex. Maneuver effort, such as coughing, can evaluate the sphincter function, which can be performed with the patient standing, with the bladder full, and where he is asked to simulate cough. From this assessment is given the goal of treatment [20-23].

One of the objectives of the intervention of the physiotherapy is to re-train the muscles of the pelvis by improving the active retention strength of the striated muscles of the pelvic floor in order to overcome the insufficiency of the injured sphincters and improve the continence of men with PCa. This level includes the awareness of the pelvic floor musculature and the coordination of the contraction-relaxation process to improve the control and the quality of the muscle contraction. Specific attention is given to the muscles of the deep plane of the pelvic floor [5, 24, 25].

To facilitate the perception of the muscles of the pelvic floor, electrotherapy is often used. This technique beyond to guide the patient to correct the contraction of muscles, depending on the type of electrical current, it also can be used other responses. Two types of electrodes can be used in the electrotherapy; internal (anal) and external electrodes [20-26].

In the case of functional electrical stimulation, which is an alternating current of low frequency, it generates muscle contractions and an increase of muscle function. In the pelvic floor muscles, electrode stimulation in the perineal body, the contraction is perceived by the patient and the physiotherapist with the apparent anal contraction. This contraction also acts by stimulating the sacral nerve roots, or specifically the pelvic and pudendal nerves, suppressing the (hyper) detrusor activity [24]

In figure 4, a patient that is undergone electrotherapy with external electrodes is shown. A correct frequency is choosen, following international studies and the intensity of electric current is selected considering the sensibility of the patient.

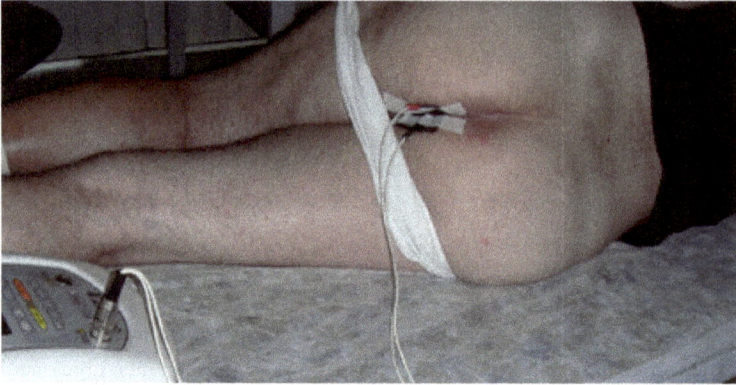

**Figure 4.** Patient after prostate cancer surgery undergoing electrotherapy

Physiotherapy also assists with postoperative respiratory recovery, early mobilization, lymphoedema prevention, education and garments if required, as well as the later management of pelvic floor re-education, continence advice and lymphoedema treatment if necessary. Men undergoing RP under a general anaesthetic will be off work for about 6 weeks. Moerover, they will stay in hospital for 5-7 days and have a urinary catheter for 2 weeks. The sphincter "valve" has gone and the urine leaks without control, day and night until the patient has learned again to use his muscles of the pelvic floor to regain his continence. Concerning ED, when a man wakes up from a RP he will almost certainly have ED initially. If there is going to be a recovery of erectile function, it may take 18-24 months to occur. Approximately 30% of men will recover erectile function and medication (Viagra or Cialis) will usually boost this recovery. However, physiotherapy procedures could be another suitable option without contraindications. In figure 3 is possible to see a man that has previously been submitted to RP and is undergoing external electrotherapy. In addition, the patient that has learned about the exercises involving the muscles of the pelvic floor can start these exercises immediately just after the surgery or after the catheter removal [20-26, 52, 53].

In the figure 5 are shown men doing exercises using a ball to increase the perception of the pelvic floor muscles, as well as to work these muscles.

In figure 5.a, the man relaxed and in 6.b, he has raising the hips and contracting the pelvic floor muscles. In figure 5.c, the man is sitting on the ball to increase the perception of the pelvic floor muscles and in 6.d, the man puts the hands together and begins to lift up the hands and feeling the contraction of the pelvic floor muscles to upward movement.

Beneficial effects of pre- and postoperative pelvic floor re-education are clear, since both the duration and degree of UI after RP can be distinguishably decreased [5, 43, 51].

Physiotherapy has responded to the improved outcomes and patient demand for quality of life improvements by instituting new treatments and education, such as informing about the possible importance of the sunlight in the prevention of the PCa and the equal need to protect against the harmful effects of the ultraviolet radiation, or about the options of physio-therapy for rehabilitation and re-integration to normal life [5, 6, 8, 9].

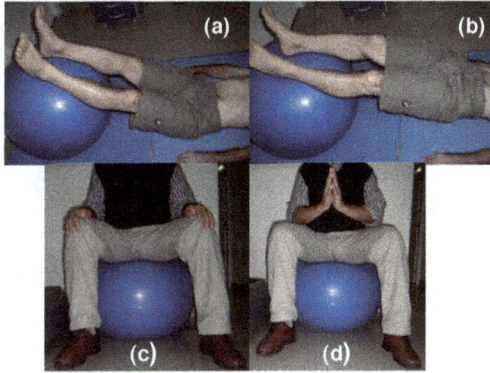

**Figure 5.** Men doing exercises with a ball to perception and to work the pelvic floor muscles.

Alternative and complementary techniques have also been considered as an option to be used for treating ED. One of these techniques that is related to the physiotherapy is the acu-puncture. Acupuncture is safe and involves the insertion of thin needles into different areas of the body known as acupuncture points. Traditionally, acupuncture has been often used to restore and maintain health through the stimulation of these specific points on the body. As this stimulation could modulate the NO, it is possible to consider that acupuncture might be effective for treating ED. Although, in some studies the acupuncture has been used success-fully to treat ED, there is sufficient evidence that acupuncture is an effective intervention for treating ED [55].

Mechanical vacuum devices cause erection by creating a partial vacuum, which draws blood into the penis, engorging and expanding it. The devices have three components. A plastic cylinder, into which the penis is placed; a pump, which draws air out of the cylinder; and an elastic band, which is placed around the base of the penis to maintain the erection after the cylinder is removed and during intercourse by preventing blood from flowing back into the body.One variation of the vacuum device involves a semirigid rubber sheath that is placed on the penis and remains there after erection is attained and during intercourse [27, 28, 50].

In general, physiotherapy management in the area of oncology have relevant contributions to patient care, including: (i) Decreasing length of stay in acute facilities (early discharge planning, outpatient follow up and education, involvement in palliative care facilities and physiotherapy services in home care); (ii) Improving functional capacity (early mobilization, management of complications of surgery, convenient manipulations of the areas submitted to RT and other treatments, as treating lymphoedema and scars); (iii) Improving lymphoe-dema management that has lead to decreased hospital admissions for cellulitis (a feature of poorly controlled lymphoedema and/or orientation of the patient) and decreased need for costly and at times uncomfortable pressure garments; (iv) Improving local and general exercise capacity (prevention of loss of body weight and managing the side effects of the disease, medication and surgery); (v) Shortening the period of time of UI after RP; and (vi) Affecting quality of life factors for all patients with cancer and their carers and families. These all provide examples where physiotherapy intervention contributes considerably to the health care provision and demonstrate how the various disciplines allied to medicine are working together to either bring the now healthy individual back to normal life and re-integration to the society, or improve the quality of life of patients that have to live with cancer as a chronic disorder and those that are in the terminal stages of the disease and life [5-7, 43, 53].

## 6. Considerations about the various prostate cancer treatments and their associated side effects

A number of side effects are associated with the various treatments available for PCa. As it was presented before, associated side effects include ED and UI amongst others, and a number of palliative care treatments and exercises have been proposed to counteract these effects [24, 52, 53]

A very important and unquestionable point is that pelvic floor muscle exercises are relevant to the treatment of ED in patients with PCa that will be submitted to RP. Most physiotherapy treatments for ED focus also on pelvic floor muscles. It is relevant to consider also the arrangement of the muscles at the base of the penis, as well as the other local structures that, with the time without erection, can lead to veno-occlusive ED. This undesirable condition is the result of a sequence of penile morphologic alterations post-RP. The physiotherapist will guide the patient to do exercises for the muscles direct related to the pelvic floor and also to the muscles indirectly related with the pelvis, such as abdominal and gluteal muscles. When they are contracted an increase of the local blood flow to the pelvic region is verified. This process seems to lead to a release of NO to the penis, acting on endothelium vasodilation and dependent on the flow, increasing in oxygen supply to the penile tissue and keeping the erectile tissue healthy [22, 24, 54].

On this same point of view about the treatment of the ED with physiotherapy, the vaccum therapy could also provide oxygen supply generated by negative pressure that distends the corporal sinusoids and increases the blood inflow to the penis. This system reduces apoptosis minimizing fibrosis of the corpora cavernosa which directly influences in the maintaining of the penile length. Differently, the use of the vacuum device (figure 6) for intercourse, the vaccum therapy does not use the ring constrictor, since it would keep in the corpora cavernosa a poorly oxygenated blood. The vaccum therapy could be combined with anothers therapies for ED, as pelvic floor muscles exercices (kinesiotherapy) and oral therapies (medications) [27, 40, 50].

UI has been also treated with the various exercises (kinesiotherapy) involving the muscles of the pelvic floor in patients submitted to RP. Prior to a pelvic floor muscle exercise program, an anal assessment is performed to grade the strength, endurance and speed of the anal sphincter and the puborectalis muscle. Pelvic floor muscle exercises are individually taught to ensure that they are being performed correctly [52],

In consequence, a number of pertinent considerations arise from the treatments and their associated side effects, which can related directly to personal circumstances and situations, clinical conditions after treatment or laboratory determinations (PSA) and medications/ procedures used after treatment [40, 41, 46, 47].

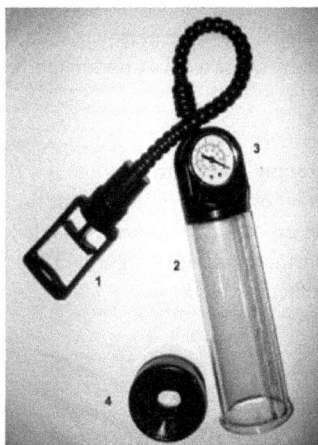

(1)Suction syringe, (2) Plexiglass cylinder, (3) Barometer,
(4) Sealing ring of silicone cylinder

**Figure 6.** A model of a vacuum device

Personal situations related with the possible treatments for PCa must be considered, as bladder irritation is common after RT, bowel complications might occur in the long-term and have high incidence during external beam RT, ED can be early in the surgery in comparison with RT, and penile shortening or fibrosis might occur after RP [6, 14].

Clinical conditions after the RP, such as pelvic pain, is common mainly in young men, UI will occur in the post operative period, erectile functioning might return slowly over years after the surgery. All these must be considered and must be explained to the patient and his family [6, 14].

The decline of the quality of the sexual activity can lead to a complicated pattern of change in quality of life and also negatively affect the psychosocial wellbeing of men and of the couple [6, 14].

Concerning the laboratory determinations as well as the medications used after the RP, it is important to consider that phosphodiesterase-5 inhibitors have limited actions in the cases of ED and the velocity is a more reliable indicator of recurrence than an isolated PSA measurement. When the available procedures to minimize the clinical complications of the RP or of the RT are considered, it is highly relevant to emphasize that the decrease of the appearance of complications occurs in patients thar have undergone physiotherapy before the RP and the improvement of the symptoms is observed due to the procedures of the physiotherapy just after the RP [6, 14].

Due to the high occurence of the PCa in the world, the high cost involved in the treatment and its impact in the quality of life of the patients with this disease, considerations about the different kinds of treatment as well as the possible complications of the treatments available are desirable [6, 14].

In addition, the questions associated with the personal situations related with the possible treatments for PCa would be relevant for a better understanding of the clinical situations of each patient [6, 14].

Finally, the knowledge of the patient about his situation as well as the involvement of the family and partner must be strongly considered. Moreover, it is also important to explain and present all the possibilities involving the treatment of the PCa. In addition, it is highly desired thal all the modalities of procedures that are available to aid in the prevention of undesirable clinical conditions. Furthermore, it is suggested that is necessary to consider the techniques related to the physiotherapy before and after the treatment of choice to the PCa.

## Acknowledgements

We. would like to acknowledge the assistance of Dr Sotiris Missailidis in the proof reading of this manuscript. We thank the support of the CNPq (Conselho Nacional de Desenvolvimento Científico e Tecnológico - "National Counsel of Technological and Scientific Development") and UERJ (Universidade do Estado do Rio de Janeiro).

## Author details

Mario Bernardo Filho[1*] and Mauro Luis Barbosa Júnior[2*]

*Address all correspondence to: bernardofilhom@gmail.com

*Address all correspondence to: maurolbarbosajr@gmail.com

1 Coordenadoria de Pesquisa, Instituto Nacional de Câncer and Departamento de Biofísica e Biometria, Instituto de Biologia Roberto Alcântara Gomes, Universidade do Estado do Rio de Janeiro, Rio de Janeiro, RJ, Brasil

2 Departamento de Medicina de Integral Familiar e Comunitária, Hospital Universitário Pedro Ernesto, Universidade do Estado do Rio de Janeiro, Rio de Janeiro, RJ, Brasil

# References

[1] Instituto Nacional do Câncer. Available: http://www2.inca.gov.br/wps/wcm/connect/inca/portal/home. Accessed 2012 July 11th.

[2] National Cancer Institute, Available: http://www.cancer.gov/cancertopics/types/prostate. Accessed 2012 July 11th.

[3] Boulikas T, Alevizopoulos N (2008) Representative Cancers, Treatment and Market. In: Missailidis S (editor) Anticancer Therapeutics.UnitedKingdon: Wiley & Sons. pp. 377-386.

[4] Perkins AC (2007) Tumour imaging and therapy. In: Missailidis S (editor) The Cancer Clock. UK: Wiley & Sons. pp. 135- 157

[5] Bernardo-Filho M, Bergmann A, Tavares A (2007) Physiotherapy in cancer patients. In: Missailidis S (editor) The Cancer Clock. United Kingdon: Wiley & Sons. pp. 245-263.

[6] Bernardo-Filho M, Missailidis S, Santos-Filho S, Fonseca A (2009) Prostate cancer therapies, complications and sixteen questions that the patients and the multidisciplinary team are interested in. Gene Ther. Mol. Biol. 13: 254-263

[7] Bennett CJ, Grant MJ (2004). Specialisation in physiotherapy: a mark of maturity. Aust. J. Physiother. 50: 3-5.

[8] Moon SJ, Fryer AA, Strange RC (2005) Ultraviolet radiation, vitamin D and risk of prostate cancer and other diseases. Photochem. Photobiol. 81: 1252–1260.

[9] Kricker A, Armstrong B (2006) Does sunlight have a benefificial influence on certain cancers? Prog. Biophys. Mol. Biol. 92: 132-139.

[10] Oyama N, Miller TR, Dehdashti F, Siegel BA, Fischer KC, Michalski JM, Kibel AS, Andriole GL, Picus J, Welch MJ (2003) 11C-Acetate PET Imaging of prostate cancer: detection of recurrent disease at PSA Relapse. J. Nucl. Med. 44: 549–555.

[11] Lee ST, Lawrentschuk N, Scott AM (2012) PET in Prostate and bladder tumors. Semin. Nucl. Med. 42: 231-246.

[12] Friedenreich CM, Neilson HK, Lynch BM (2010) State of the epidemiological evidence on physical activity and cancer prevention. Eur. J. Cancer. 46: 2593-2604

[13] Johnson BK (2004) Prostate Cancer and Sexuality: Implications for Nursing. Geriatr. Nurs. 25: 341-347.

[14] Katz A, Katz A (2008) The top 13: what family physicians should know about prostate cancer. Can. Fam. Physician. 54: 198-203.

[15] Wolin KY, Schwartz AL, Matthews CE, CourneyaKS, Schmitz KH (2012) Implementing the Exercise Guidelines for Cancer Survivors. J. Support. Oncol. May 10

[16]  Sternberg CN, Krainer M, Oh WK, Bracarda S, Bellmunt J, Ozen H, Zlotta A, Beer TM, Oudard S, Rauchenwald M, Skoneczna I, Borner MM, Fitzpatrick JM (2006) The medical management of prostate cancer: a multidisciplinary team approach. BJU Int. 99: 22-27.

[17]  Pinto NS, MonteiroMB, Santos-FilhoSD, Paiva D, Tavares A, Missailidis S, Marin PJ, Bernardo-Filho M (2010) Postmenopausal/menopause, bone mineral density and whole body vibration: a short review. J. Med. Med. Sci. 1: 516-525.

[18]  Santos-Filho SD, PintoNS, MonteiroMB, Arthur AP, Misssailidis S, Marín PJ, Bernardo-Filho M (2011) The ageing, the decline of hormones and the whole-body vibration exercises in vibratory platforms: a review and a case report. J. Med. Med. Sci. 2: 925-931.

[19]  Cardinale M, Wakeling J (2005) Whole body vibration exercises: are vibrations good for you? Br. J. Sports Med. 39: 585-589.

[20]  Cornel EB, de Wit R, Witjes JA (2005) Evaluation of early pelvic floor physiotherapy on the duration and degree of urinary incontinence after radical retropubic prostatectomy in a non-teaching hospital. World J. Urol. 23: 353-355.

[21]  Dorey G, Speakman M, Feneley R, Dunn C, Swinkels A, Ewings P. (2004a) Randomised controlled trial of pelvic floor muscle exercises and manometric biofeedback for post-micturition dribble. Urol. Nurs. 24: 490-512

[22]  Dorey G, Speakman M, Feneley R, Dunn C, Swinkels A, Ewings P (2004b) Randomised controlled trial of pelvic floor muscle exercises and manometric biofeedback for erectile dysfunction. Br. J. Gen. Pract. 54: 819-825

[23]  Dorey G, Speakman MJ, Feneley RCL, Swinkels A, Dunn CDR (2005) Pelvic floor exercises for erectile dysfunction. BJU Int. 96: 595-597.

[24]  Dorey G (2006) Pelvic Dysfunction in men: Diagnosis and Therapy of Male Incontinence and Erectile Dysfunction.Chichester: John Wiley & Sons. pp. 1-221.

[25]  Dorey G (2007) Why men need to perform pelvic floor exercises? Nurs. Times. 103: 40-43.

[26]  Feys H, Baert L (2000) Effect of physiotherapy on duration and degree of incontinence after radical prostatectomy: a randomised controlled study. Lancet. 355: 98-102.

[27]  Miner MM, Seftel AD (2007) Centrally Acting Mechanisms for the Treatment of Male Sexual Dysfunction. Urol. Clin. North Am. 34: 483-496.

[28]  Mulhall JP, Morgentaler A (2007) Penile rehabilitation should become the norm for radical prostatectomy patients. J. Sex. Med. 4: 538-543.

[29]  World Health Organization, Defining sexual health, Sexual health document series, Available:        http://www.who.int/reproductivehealth/topics/gender_rights/defining_sexual_health.pdf, 2006. Accessed 2012 July 24th

[30]   Mello AS, Carvalho EC, PeláNT (2006) The sexuality of patients with onco-hemato-logical diseases. Rev. Lat. Am. Enfermagem.14: 227-232.

[31]   World Health Organization (WHO), http://www.who.int/cancer/en/, accessed 2012 July 24th

[32]   PubMed, http://www.ncbi.nlm.nih.gov/pubmed/, accessed 2012 July,

[33]   Center MM, Jemal A, Lortet-Tieulent J, Ward E, Ferlay J, Brawley O, Bray F (2012) International Variation in Prostate Cancer Incidence and Mortality Rates. Eur. Urol. 61: 1079-1092.

[34]   National Institutes of Health. Publication No. 06-3923 December 2005, National Kidney and Urologic Diseases Information Clearinghouse

[35]   Wolf AMD, WenderRC, Etzioni RB, Thompson IM, D'Amico AV, Volk, RJ,Brooks DD, Dash C, Guessous I, Andrews K, DeSantis C, Smith RA (2010). American Cancer Society Guideline for the Early Detection of Prostate Cancer Update 2010. CA: Cancer J. Clin. 60: 70–98.

[36]   Greene KL, Albertsen PC, Babaian RJ, Carter HB, Gann PH, Han M, Kuban DA, Sartor AO, Stanford JL, Zietman A, Carroll P (2009) Prostate specific antigen best practice statement. J. Urol. 182: 2232–2241.

[37]   Imamura T, Yasunaga H (2008) Economic evaluation of prostate cancer screening with prostate-specific antigen. Int. J. Urol. 15: 285-288.

[38]   Kendirci M, Bejma J, Hellstrom WJ (2006) Update on erectile dysfunction in prostate cancer patients. Curr. Opin. Urol. 16: 186-195.

[39]   McCullough AR (2008) Rehabilitation of erectile function following radical prostatectomy. Asian J. Androl.10: 61-74.

[40]   Seftel AD, Mohammed MA, Althof SE (2004) Erectile dysfunction: etiology, evaluation, and treatment options. Med. Clin. North. Am. 88: 387-416.

[41]   Sivalingam S, Hashim H, Schwaibold H (2006) An overview of the diagnosis and treatment of erectile dysfunction. Drugs. 66: 2339-2355.

[42]   Weber BA, Roberts BL, Yarandi H, Mills TL, Chumbler NR, Algood C (2007). Dyadic support and quality-of-life after radical prostatectomy. J. Mens. Health Gend. 4: 156–164.

[43]   Filocamo MT, Marzi VL, Del Popolo G, Cecconi F, Marzocco M, Tosto A, Nicita G (2005) Effectiveness of early pelvic floor rehabilitation for post-prostatectomy incontinence. Eur. Urol. 48: 734-738.

[44]   Musicki B, Burnett AL (2006) eNOS Function and Dysfunction in the Penis. Exp. Biol. Med. 231: 154-165.

[45]   Priviero FBM, Leite R, Webb RC, Teixeira CE (2007) Neurophysiological basis of penile erection. ActaPharmacol. Sin. 28: 751-755.

[46] Andersson KE (2011). Mechanisms of penile erection and basis for pharmacological treatment of erectile dysfunction. Pharmacol. Rev. 63: 811-859.

[47] National Institutes of Health (2003) Consensus Development Panel on Impotence. JAMA.270:83-90.

[48] Ribeiro CG, Moura R, Neves RF, Spinosa JP, Bernardo-Filho M (2007) Nuclear medicine imaging technique in the erectile dysfunction evaluation: a mini-review. Braz. Arch. Biol. Technol. 50: 91-96.

[49] Santos-Filho SD, Paoli S, Vicentini SC, Pinto NS, Oliveira MP, Tavares A, Bernardo-Filho M (2012) Erectile dysfunction: The interest of the scientific community. J. Med. Med. Sci. 3: 70-76.

[50] Yuan J, Hoang AN, Romero CA, Lin H, Dai Y, Wang R (2010) Vacuum therapy in erectile dysfunction - Science and clinical evidence. Int. J. Impot. Res. 22: 211-219.

[51] Burgio KL, Goode PS, Urban DA, Umlauf MG, Locher JL, Bueschen A, Redden DT (2006) Preoperative biofeedback assisted behavioral training to decrease post-prostatectomy incontinence: a randomized controlled trial. J. Urol. 175: 196-20.1

[52] Parekh AR, Feng MI, Kirages D, Bremner H, Kaswick J, Aboseif S (2003) The role of pelvic floor exercises on postprostatectomy incontinence. J. Urol. 170: 130-133.

[53] Serdà BC, Vesa J, del Valle A, Monreal P (2010) Urinary incontinence and prostate cancer: A rehabilitation program design. Actas Urol. Esp. 34: 522-530.

[54] Claes H, Van Kampen M, Lysens R, Baert L (1995) Pelvic floor exercises in the treatment of impotence. Eur. J. Phys. Rehabil. Med. 5: 135-140.

[55] Lee MS, Shin B, Ernst E (2009) Acupuncture for treating erectile dysfunction: a systematic review. BJU Int. 104: 366-370.

# Chapter 4

# Psychological and Social Factors influencing Patients' Treatment Selection for Localised Prostate Cancer

Luke A Robles, Shihning Chou, Owen J Cole,
Akhlil Hamid, Amanda Griffiths and Kavita Vedhara

Additional information is available at the end of the chapter

## 1. Introduction

Prostate cancer is the most common form of cancer in men in the United Kingdom (UK). A quarter of all new cases of cancer diagnosed in men are prostate cancers. In 2009, over 40,000 cases of prostate cancer were reported in the UK and more than 10,000 men die from the disease each year [1]. Prostate cancer is also a major concern worldwide. Its highest incidence rates are found in Australia and New Zealand with its lowest in South-Central Asia [2].

The rate of men being diagnosed with prostate cancer has significantly increased worldwide in recent decades [3]. This is likely due to the prostate-specific antigen test being performed among younger men and resulting in the majority of men being diagnosed with localised prostate cancer (LPCa) [4, 5]. These men are usually presented with treatment options, which most commonly include: (1) active surveillance (i. e. , regular monitoring of disease activity for those intended to be treated with subsequent curative treatment), (2) radical prostatectomy, (3) external beam radiation therapy, and (4) brachytherapy, and are asked to consider and select their preferred treatment. The situation that patients with LPCa face is somewhat unique. They have to decide between treatments because there is no substantial evidence to suggest that one treatment modality differs from other treatments, in terms of overall survival rate [6, 7]. However, there are considerable differences in the side-effects associated with each treatment option.

## 2. Treatment side-effects and their psychological impact

Men confronted with this treatment decision often need to take into consideration a range of factors, including the potential physical side effects of treatments and their psychological, social and emotional consequences. For example, patients being treated with radical therapies can experience severe side-effects, such as urinary incontinence (UI) and erectile dysfunction (ED), as a result of treatment. UI symptoms can persist years after treatment [8] and this can have an impact on all aspects of an individual's functioning. Men with UI often avoid social situations due to the risk of their incontinence becoming apparent to other people. They can feel embarrassed by their inability to self-control their bodily functions and by the lack of empathy from other people within social situations [9].

Relatively little research has been conducted to examine the relationship between ED and psychological morbidity among men with prostate cancer. Nevertheless, ED has been reported to have a profound effect on a patient's quality of life post-treatment. Nelson et al. [10] examined the relationship between depressive symptoms and erectile function. A group of men, who did not receive any treatment for their prostate cancer, completed self-report questionnaires measuring anxiety and depression symptoms and erectile function approximately 4-years post-diagnosis. Erectile dysfunction was found to be a significant predictor of depression independent of other influential factors of depression, such as anxiety and marital status. This finding suggests that men can experience lasting psychological effects from their disease. Another study by Nelson et al. [11] examined men's responses to ED affecting their sexual function and their adjustment to diminished erections after having undergone a radical prostatectomy. These men completed self-report questionnaires measuring erectile function and sexual satisfaction pre-operatively, 12 and 24 months post-operatively. The findings revealed that sexual satisfaction decreased after surgery with patients feeling ashamed and embarrassed by their difficulty to perform sexually with their partners. Sexual dissatisfaction persisted over the period of 24-months, even in men who reported good erectile function post-operatively. Thus, it appears that men do not seem to adjust well to the consequences of their treatment.

ED is a condition which not only affects the individual but also affects couples. There have been differences in the perceptions held by men with ED due to treatment for prostate cancer and their partners. Men with ED have reported an "all or nothing" approach to their sexual relationship with their partner; in that if they are unable to 'perform' sexually then it is pointless to engage in sexual contact. This can lead to men withdrawing from intimate contact with their partners causing strain on the relationship [12]. Women partners have reported to be less concerned about treatments to help the physical functioning of their partners with ED, and are more focused on finding alternative ways to maintain intimacy and sexual stimulation [13].

The option of active surveillance as a management plan for LPCa can also affect the quality of life of men diagnosed with the disease. Although no active treatment is administered, active surveillance can have a psychological impact. Qualitative studies have provided some insight into the experiences of living with prostate cancer. For instance,

Hedestig et al. [14] conducted interviews with patient with untreated LPCa and analysed the interview transcripts using in-depth qualitative narrative analysis. Their findings revealed that men perceived their disease as life-threatening, experienced uncertainty, fear and worry about their cancer progression, and a repressed sense of manhood due to sexual dysfunctions.

## 3. Personal beliefs and treatment selection

The decision on a treatment modality for LPCa could, therefore, be described as a challenging one requiring patients to weigh up a range of physical and psychological outcomes of treatments. Indeed, it has been shown that patients can experience decision-related distress at diagnosis, which can persist over time and lead to poorly informed treatment decisions [15]. The difficulties associated with making a treatment choice can be further magnified by patients making their decisions based on their personal beliefs. These personal beliefs can help patients construct a mental representation about their disease and its treatment, which can guide their adjustment to their disease. Such beliefs are of particular importance to treatment decisions when there is great uncertainty around the long-term effects of treatment.

Extensive research has found that personal beliefs can predict a range of outcomes, including quality of life, help-seeking behaviour and treatment adherence [16-18]. These beliefs have also been shown to affect treatment choice, mainly by way of selecting between conventional treatment and complementary and alternative medicines (CAM) for conditions, such as chronic pain, hypertension, and both localised and advanced prostate cancer [19-22]. These studies reported that patients who used CAM were more likely to hold negative beliefs about their illness (i. e. , that their illness was chronic and that they had little personal control over its management); and about conventional treatments (i. e. , believed the treatments would result in significant undesirable side-effects). In contrast, patients who were less likely to favour CAM held positive beliefs about their illness and its treatment (i. e. , believed the condition was not severe and would easily be controlled with conventional treatment). Indeed, patients' positive beliefs about their illness were also shown to increase the likelihood of choosing generic rather than branded medicines, as well as reduce the amount of drugs they consumed to manage their conditions [20, 23].

It is not well-understood how patients, who are diagnosed with LPCa and offered conventional treatments, make sense of their disease and their treatment decisions through examining personal beliefs. Patients with LPCa can make treatment decisions that may not necessarily be in accordance with the treatment-related information provided by urologists [24]. Thus, patients may choose a treatment based on confounding information derived from their own experience and from other sources available to them. By gaining a better understanding of patients' personal beliefs may help both patients and urologists make more informed decisions about treatments.

## 4. A systematic review of the literature

An initial scope for existing literature reviews in prostate cancer research yielded two reviews [25, 26]. The more recent review [26] was conducted five years ago and restricted its search period to a 14 year time span, used a small number of literature databases and only searched for original, peer-reviewed studies to explore broadly the personal (not just beliefs specifically) and external factors pertaining to the decision-making process of patients. It concluded that there is a general lack of understanding about the role of patients' beliefs in treatment selection and that this was an area worthy of enquiry. Our aim was, therefore, to provide an updated review on factors influencing treatment selection for LPCa, as well as specifically examine the literature pertaining to patients' personal beliefs about LPCa and/or its treatments.

A systematic search of the literature was conducted in electronic databases to retrieve relevant published papers from 1980 – 2010, which included: MEDLINE (1950-present); CINAHL; ScienceDirect and CancerLIT (PubMed). Searches were conducted by exploding and combining the medical subject term 'prostate cancer' and free-text words, such as 'beliefs, cognitions, choices, treatment options'. A language restriction was not set whilst searching for the papers.

Non-scholarly literature was searched using the following charity databases: The Prostate Cancer Charity (Jan-April 2010) and Cancer Research UK. The following Government websites were also searched: World Health Organisation (WHO) and the National Institute of Health and Clinical Excellence (NICE). The Networked Digital Library of Theses and Dissertations was searched for theses discussing relevant work and studies.

The reference lists of literature reviews were hand-searched and key authors identified from the search procedure were contacted for any other relevant studies.

The studies retrieved from the literature searches were screened against the inclusion criteria, which included: (i) samples of men diagnosed with, and being treated for, LPCa, and (ii) studies examining patients' beliefs about their LPCa and treatment options. All study designs except reviews, opinion papers and single case studies, were considered for inclusion into the present review.

The titles and abstracts of the references yielded from the search procedure were screened against the inclusion criteria. The full text of the potentially relevant papers were retrieved and read for consideration into the review. The papers that met the inclusion criteria were assessed for their methodological quality.

## 5. Synthesis of findings

The search procedure yielded ten papers, which are summarised in Tables 1 and 2. It was inappropriate to combine findings statistically to produce meaningful outcomes. This was partly due to the small number of quantitative studies identified for inclusion into the review. Primarily, the assessment of the included studies revealed there to be many methodological differences that existed between the studies. This made it difficult to pool studies to determine the effect of perceptions on treatment selection. Therefore, a qualitative synthesis of the findings was undertaking with studies being grouped according to treatment modality and those factors affecting decision-making. Statistical findings from the quantitative studies were used to support the observed findings from the qualitative studies.

## 5.1. Beliefs underpinning treatment selection for localised prostate cancer

### 5.1.1. Radical prostatectomy

Patients' beliefs and other influences in selecting to undergo a radical prostatectomy were clearly reported in nine of the studies [27-35]. Many of the patients perceived their cancer as a localised problem and that the most tangible and definitive method of curing or preventing the disease from spreading was to remove the tumour [27-29, 31, 35]. These findings were also replicated in three of the quantitative studies, which reported that beliefs about the effectiveness of surgery and complete tumour removal were statistically associated with selecting surgery [33-35]. Surgery would also allow for surgeons to be more informed about the nature and extent of the cancer and would provide the patients with more information about their disease [27, 28]. Surgery was considered to have the best evidence base in terms of its efficacy in combating cancer compared to other curative treatment options [31, 32]. Overall, patients believed surgery to be the best and most effective form of treatment. This corresponds with current treatment rates, which show that the majority of patients with LPCa opt for surgery [36].

### 5.1.2. External beam radiation therapy and brachytherapy

External beam radiation therapy (EBRT) was regarded by most patients as being an inferior treatment option to a radical prostatectomy. This was based on their belief that EBRT provided uncertainty surrounding its ability to cure their cancer [27, 28, 30, 31] through treatment administered externally to the body. Unlike a radical prostatectomy, EBRT was believed to disadvantage the patient by being time-consuming and disruptive to daily life with severe consequential side-effects [27, 28]. Interestingly, some of these side-effects were mistaken for side-effects associated with chemotherapy (e. g. , hair loss, weight loss, vomiting) [27, 28, 30]. It appeared that when patients selected EBRT as their preferred treatment, it was to avoid the negative effects of surgery, i. e. , being less invasive and resulting in fewer side-effects [31, 35]. These beliefs were similar to those held by patients who selected brachytherapy as their preferred treatment. However, like a radical prostatectomy, brachytherapy was believed to provide a 'direct' and, therefore, more effective and convenient form of treatment to cure their cancer [31, 34].

### 5.1.3. Active surveillance / watchful waiting

The terms 'watchful waiting' were used in some of the papers along with the other active treatment options. Watchful waiting usually refers to a less intense management plan where palliative care is usually provided. These options were rarely considered by patients as a management option for their cancer. They were typically rejected due to patients' fear about the cancer spreading [31, 33] and their need to be "doing something" active to combat their prostate cancer [28, 31]. Holmboe and Concato [31] suggested that other possible explanations for patients rejecting watchful waiting included fear of death or the inability to monitor cancer progression. Patients who opted for active surveillance perceived their cancer as 'a very small growth' and a common disease among men as they get older. These men were accepting of the uncertainty surrounding their disease progression and believed it would be best to endure the severe side-effects of curative treatment only when it was evident that treatment was required [37]. However, this willingness to accept active surveillance as a management option appeared to occur in men whose urologists advocated the view that the disease was not severe and would progress slowly [37].

| Study Ref | Authors, year, & study location | Design | Characteristics of sample | Major findings |
|---|---|---|---|---|
| [27] | Denberg et al. (2006) Denver, USA | Perspective cohort (follow-up 6-8 months) using semi-structured interviews | 20 men newly diagnosed with LPCa considering treatment options Age range 53-80 years 70% (white); 25% (African American); 5% (Latino) | 40% perceived surgery as a definitive treatment Surgery offered crucial knowledge about tumour 55% perceived surgery as undesirable regarding invasiveness |
| [28] | O'Rourke (1999) North Carolina, USA | Perspective cohort (follow-up 3 & 12 months) using couple & individual semi-structured interviews | 18 men newly diagnosed with LPCa who have made a treatment decision 18 spouses recruited Mean age 67.6 (range 52-78 years) (patient) Mean age 62.1 (range 49-74 years) (partner) 13% white (patient), 5% African American; 72% white, 28% African American (spouse) | Couples believed cancer is only curable through surgery Perceived uncertainty about radiotherapy regarding efficacy & outcome Men more concerned about side-effects than wives |

| Study Ref | Authors, year, & study location | Design | Characteristics of sample | Major findings |
|---|---|---|---|---|
| [29] | O'Rourke & Germino. (1998) North Carolina, USA | Retrospective cross-sectional study using unstructured focus groups | 11 men diagnosed with LPCa, who have made a treatment decision 6 spouses recruited Age range 58-72 years (patients) Age range 51-64 years (spouses) 99% white; 1% African American | Surgery perceived as a first line choice Prior bias toward surgery due to perceived association with cure Radiotherapy perceived inferior to surgery due to its efficacy & side-effects |
| [30] | Steginga et al. (2002) Queensland, Australia | Cross-sectional study using semi-structured interviews | 108 men diagnosed with LPCa considering curative treatment options Mean age 62 years (range 39-80 years) Ethnicity not specified | 47% described other patients' treatment experiences used in their decision-making 34% held lay belief that surgery was the best way to cure their cancer 12% were uncertain about radiotherapy as a way to cure their cancer |
| [31] | Holmboe & Concato. (2000) New Haven, USA | Cross-sectional study using interviews with open-ended questions | 102 men newly diagnosed with LPCa, who have made a treatment decision Mean age 66.4 years Majority white (89%) | Majority influenced by external information (i.e., 30% for physician recommendation) Classified likes & dislikes of treatments Removal of tumour & evidence of efficacy as main likes for surgery Fear of future consequences was the most common reason to reject watchful waiting |
| [37] | Davison et al. (2009) Vancouver, Canada | Retrospective cross-sectional study using interviews with semi-structured interviews | 25 men with low-risk prostate cancer on active surveillance Mean age 66 years (range 48-77 years) Majority white (92%); 8% South Asian | Men perceived their cancer as a common disease & exaggerated the potential incidence Realised treatment might be necessary, but viewed as "a grey zone" |

**Table 1.** Description of the Qualitative Studies included in the Systematic Review

| Study ID reference | Authors, year, & study location | Design | Characteristics of sample | Major findings |
|---|---|---|---|---|
| [32] | Hall et al. (2003) Virginia, USA | Retrospective cross-sectional study using self-report questionnaires developed from literature review & clinical impressions | 351 men with LPCa treated with surgery or brachytherapy Mean age 62±5 years (radical prostatectomy); 66±8 years (brachytherapy); 70±7 years (combination of brachytherapy & radiotherapy) Ethnicity not specified | 42.9% brachytherapy patients & 97.5% radical prostatectomy patients chose treatment based on evidence shown to cure the cancer Side-effects were an important motivator Urologists were the most important source of information and a major factor in decision-making process |
| [33] | Zeliadt et al. (2010) USA | Cross-sectional study using self-report questionnaires developed from preliminary focus groups & cognitive interviews | 198 newly diagnosed patients considering surgery only & patients considering other treatment options Mean age 63 years 72% white, 11% black, 16% Hispanic/Asian (surgery); 68% white, 26% Black, 6% Hispanic/Asian (other options) | Treatment efficacy influenced preference for surgery Personal burden influenced nonsurgical options |
| [34] | Gwede et al. (2005) Florida, USA | Cross-sectional study using questions derived from previous study | 69 men diagnosed with LPCa, who have made a decision about treatment Mean age: 57.7 years (range 39.6-71.1) (surgery); 65.2 years (range 45.7-89.2) (brachytherapy) 86.5% (surgery); 97% (brachytherapy) white | Cure and complete tumour removal were the main motivations for surgery (74%) Brachytherapy related to quality-of-life issues |
| [35] | Teramoto et al. 2006 Kamogawa, Japan | Cross-sectional study using self-report questionnaires | 51 men diagnosed with LPCa treated with radical prostatectomy or external beam radiation therapy Overall mean age: 68.2 (range 56–75 years) Japanese sample | Physician was the major factor influencing treatment decisions in both treatment groups (>90%) Family and others was a more important factor for patients undergoing surgery than patients undergoing radiation therapy Surgery was desired for cancer control Radiation therapy favoured concerning side-effects |

**Table 2.** Description of the Quantitative Studies included in the Systematic Review

*5.1.4. The role of urologists and partners in informing patient beliefs*

The recommendations made by urologists emerged in many of the papers [28, 29, 31-33, 37] as being influential in shaping patients' beliefs regarding their treatment choice. A high percentage of patients (48-65%) said they would selected the treatments recommended by their urologist [30, 32]. Consequently, seeking a second opinion was unnecessary serving only to delay treatment and provide potentially more conflicting information to process [27, 28].

Partners, who often experience considerable emotional distress themselves on hearing the diagnosis [25, 38], have also been found to exert an important influence on patients' beliefs. Three studies reported the role of the partners to be a source of information or a mediator in helping men to process their treatment information [27, 32, 34]. However, it was also reported in two studies that, ultimately, it is the patients themselves who reported ownership of their treatment decision [29, 37].

*5.1.5. The role of patients' information seeking behavior in informing beliefs*

Another major factor influencing patients' beliefs was their own information-seeking behaviour. Patients and their partners are often actively engaged in learning about their treatment options, side-effects and the background of their urologists [29]. The evidence suggested that they made use of a variety of resources, including health care professions (HCPs) (i. e. , urologists, radiation oncologist), the internet, books, magazines, friends and family [27, 29, 30, 32, 34, 37]. Processing such large amounts of advice and potential contradictory information was suggested to be an explanation for the misconceptions about treatments reported by the patients (i. e. , associating the effects of chemotherapy with radiotherapy) [27, 30].

*5.1.6. The role of other patients' treatment experiences in informing patient beliefs*

In four studies, there was evidence that patients [27, 28, 30, 33] and their partners used the experiences of other people with cancer in their decisions about treatment. Denberg et al. [27] described that these experiences influenced patients' beliefs regarding LPCa, its treatment and treatment side-effects. Steginga et al. [30] reported that 47% of men described considering other people they knew (not just those with prostate cancer), who had negative experiences with cancer or cancer treatment, in their decision-making. O'Rourke [28] reported that comparisons with other patients, who had a positive outcome from treatment, were mostly related to surgery and that comparisons were usually made between friends and family members, who had undergone surgery and were making a good recovery. It has been suggested that patients may pay more attention to the experiences of other patients with cancer than to the risk information presented to them by their urologists and specialist nurses [27]. The reliability of their findings was supported by the quantitative findings of Zeliadt et al. [33], who reported a statistically significant association between the experiences from other patients and treatment selection for patients who only considered surgery as a viable treatment.

## 6. Discussion

The findings synthesised in the present review have demonstrated that patients select a treatment or management option based on their beliefs about their cancer, the perceived effectiveness of the treatment and their beliefs regarding the side-effects of the treatment. With regards to the present findings, the majority of patients select active surveillance because of their belief that their cancer was not aggressive, selected to undergo a radical prostatectomy because they believed it to be most effective at curing their cancer, and selected EBRT because of the reduced risk of side-effects. A range of factors external to the patient, which inform these beliefs, were also identified. These included the patients' high regard of the urologists' treatment recommendation, the emotional distress experienced by partners, the various modes of seeking information about treatments, and other peoples' experiences of treatment.

It is, however, also very clear that the evidence base on patients' beliefs in the context of LPCa remains limited. This is an area in need of high quality prospective studies to gain a greater understanding of the factors that influence treatment decisions. This understanding could help develop interventions designed to support men in these decisions and to assist with their long-term adjustment to prostate cancer and its treatment.

The limited evidence that has been synthesised in this review does, however, enable some clear recommendations to be made how this area of research and, ultimately, clinical practice may move forward. In particular, it is clear that the existing findings relate well to two theoretical frameworks, which have been developed to understand patients' beliefs regarding illness and treatment; and which have also been the basis of therapeutic interventions [39, 40]. These are the self-regulatory model (SRM) [41, 42] and the Necessity Concerns Framework (NCF) [17, 43]. The SRM describes that individuals' personal beliefs allow them to make sense of their disease and enable them to reach their illness goals (e. g. , in LPCa these could be survival, reducing the risk of side effects, etc. ). These beliefs cluster around 5 domains: (1) identity (the way patients describe their disease and its symptoms); (2) cause (what caused the disease); (3) timeline (how long the disease is going to last); (4) consequence (how will the disease and/or its treatment affect me?); and (5) controllability (whether the disease is believed to be preventable, curable, or controllable). Similarly, the NCF also focuses on personal beliefs, but those specifically related to treatment. Previous research has shown that patients' beliefs regarding treatment tend to focus on two domains: beliefs regarding how necessary/important the treatment is to their future well-being and beliefs regarding concerns (i. e. , what are the potential adverse consequences of the treatment?).

There was clear evidence in the studies included in this review of the beliefs specified by both the SRM and NCF. For example, patients believed their cancer to be a mass within the body (akin to identity beliefs) and that removing this mass would cure their cancer (akin to controllability beliefs). Similarly, patients believed curative treatment would offer them the best outcome in terms of survival (akin to necessity beliefs) because their cancer could potentially re-occur (akin to concern beliefs). Furthermore, the importance of factors external to the patient in shaping their beliefs is also specified by the SRM. Thus, it was suggested that the results of this review provide strong evidence to support the use of these theoretical frameworks in future research.

# 7. Recommendation for health care

It is clear that the use of patients' beliefs in their decisions on a treatment modality has led them to base their decisions on misconceptions rather than on evidential information. HCPs may need to challenge misinformed beliefs held by patients to help them make more informed decisions regarding their treatment. In order to make more conclusive recommendations for health care practice, further research is required to establish the extent to which personal beliefs alter treatment selection.

# 8. Recommendations for further research

The majority of the studies included in this review used a qualitative approach. Such methods explore a topic area in-depth and provide a descriptive account of findings. While this approach can provide very rich data in specific domains, these data are not intended to be generalisable. Thus, quantitative studies (preferably with prospective designs) are required in the future to ascertain, not only the salient beliefs influencing treatment choices but also, how these beliefs affect long-term adjustment to the disease and its treatment.

With regards to the studies which employed quantitative methodologies, none used standardised and validated measures for examining illness or treatment beliefs. Two of the quantitative studies [32, 34] developed their measures of beliefs from previous published work. The remaining study developed its measure from preliminary focus groups and interviews [33]. It could be suggested that further validation of these measures is required before any strong conclusions can be drawn.

The time at which illness and treatment beliefs were measured is another shortcoming of the included studies. Some of the studies included those patients who had already made a treatment decision or who had already started treatment. This may have affected the reliability of the findings due to the potential bias of patients recalling what they believed about their illness and its treatment at these times in the treatment process. Prospective designs involving the assessment of beliefs before a treatment choice is made would offer a more robust approach.

A further limitation concerned the majority of the patient samples being predominantly white and from North America. Therefore, the experiences of other groups, such as men of Afro-Caribbean origin in whom the risk of prostate cancer is greater, were not represented. Further research is required across a range of ethnic and cultural groups.

## 9. Conclusion

The present review has revealed that our understanding of the role played by the personal beliefs of men regarding their LPCa and its treatment is still limited. The existing evidence has been dominated by qualitative methods, cross-sectional designs and the use of non-validated instruments. However, it is also clear from existing findings that the adoption of the SRM and NCF, with their associated validated instruments, could provide a greater understanding of the factors that influence treatment decisions. Further research using psychological frameworks could also help develop interventions to support men in their treatment decisions, and assist with their long-term adjustment to LPCa and its treatment.

## Acknowledgements

The authors would like to thank Dr Chris Bridle for his help and support with this review.

## Author details

Luke A Robles[1], Shihning Chou[1], Owen J Cole[2], Akhlil Hamid[3], Amanda Griffiths[1] and Kavita Vedhara[4]

*Address all correspondence to: lwxlar@nottingham. ac. uk

1 Institute of Work, Health & Organisation, The University of Nottingham, Nottingham, UK

2 Department of Urology, The Medical Specialist Group, Guernsey

3 Department of Urology and University of Western Australia, Royal Perth Hospital, Western Australia

4 Division of Primary Care, The University of Nottingham, Nottingham, UK

## References

[1] Cancer Research UK. *Prostate cancer key Facts.* http://info.cancerresearchuk.org/cancerstats/keyfacts/prostate-cancer/cancerstats-key-facts-on-prostate-cancer (accessed 23 July 2012).

[2] World Cancer Research Fund International. *The incidence of prostate cancer is 25 times higher in Australia and New Zealand then in South-Central Asia.* http://www.wcrf.org/cancer_facts/prostate-cancer-worldwide.php (accessed 23 July 2012).

[3]  Albertsen PC. When is active surveillance the appropriate treatment for prostate cancer? *Acta Oncologica* 2011; 50(1): 120-6.

[4]  Moore AL, Dimitropoulou P, Lane A, Powell PH, Greenberg DC, Brown CH, et al. Population-based prostate-specific antigen testing in the UK leads to a stage migration of prostate cancer. *British Journal of Urology International* 2009; 104(11): 1592-8.

[5]  McGregor M, Hanley J, Boivin J, McLean R. Screening for prostate cancer: estimating the magnitude of overdetection. *Canadian Medical Association Journal* 1998; 159(11): 1368-72.

[6]  O'Rourke ME. Choose wisely: therapeutic decisions and quality of life in patients with prostate cancer. *Clinical Journal of Oncology Nursing* 2007; 11(3): 401-8.

[7]  Neal DE, Donovan J. Prostate cancer: to screen or not to screen. *Lancet Oncology* 2000; 1: 17-24.

[8]  Ponholzer A, Brössner C, Struhal G, Marszalek M, Madersbacher S. Lower urinary tract symptoms, urinary incontinence, sexual function and quality of life after radical prostatectomy and external beam radiation therapy: real life experience in Austria. *World Journal of Urology* 2006; 24(3): 325-30.

[9]  Palmer MH, Fogarty LA, Somerfield MR, Powel LL. Incontinence after prostatectomy: coping with incontinence after prostate cancer surgery. *Oncology Nursing Forum* 2003; 30(2): 229-38.

[10]  Nelson C, Mulhall J, Roth A. The association between erectile dysfunction and depressive symptoms in men treated for prostate cancer. *Journal of Sexual Medicine* 2011; 8(2): 560-6.

[11]  Nelson C, Deveci S, Stasi J, Scardino P, Mulhall J. Sexual bother following radical prostatectomyjsm. *Journal of Sexual Medicine* 2010; 7(1): 129-35.

[12]  Sand MS, Fisher W, Rosen R, Heiman J, Eardley I. Erectile dysfunction and constructs of masculinity and quality of life in the multinational Men's Attitudes to Life Events and Sexuality (MALES) study. *Journal of Sexual Medicine* 2008; 5(3): 583-94.

[13]  Chambers SK, Schover L, Halford K, Clutton S, Ferguson M, Gordon L, et al. ProsCan for Couples: randomised controlled trial of a couples-based sexuality intervention for men with localised prostate cancer who receive radical prostatectomy. *BMC Cancer* 2008; 8: 226.

[14]  Hedestig O, Sandman PO, Widmark A. Living with untreated localized prostate cancer: a qualitative analysis of patient narratives. *Cancer Nursing* 2003; 26(1): 55-60.

[15]  Steginga S, Turner E, Donovan J. The decision-related psychosocial concerns of men with localised prostate cancer: targets for intervention and research. *World Journal of Urology* 2008; 26: 469-74.

[16]  Karamanidou C, Clatworthy J, Weinman J, Horne R. A systematic review of the prevalence and determinants of nonadherence to phosphate binding medication in patients with end-stage renal disease. *BMC Nephrology* 2008; 9: 2.

[17]  Horne R, Weinman J. Patients' beliefs about prescribed medicines and their role in adherence to treatment in chronic physical illness. *Journal of Psychosomatic Research* 1999; 47(6): 555-67.

[18]  Petrie KJ, Jago LA, Devcich DA. The role of illness perceptions in patients with medical conditions. *Current Opinion in Psychiatry* 2007; 20(2): 163-7.

[19]  Brown M, Dean S, Hay-Smith EJC, Taylor W, Baxter GD. Musculoskeletal pain and treatment choice: an exploration of illness perceptions and choices of conventional or complementary therapies. *Disability and Rehabilitation* 2010; 32(20): 1645-57.

[20]  Figueiras M, Marcelino DS, Claudino A, Cortes MA, Maroco J, Weinman J. Patients' illness schemata of hypertension: The role of beliefs for the choice of treatment. *Psychology & Health* 2010; 25(4): 507-17.

[21]  Boon H, Brown JB, Gavin A, Westlake K. Men with prostate cancer: making decisions about complementary/alternative medicine. *Medical Decision Making* 2003; 23(6): 471-9.

[22]  Porter MC, Diefenbach MA. Pushed and Pulled: The Role of Affect and Cognition in Shaping CAM Attitudes and Behavior among Men Treated for Prostate Cancer. *Journal of Health Psychology* 2009; 14(2): 288-96.

[23]  Al Anbar NN, Dardennes RM, Prado-Netto A, Kaye K, Contejean Y. Treatment choices in autism spectrum disorder: The role of parental illness perceptions. *Research in Developmental Disabilities* 2010; 31(3): 817-28.

[24]  Berry D, Ellis W, Woods N, Schwien C, Mullen K, Yang C. Treatment decision-making by men with localized prostate cancer: the influence of personal factors. *Urologic Oncology* 2003; 21(2): 93-100.

[25]  O'Rourke ME. Decision Making and Prostate Cancer Treatment Selection: A Review. *Seminars in Oncology Nursing* 2001; 17(2): 108-17.

[26]  Zeliadt SB, Ramsey SD, Penson DF, Hall IJ, Ekwueme DU, Stroud L, et al. Why do men choose one treatment over another?: a review of patient decision making for localized prostate cancer. *Cancer* 2006; 106(9): 1865-74.

[27]  Denberg TD, Melhado TV, Steiner JF. Patient treatment preferences in localized prostate carcinoma: The influence of emotion, misconception, and anecdote. *Cancer* 2006; 107(3): 620-30.

[28]  O'Rourke ME. Narrowing the options: the process of deciding on prostate cancer treatment. *Cancer Investigation* 1999; 17(5): 349-59.

[29]  O'Rourke ME, Germino BB. Prostate cancer treatment decisions: a focus group exploration. *Oncology Nursing Forum* 1998; 25(1): 97-104.

[30] Steginga SK, Occhipinti S, Gardiner RA, Yaxley J, Heathcote P. Making decisions about treatment for localized prostate cancer. *British Journal of Urology International* 2002; 89(3): 255-60.

[31] Holmboe ES, Concato J. Treatment decisions for localized prostate cancer: asking men what's important. *Journal of General Internal Medicine* 2000; 15(10): 694-701.

[32] Hall JD, Boyd JC, Lippert MC, Theodorescu D. Why patients choose prostatectomy or brachytherapy for localized prostate cancer: results of a descriptive survey. *Urology* 2003; 61(2): 402-7.

[33] Zeliadt SB, Moinpour CM, Blough DK, Penson DF, Hall IJ, Smith JL, et al. Preliminary treatment considerations among men with newly diagnosed prostate cancer. *American Journal of Managed Care* 2010; 16(5): 121-30.

[34] Gwede CK, Pow-Sang J, Seigne J, Heysek R, Helal M, Shade K, et al. Treatment decision-making strategies and influences in patients with localized prostate carcinoma. *Cancer* 2005; 104(7): 1381-90.

[35] Teramoto S, Ota T, Itaya N, Maniwa A, Matsui T, Nishimura Y, et al. [Survey of factors underlying treatment choice for patients with localized prostate cancer (radical prostatectomy vs extrabeam radiotherapy)]. *Nippon Hinyokika Gakkai Zasshi - Japanese Journal of Urology* 2006; 97(7): 823-9.

[36] McVey GP, McPhail S, Fowler S, McIntosh G, Gillatt D, Parker CC. Initial management of low-risk localized prostate cancer in the UK: analysis of the British Association of Urological Surgeons Cancer Registry. *British Journal of Urology International* 2010; 106(8): 1161-4.

[37] Davison BJ, Oliffe JL, Pickles T, Mroz L. Factors influencing men undertaking active surveillance for the management of low-risk prostate cancer. *Oncology Nursing Forum* 2009; 36(1): 89-96.

[38] Kirby R, Holmes K, Amoroso P. Supporting the supporter: helping the partner of patients newly diagnosed with prostate cancer. *British Journal of Urology International* 2010; 105(11): 1489-90.

[39] Petrie KJ, Cameron LD, Ellis CJ, Buick D, Weinman J. Changing illness perceptions after myocardial infarction: an early intervention randomized controlled trial. *Psychosomatic Medicine* 2002; 64(4): 580-6.

[40] Petrie KJ, Jago LA, Devich DA. The role of illness perceptions in patients with medical conditions. *Current Opinion in Psychiatry* 2007; 20(2): 163-7.

[41] Leventhal H, Brissette I, Leventhal EA. The common-sense model of self-regulation of health and illness. In: Cameron LD, Leventhal, H. (ed.) *The self-regulation of health and illness behaviour.* New York: Routledge; 2003. p42-65.

[42] Meyer D, Leventhal H, Gutmann M. Common-sense models of illness: the example of hypertension. *Health Psychology* 1985; 4(2): 115-35.

[43]  Horne R, Cooper V, Gellaitry G, Date HL, Fisher M. Patients' perceptions of highly active antiretroviral therapy in relation to treatment uptake and adherence: the utility of the necessity-concerns framework. *Journal of Acquired Immune Deficiency Syndromes* 2007; 45(3): 334-41.

# Surgical Care and Radiation Therapy

# Chapter 5

# Radiation Therapy for Prostate Cancer

Shinji Kariya

Additional information is available at the end of the chapter

## 1. Introduction

Public concern on the radiation therapy for prostate cancer has increased recently. The leading causes of this phenomenon are thought of as popularization of prostate-specific antigen (PSA) measurement and having been able to tell the curable patients apart by means of the accomplished risk classifications. Massive development of radiation therapy technology also seems to be one of the leading causes. This chapter focuses on the variety of curative radiation therapy for clinically localized prostate cancer.

## 2. External beam radiation therapy

### 2.1. Conventional External Beam Radiation Therapy (EBRT)

In the 1970s, the treatment field size and portal configuration for radiation therapy were based on estimations of the anatomic boundaries of the prostate defined by plain-film radiography and by the digital rectal examination. At that time, a variety of treatment techniques were used. In general, four fields were used to treat the pelvis and prostate to an initial dose of 45 Gy, with a boost to 70 Gy to the prostate only [1, 2]. Early conventional external beam radiation therapy used total doses in the range of 60 to 70 Gy, because it was believed that this dose was close to the maximum dose allowed by the surrounding normal tissues, especially rectum. Today, it is obvious that this dose is not sufficient to get an adequate local control rate.

### 2.2. Three-Dimensional Conformal Radiation Therapy (3D-CRT)

In the early to mid-1908s, three-dimensional conformal treatment techniques became increasingly available. Although these techniques vary in some aspects, they share certain common principles that offer significant advantages over conventional external beam radiation therapy techniques. CT-based images referenced to a reproducible patient position are used to localize the prostate and normal organs and to generate high resolution 3D reconstructions of the patient. Treatment field directions are selected using beam's-eye-view techniques and the fields are shaped to conform to the patient's CT-defined target volume, thereby minimizing the volume of normal tissue irradiated. Compared with treating a patient by conventional external beam radiation therapy technique, 3D-CRT is associated with a nearly 30% reduction in the dose received by 50% of the rectum. Based on this kind of analysis, it greater than or equal to 10% should be possible without an increase in acute or chronic toxicity [3].

### 2.3. Intensity Modulated Radiation Therapy (IMRT)

IMRT is a relatively recent refinement of three-dimensional conformal techniques that uses treatment fields with highly irregular radiation intensity patterns to deliver exquisitely conformal radiation distributions. These intensity patterns are created using special inverse and optimization computer planning systems. Rather than define each shape and weight as is done in conventional treatment planning, planners of IMRT treatment specify the desired dose to the target and normal tissues using mathematical descriptions referred to as constraints or objectives [4]. Sophisticated optimization methods are then used to determine the intensity pattern for each treatment field that results in a dose distribution as close to the user-defined constraints as possible. IMRT delivery is significantly more complex than conformal delivery as well. Delivery of an IMRT intensity pattern requires a computer-controlled beam-shaping apparatus on the linear accelerator known as a multi-leaf collimator (MLC). The MLC consists of many small individually moving leaves or fingers that can create arbitrary beam shapes. The MLC is used for IMRT delivery in either a static mode referred to as step and shoot, which consists of multiple small, irregularly shaped fields delivered in sequence, or a dynamic mode with the leaves moving during treatment to create the required irregular intensity patterns [5]. Since its inception, IMRT has become a common and important method for treating prostate cancer and has facilitated an escalation in dose.

### 2.4. Clinical results of EBRT

#### 2.4.1. Clinical results of conventional EBRT

The results of several large single-institution comparison between radical prostatectomy (RP) and EBRT were reported.

Investigators from Cleveland Clinic Foundation, USA analyzed 1,682 patients with clinical stage T1 and T2 disease treated with either RP or RT. They reported that the 8-year biochemical relapse free survival (bRFS) rates for RP and conventional EBRT less than 72 Gy were 72% and 34%, respectively, and conventional EBRT less than 72 Gy was inferior to RP in the 8-year bRFS rate (Fig 1)[6].

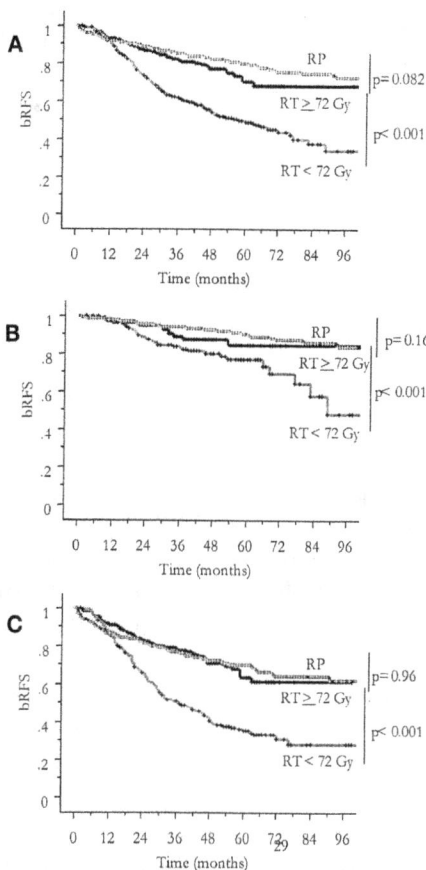

(Cited from Kupelian PA et al.[5])

**Figure 1.** Biochemical relapse-free survival by treatment modality: RT to doses < 72 Gy, RT to doses > or = 72 Gy, and RP for all (A), favorable (B), and unfavorable patients(C).

D'Amico et al. reported a retrospective cohort study of 2635 patients with either RP or RT of median dose to 70.4 Gy (95% CI, 69.3-70.4 Gy) [7]. Eight-year bRFS rates for low-risk (T1c, T2a, PSA < or = 10 ng/ml, and Gleason score (GS) < or = 6) patients were 88% and 78% for RP and RT, respectively. Eight-year bRFS rates for intermediate-risk (T2b or GS 7 or PSA > 10 and < or = 20 ng/ml) patients with < 34% positive prostate biopsies were 79% and 65% for PR and RT, respectively. Eight-year bRFS rates were 36% versus 35% for intermediate-risk patients with at least 34% positive prostate biopsies and 33% versus 40% for high-risk (T2c or PSA > 20ng/ml or GS > or = 8) patients treated with RP versus those treated with RT, respectively. In conclusion, in their retrospective cohort study, intermediate-risk and low-risk patients with a low biopsy tumor volume who were treated with RP appeared to fare significantly better compared with patients who were treated using conventional-dose RT. For the meanwhile, Intermediate-risk and high-risk patients with a high biopsy tumor volume who were treated with RP or RT had long-term estimates of bRFS that were not found to be significantly different.

### 2.4.2. Clinical results of 3D-CRT

Above-mentioned investigators from Cleveland Clinic Foundation reported that 3D-CRT more than 72 Gy was superior to Conventional EBRT less than 72 Gy and very similar to RP in the 8-year bRFS (6). Eight-year bRFS rate were 86% versus 86% (p = 0.16) for favorable-risk (T1 to T2a, GS < or = 6, PSA < or = 10 ng/ml) patients and 62% versus 61% (p = 0.96) for unfavorable-risk (T2b to T2c, GS > or = 7, PSA > 10 ng/ml) patients with RP versus those treated with RT > or = 72 Gy (Fig 1). Several study also have demonstrated that doses in excess of 70 to 72 Gy are associated with a reduction in the risk of recurrence compared with lower doses [8-12].

### 2.4.3. Clinical results of IMRT

Investigators from Memorial Sloan Kettering Cancer Center (MSKCC) reported their experience in 1002 patients treated with IMRT of 86.4 Gy [13]. They reported 7-year bRFS rates for low, intermediate, and unfavorable risk group patients as 98.8%, 85.6%, and 67.9%, respectively. In this report, they concluded that high dose IMRT to 86.4 Gy for localized prostate cancer resulted in excellent clinical outcomes with acceptable toxicity.

### 2.4.4. Clinical results of combined with Androgen Deprivation Therapy (ADT) and EBRT

Thus far, there have been five phase III randomized controlled trials for high-risk prostate cancer that compared radiotherapy alone with radiotherapy and ADT [14-18]. In all of these trials, ADT improved bRFS. In three of these four trials, ADT improved both overall survival (OS) and cause-specific survival (CSS).

From above-mentioned results, combining ADT with radiotherapy should be recommended in the high-risk group.

For intermediate-risk prostate cancer, two studies were published. Investigators from Brigham and Women's Hospital reported their randomized trial that consisted of 206 patients [19]. Two months each of total androgen blockade given before, during, and after radiotherapy for a total of 6 months. After a median follow-up of 4.52 years, ADT had improved 5-year bRFS, CSS, and OS. The Trans-Tasman Radiation Oncology Group (TROG) 96.01 study consisted of 802 patients, who were randomized to radiotherapy alone, 3 months, or 6 months of neoadjuvant hormones with radiotherapy. Five-year bRFS was significantly improved in the 3-month and 6-month arms as compared to the control arm. Although the 6-months arm showed significantly improved 5-year CSS, the 3-month arm was not significantly improved.

The thing to note is that these trials used doses less than 72 Gy that would be considered suboptimal by today's standard. Whether the benefit of ADT remains in the current era of dose escalation is currently unclear.

## 2.5. Acute and late adverse events

### 2.5.1. Acute and late adverse events of conventional EBRT

EBRT delivered with conventional techniques is fairly well tolerated, although grade 2 or higher acute rectal morbidity (discomfort, tenesmus, diarrhea) or urinary symptoms (frequency, nocturia, urgency, dysuria) requiring medication occur in approximately 60% of patients. Symptoms usually appear during the third week of treatment and resolve within days to weeks after treatment is completed. The incidence of late complications that develop > or = 6 months after completion of treatment is significantly lower, whereas serious complications that require corrective surgical intervention are rare. An analysis of 1,020 patients treated in two large Radiation Therapy Oncology Group (RTOG) trials 7506 and 7706 demonstrated an incidence of chronic urinary sequelae, such as cystitis, hematuria, urethral stricture, or bladder contracture, requiring hospitalization in 7.7% of cases, but the incidence of urinary toxicities requiring major surgical interventions such as laparotomy, cystectomy, or prolonged hospitalization was only 0.5% [20]. More than half of chronic urinary complications were urethral strictures, occurring mostly in patients who had undergone a previous transurethral resection of the prostate (TURP). The incidence of chronic intestinal sequelae, such as chronic diarrhea, proctitis, rectal and anal stricture, rectal bleeding or ulcer, requiring hospitalization for diagnosis and minor intervention was 3.3%, with 0.6% of patients experiencing bowel obstruction or perforation. Fatal complications were rare (0.2%). Most complications attributed to radiation therapy are observed within the first 3 to 4 years after treatment, and the likelihood of complications developing after 5 years in low. The risk of complications is increased when radiation doses exceed 70 Gy. The risk of rectal toxicity has been correlated with the volume of the anterior wall exposed to the higher doses of irradiation

### 2.5.2. Acute and late adverse events of CRT

Michalski et al. reported the toxicity outcomes of Stages T1-T2 prostate cancer in RTOG 9406, a phase I-II dose escalation study [21]. Two hundred twenty five patients were treated to 78 Gy (2 Gy fractions). The median follow-up was 2.2 years. Only 3% of patients had grade 3 acute toxicity. No grade 4 or 5 acute toxicity was reported. The late grade 2 and 3 bowel toxicity rates were 18% and 2%, respectively. 2 had grade 4 bowel toxicity. The late grade 2 and 3 bladder toxicity rates were 17% and 4%, respectively. No grade 4 or 5 late bladder toxicity was reported.

Zietman et al. reported acute and late genitourinary (GU) and gastrointestinal (GI) toxicity among patients treated on a randomized controlled trial [22]. The median follow-up was 5.5 years. The acute GU grade 3 toxicity for both the 70.2 Gy (1.8 Gy fractions) and 79.2 Gy dose arms in 2 Gy per fraction were 1%. The acute GI grade 3 toxicity for the 70.2 Gy and 79.2 Gy dose arms were 1% and 0%, respectively. The late GU grade 2 and 3 toxicity were 18% and 2%, respectively, for the 70.2 Gy dose arm, and 20% and 1%, respectively, for the 79.2 Gy dose arm (difference not significant between two arms). The late GI grade 2 for the 70.2 Gy and 79.2 Gy arms were 8% and 17%, respectively (p = 0.005). The late GI grade 3 toxicity, however, was 1% for both arms.

Zelefsky et al. reported the long-term tolerance of high-dose 3D-CRT at MSKCC [23]. The 5-year actuarial rate of grade 2 rectal toxicity for patients receiving 64.8 to 70.2 Gy was 7%, compared with 16% for those treated to 75.6 Gy and 15% for those who treated to 81 Gy (70.2 vs. 75.6 or 81 Gy, p <0.001). The 5-year actuarial rate of grade 3 or higher rectal toxicity was 0.85%, and no correlation between dose and the development of grade 3 complications was found within the range of 64.8 to 81 Gy. Multivariable analysis demonstrated the following variables as predictors of late grade 2 or higher GI toxicity: prescription doses >75.6 Gy (p < 0.001), history of diabetes mellitus (p = 0.01), and the presence of acute GI symptoms during treatment (p = 0.02). The 5-year actuarial likelihood of Grade 2 or higher late GU toxicity for patients who receiving 75.6 to 81 Gy was 15%, compared with 8% for those treated to 64.8 to 70.2 Gy (p = 0.008). The 5-year actuarial likelihood of the development of a urethral stricture (Grade 3 toxicity) for patients who had a prior TURP was 4%, compared with 1% for those who did not have a prior TURP (p = 0.03). No correlation was observed between higher radiation doses and the development of a urethral stricture. Multivariable analysis demonstrated the following variables as predictors of late Grade 2 or higher GU toxicity: prescription doses >75.6 Gy (p = 0.008) and the presence of acute GU symptoms during treatment (p <0.001).

Peeters et al. reported on the incidence of acute and late complications in a multicenter randomized trial comparing 68 Gy to 78 Gy 3D-CRT [24]. The median follow-up was 31 months. For acute toxicity, no significant differences were seen between the two arms. GI toxicity Grade 2 and 3 was reported as the maximum acute toxicity in 44% and 5%, respectively. For acute GU toxicity, these figures were 41% and 13%. The 3-year in incidence of grade 2 and higher GI and GU toxicities for the 68 Gy dose arm was 23.2% and 28.5%, respectively. The 3-year incidence of grade 2 and higher GI and GU toxicities for the 78 Gy dose arm was 26.5% and 30.2%, respectively. The differences were not significant. However, the authors did note a significant increase in grade 3 rectal bleeding at 3 years was 10% for the 78 Gy arm, compared to 2% for the 68 Gy arm (p = 0.007), and in nocturia (p = 0.05). The factors related to acute GI toxicity were hormone therapy (HT) (p < 0.001), a higher dose-volume group (p = 0.01), and pretreatment GI symptoms (p = 0.04). For acute GU toxicity, prognostic factors were: pretreatment GU symptoms (p < 0.001), ADT (p = 0.003), and prior TURP (p = 0.02). The following variables were found to be predictive of late GI toxicity: a history of abdominal surgery (p <0.001), and the presence of pretreatment GI symptoms (p = 0.001). The following variables were predictive of late GU toxicity: pretreatment urinary symptoms (p <0.001), the use of neoadjuvant ADT (p <0.001), and prior TURP (p = 0.006).

Sabdhu et al. reported that urethral strictures for 1,100 patients treated with 3D-CRT [25]. The 5-year actuarial likelihood of developing urethral stricture was 4% for 120 patients with a prior history or TURP compared to 1% for 980 patients with no history of TURP (p = 0.01). Other late urinary toxicities were not observed among patients with a prior history of a TURP. Lee et al. observed a 2% incontinence rate among patients with a prior history of TURP who were treated with EBRT compared with a 0.2% rate in patients without a prior TURP[26].

### 2.5.3. Acute and late adverse events of IMRT

In an attempt to improve further the conformality of the high-dose therapy plans and decrease the rate of grade 2 and higher toxicity, an IMRT approach was introduced for the treatment of clinically localized disease.

Zelefsky et al. reported their experience in 1571 patients treated with 3D-CRT or IMRT with dose raging from 66 to 81 Gy [27]. The median follow-up was 10 years. In this experience, IMRT significantly reduced the risk of grade 2 and higher late GI toxicities compared with conventional 3D-CRT (5% vs. 13%, p < 0.001), although IMRT delivered higher dose than 3D-CRT. However, IMRT increased the risk of acute and late grade 2 and higher GU toxicities and acute grade 2 and higher GI toxicities compared with conventional 3D-CRT (37% vs. 22%, p = 0.001, 20% vs. 12%, p = 0.01, and 3% vs. 1%, p = 0.04, respectively).

According to the latest report from MSKCC, actuarial 7-year grade 2 or higher late GI and GU toxicities with the use of IMRT to 86.4 Gy were 4.4% and 21.1%, respectively. Late grade 3 GI and GU toxicities were 0.7% and 2.2%, respectively [13].

Mamgani et al. compared the toxicity of 41 prostate cancer patients treated with IMRT to 78 Gy with that of 37 patients treated with the 3D-CRT approach at the same dose level within the Dutch dose-escalation trial [28]. They reported that IMRT significantly reduced the incidence of acute grade 2 or higher GI toxicity compared with 3D-CRT (20% vs. 61%, p = 0.001). For acute GU toxicity and late GI and GU toxicities, the incidence was lower after IMRT, although these differences were not statistically significant (53% vs. 69%, p = 0.3, 21% vs. 37%, p = 0.16, and 43% vs. 45%, p = 1.0, respectively).

# 3. Low-Dose-Rate (LDR) brachytherapy (Permanent implants)

### 3.1. Introduction to permanent implants

Interstitial prostate brachytherapy was first performed by Barringer in 1915 [29-31]. Its first widespread adoption occurred in the 1970s, when the retropubic method was popularized [32]. A laparotomy was done for lymph node dissection and exposure of the prostate. Iodine-125 sources were implanted under direct visualization. The procedure was technically difficult to perform, in part because of limited working space in the pelvis. As a result, retropubic implantation lost popularity in the 1980s [33]. Instead, ultrasound-guided permanent prostatic implantation emerged in the early 1980s and has spread all over the world. The ultrasound-guided transperineal technique was initially described by Holm and coworkers in 1983 [34]. Transrectal ultrasound (TRUS) allowed visualization of the needle location within the prostate, facilitating real-time read-justments of needle position as necessary. Implants could be computer preplanned using transverse ultrasound images. Transperineal implants also could be done percutaneously on an outpatient basis, without laparotomy. Combined with modern, computer-based treatment planning, technological advances allowed for higher quality outpatient prostate brachytherapy [35].

Brachytherapy offers substantial biologic advantages over EBRT in terms of dose localization and higher biologic doses. A modification of the time, dose, and fractionation tables has been made to allow interconvertability between beam radiation and low-dose-rate brachytherapy [36]. There are also substantial practical advantages of brachytherapy, including vastly shorter treatment times and lower costs. These practical advantages have helped maintain widespread interest in brachytherapy, despite continuous improvements in beam radiation. Although enthusiasm remains high in some quarters, there are still vexing discrepancies in reported cure rates and morbidities. It is becoming clearer that such discrepancies result partly from different technical expertise and patient management policies [37]. Brachytherapy, like surgery, is operator-dependent and outcomes vary with skill and experience.

### 3.2. Patient selection

Contraindications to brachytherapy include metastatic disease (including lymph node involvement), gross seminal vesicle involvement because that radioactive seeds are unlikely to be capable of sterilizing more than the most proximal 1 cm of seminal vesicle tissue, or large T3 disease that cannot be adequately implanted because of geometrical impediments to adequate tumor mass implantation (an unusual presentation).

Large prostate size can be often contraindication to brachytherapy because that the anterior and lateral portion of the gland may be inadequately covered because of pubic arch interference of needle placement. When a patient has a prostate > 60 cc, and pubic arch interference is a concern, a short course of ADT will reduce prostate volume by an average of approximately 30% in 3-4 months [38, 39]

Patients with a high International Prostate Symptom Score (IPSS) for urinary irritative and obstructive symptoms are at increased risk of developing postimplant urinary retention [40-43]. Terk et al. [44] and Gutman et al. [45] reported that patients with IPSS had a high risk of urinary retention.

Patients with prior pelvic radiotherapy may be at increased risk of developing late GI or GU toxicity. In such patients, the dose delivered to the prostate, rectum, and bladder should be considered.

In patients with prior TURP, a large TURP defect may disturb implantation of seed throughout the entire gland, resulting in unacceptable dosimetry.

Early-stage prostate cancer with T < or = 2a, initial PSA < or = 10ng/ml, and GS < or = 6 is suitable for brachytherapy without supplemental EBRT. Meanwhile, the generally accepted policy has been to add EBRT for the prostate cancer with T > 2a, initial PSA > 10ng/ml, or GS > 6. However, patients with intermediate-risk disease (T = 2b, GS = 7, or PSA > 10 and < or = 20 ng/ml) represent a heterogeneous patient population some of whom may benefit from monotherapy. Some investigators reported their experiences to perform monotherapy for patients with intermediate- and high-risk disease [46 – 51].

### 3.3. Treatment techniques

#### 3.3.1. Preplanned transperineal implantation techniques

First of all, TRUS imaging is obtained before planned procedure to assess the prostate volume. A computerized plan is generated from the ultrasound images, producing isodose distributions and the ideal location of seeds within the gland to deliver the prescription dose to the prostate. Several days to weeks later, the implantation procedure is performed. Needles are then placed under ultrasonographic guidance through a perineal template according to the coordinates determined by the preplan. Radioactive seeds are individually deposited in the needle with the aid of an applicator or with preloaded seeds on a semirigid strand containing the preplanned number of seeds. In the latter case, this is accomplished by stabilizing the needle obturator that holds the seed column in a fixed position while the needle is withdrawn slowly, depositing a row or series of seeds within the gland.

In general most brachytherapists use a modified peripheral loading technique for permanent interstitial implantation. This approach can reduce the urethral doses more than a homogenous loading technique. The portion of the urethra receiving 150% dose ($UV_{150}$) should be limited [52]. Likewise, the volume of the rectum ($RV_{100}$) receiving the prescription dose ideally should be < 1 cc [53].

### 3.3.2. Intraoperative planning techniques

Intraoperative planning takes advantage of the opportunity of using real-time measurements of the prostate during the procedure while preplanning is often preformed several weeks before implantation, frequently under different conditions than the actual operative procedure. Subtle changes in the position of the ultrasound probe as well as the distortion of the prostate associated with needle placement and subsequent edema can result in profound changes in the shape of the gland compared with the preplanned prostatic contour.

### 3.4. Dose selection

Numerous studies have confirmed $D_{90}$ (the minimum dose received by 90% of the prostate volume) and $V_{100}$ (percentage of the prostate volume receiving 100% of the prescribed dose) are correlated with outcome [54-56].

Prescription doses for I-125 or palladium-103 ($^{103}Pd$) are typically 140 to 160 Gy or 110 to 130 Gy, respectively. In practice, many brachytherapists plan a dose higher than the above mentioned doses to compensate for edema, seed misplacement, and so on. Merrick et al. [57] examined variability in permanent prostate brachytherapy preimplant dosimetry among eight experienced brachytherapy teams. A range of $D_{90}$ values from 112% to 151% of the prescription dose was planned. Several investigations suggest that an acceptable dose range for postimplant $D_{90}$ for I-125 may be 130 to 180 Gy as long as normal structures are not overdosed. Zelefsky et al. [58] reported that $D_{90} < 130$ Gy was associated with and increased risk of failure. Meanwhile, Gomez-Iturriaga Pina et al. [59] reported that $D_{90}$ from 180 Gy to 200 Gy was associated with excellent biochemical disease-free survival and acceptable toxicity.

When combined EBRT and brachytherapy, a wide variety of implant and beam radiation dose combinations are used. Implant prescription doses area generally dropped to approximately 70% to 80% of monotherapy doses, ranging from 110 to 120 Gy with I-125 and 90 to 100 Gy with Pd-103. External beam doses of 40 to 50 Gy area typically used. No studies have investigated either the sequencing of EBRT and brachytherapy, or the time interval between the two.

5

A wide variety of seed activities, seed numbers, or total activities have been used because of no clinical evidence of any effect outcome. Seed activities typically vary from 0.3 to 0.6 mCi for I-125 and 1.2 to 2.2 mCi for Pd-103.

## 3.5. Clinical results

### 3.5.1. Clinical results of LDR brachytherapy as monotherapy

It is generally accepted that patients with low-risk disease are excellent candidate for LDR monotherapy. There is no randomized data comparing therapeutic outcomes between LDR monotherapy, surgery, and EBRT. However, multiple reports of low-risk patients treated with LDR monotherapy have demonstrated excellent long-term biochemical control rates of 80 – 95% (Table 1).

Patients with intermediate-risk disease represent a heterogeneous patient population. Some of them seem to benefit from LDR monotherapy, whereas others may require combined modality approaches with EBRT and/or ADT. D'Amico et al [65] reported that percentage of positive prostate biopsy cores is a predicting factor of biochemical outcome following EBRT, particularly for intermediate-risk patients. In their report, patients with > 50% of biopsy cores positive had PSA relapse rates comparable to those of high-risk patients, whereas patients with < 34% of biopsy cores positive had favorable biochemical outcomes similar to those of low risk patients. Long-term biochemical control rate for intermediate-risk patients treated with LDR monotherapy is also favorable, ranging from 70% to 90% (Table 1).

| Authors | N | Mean/Median Follow-up | Adjuvant Hormone Therapy | bRFS rate | | |
|---------|---|-----------------------|--------------------------|-----------|------------------|------------|
| | | | | Low-risk | Intermediate-risk | High-risk |
| Sylvester et al [60] | 215 | 11.7 years | NO | 15-year | | |
| | | | | 85.90% | 79.90% | 62.20% |
| Prade et al [61] | 734 | 55 months | YES | 10-year | | |
| | | | | 92.00% | 84% | 65% |
| Henry et al [62] | 1298 | 4.9 years | YES | 10-year | | |
| | | | | 86.40% | 76.70% | 60.60% |
| Zelefsky et al [63] | 2693 | 63 months | NO | 8-year | | |
| | | | | 82% | 70% | 48% |
| Zelefsky et al [64] | 367 | 63 months | YES | 5-year | | |
| | | | | 96% | 89% | - |

**Table 1.** LDR brachytherapy as monotherapy

For patients with high-risk disease, the use of supplemental beam radiation to cover the periprostatic prostate tissue has been widely practiced. However, LDR monotherapy has been good results comparable to combination of monotherapy and EBRT even in patients with high-risk disease.

### 3.5.2. Clinical results of combination of LDR brachytherapy and EBRT

Outcomes (bRFS rates) for a combination of LDR brachytherapy and EBRT are shown in Table 2.

| Authors | N | Mean/Median Follow-up | Adjuvant Hormone Therapy | bRFS rate | | |
|---|---|---|---|---|---|---|
| | | | | Low-risk | Intermediate-risk | High-risk |
| Critz et al [66] | 1469 | 6 years | NO | 10-year | | |
| | | | | 93% | 80% | 61% |
| Merrick et al [67] | 204 | 7 years | YES | 10-year | | |
| | | | | | | 86.60% |
| Sylvester et al [68] | 223 | 9.43 years | NO | 15-year | | |
| | | | | 85.60% | 80.30% | 67.80% |
| Stock et al [69] | 181 | 65 months | YES | 8-year | | |
| | | | | | | 73% |
| Wernicke et al [70] | 242 | 10 years | NO | 10-year | | |
| | | | | 77.30% | | - |

**Table 2.** Combination of LDR brachytherapy and EBRT

## 3.6. Acute and late adverse events of LDR brachytherapy

### 3.6.1. Urinary toxicity

Almost all patients after LDR brachytherapy develop some kind of acute urinary symptoms, for example, urinary frequency, urgency, and occasional urge incontinence. These symptoms often peak at about 3 months after brachytherapy, subsequently gradually decline over the ensuing 3 to 6 months, and resolve with in 1 year (71). Most patients benefit with the use of an

$\alpha$-blocker. However, Brown et al [71] reported that 22% of patients experienced persistent urinary symptoms even after 12 months.

Acute urinary retention (AUR) is a common complication of modern brachytherapy, but can occur immediately after LDR brachytherapy. Crook et al. [72] demonstrated on the basis of a multivariate analysis that larger prostate volumes and prior hormone therapy were each independent predictors of AUR. AUR should be managed by intermittent or continuous bladder drainage. If AUR persists more than a few days, clean intermittent self-catheterization is preferred to continuous drainage by a Foley catheter. The use of transurethral incision of prostate should be avoided in the first 6 months, but if retention persists, transurethral incision of prostate or minimal TURP may be considered, recognizing the risk of urinary incontinence after these procedures [73-75].

### 3.6.2. Rectal toxicity

Grade 2 rectal toxicity symptoms, which manifest as rectal bleeding or increased mucous discharge, occur in 2 to 10% of patients, nearly always manifests between 6 and 18 months of implantation [76]. It is partly related to rectal dose and its volume exposed to a particular dose. The incidence of grade 3 or 4 rectal toxicity, which symptoms manifest rectal ulceration or fistula, is unusual (< 1.0%), providing that the volume of rectal wall receiving the prescription dose is kept below 0.5 cc on day 0 or 1 cc on day 30 dosimetry [77]. Most cases of rectal bleeding do not progress to rectal ulceration or fistula and are self-limited in nature. However, healing is typically slow. With the ineffectiveness of medical therapies, more invasive therapies with argon plasma coagulation or topical formalin have been highly effective therapy for rectal bleeding [78]. Invasive therapies, however, might exacerbate radiation damage, so they should be undertaken with caution. Rectal wall biopsy in the course of evaluation for rectal toxicity should avoid as much as possible because it may result in the development of rectal ulceration or fistula.

### 3.6.3. Sexual dysfunction

Erectile impotence occurs from 20% to 80% after implantation. According to Zelefsky et al [79], whereas the incidence of impotence at 2 years after implantation was 21%, the rate increased to 42% at 5 years after. Merrick et al. [80] reported that there is a strong correlation between radiation-induced impotence and the dose to the penile bulb and proximal penis. They recommend that with day 0 dosimetric evaluation, the minimum dose delivered to 50% and 25% of the bulb should be maintained below 40% and 60% of prescribed minimum peripheral dose, respectively, whereas the minimum dose delivered to 50% and 25% of the crura should be maintained below 40% and 28% of prescribed minimum peripheral dose, respectively, to maximize posttreatment potency.

Several reports suggest that sildenafil citrate have good response to impotence after implantation[81, 82]. Potters et al. [83] reported that the addition of neoadjuvant androgen deprivation had a significant impact on the potency preservation rate after implantation.

The response to sildenafil was significantly better in those patients not treated with neo-adjuvant ADT.

## 4. High-Dose-Rate (HDR) brachytherapy (Temporary implants)

### 4.1. Introduction to HDR brachytherapy

HDR brachytherapy has been used as the brachytherapy component in combination with EBRT for the treatment of prostate cancer [84-90]. In general, for this approach patients undergo transperineal placement of afterloading catheters in the prostate under ultrasonographic guidance. After CT-based treatment planning, several high-dose fractions are administered during an interval of 24 to 36 hours using [192]Ir. This treatment is followed by supplemental EBRT directed to the prostate and periprostatic tissues to a dose of 40 to 50.4 Gy using conventional fractionation. Recently, dose-escalation studies have been implemented to increase gradually the dose per fraction delivered with the HDR boost [91]. Improved outcomes with higher HDR boost doses were observed compared with outcomes achieved using lower dose level. Single higher dose fraction also becomes used for dealing with the issue of needle displacement between each fraction [92]. More recently, several institutes have used HDR brachytherapy as monotherapy without the addition of EBRT, largely for low-risk, but also for intermediate- and high-risk patients [93-99].

HDR brachytherapy offers several potential advantages over other techniques. Taking advantage of an afterloading approach, the radiation oncologist and physicist can more easily optimize the delivery of radiation therapy to the prostate and compensate for potential regions of underdosage that may be present with permanent interstitial implantation. Further, this technique reduces involved in the procedure compared with permanent interstitial implantation. Finally, HDR brachytherapy boosts may be radiobiologically more efficacious in terms of tumor cell kill for patients with increased tumor bulk or adverse prognostic features compared with low-dose-rate boost such as [125]I or [103]Pd.

### 4.2. Clinical results of HDR brachytherapy

The reported outcomes of combination of HDR brachytherapy and EBRT are favorable (Table 3). Multiple reports of low- and intermediate-risk patients treated with combination of HDR brachytherapy and EBRT have demonstrated excellent long-term biochemical control rates of 90-100% and 87-98%, respectively (Table 3). Long-term biochemical control rate for high-risk patients treated with combination of HDR brachytherapy and EBRT is also favorable.

Yoshioka et al. [99] have performed HDR brachytherapy as monotherapy for localized prostate cancer since 1996. The 5-year bRFS rate for low-, intermediate-, and high-risk patients was 85%, 93%, and 79%, respectively.

| Authors | N | Mean/Median Follow-up | HDR dose | bRFS rate | | |
|---|---|---|---|---|---|---|
| | | | | Low-risk | Intermediate-risk | High-risk |
| Boost | | | | | | |
| Astrom et al. [100] | 214 | 4 years | 10 Gy x 2 | | 5-year | |
| | | | | 92% | 88% | 61% |
| Bachand et al. [101] | 153 | 44 months | 9 Gy x 2/ 10 Gy x 2 | | 5-year | |
| | | | | | 95.9% | 95.5% |
| Chen et al. [84] | 85 | 40 months | 5.5 Gy x 3 | | 4-year | |
| | | | | 100% | 91% | 81% |
| Demanes et al. [85] | 209 | 6.4 years | 5.5 Gy x 4/ 6.0 Gy x 4 | | 10-year | |
| | | | | 92% | 87% | 63% |
| Yamada et a.l [86] | 105 | 44 months | 5.5 Gy x 3/ 7.0 Gy x 3 | | 5-year | |
| | | | | 100% | 98% | 92% |
| Phan et al. [89] | 309 | 59 months | 6 Gy x 4 | | 5-year | |
| | | | | 98% | 90% | 78% |
| Prada et al. [102] | 313 | 71 months | 11.5 Gy x 2 | | 10-year | |
| | | | | 100% | 91%/88% | 79% |
| Monotherapy | | | | | | |
| Yoshioka et al. [99] | 112 | 5.4 years | 6 Gy x 9 | | 5-year | |
| | | | | 85% | 93% | 79% |
| Rogers CL et al. [103] | 284 | 35.1 months | 6.5 Gy x 6 | | 5-year | |
| | | | | | 94.40% | |

**Table 3.** HDR brachytherapy

## 4.3. Acute and late adverse events of HDR brachytherapy

### 4.3.1. Urinary toxicity

Acute urinary symptoms such as urinary urgency and frequency are common and usually resolve within a few months. Urinary retention occurs in less than 5% of patients treated with combination of HDR brachytherapy and EBRT [89, 94, 104, 105]. Urinary strictures are reported in up to 15% of patients, and most commonly seen in the bulbomembranous urethra [106, 107]. Urinary incontinence is extremely rare, and seen in less than 2% of patients [107, 108].

*4.3.2. Rectal toxicity*

Transient rectal symptoms such as rectal urgency or frequency often occur. Late rectal bleeding may occur and is usually not clinically significant. Rectal fistula is extremely rare, and seen in less than 1% of patients[89].

*4.3.3. Sexual toxicity*

Erectile dysfunction has been reported in up to 40% of patients, but approximately 80% will respond to phosphodiesterase-5 inhibitors (86).

# 5. Particle beam radiation therapy

Particle beam radiation therapy is the cancer therapy to deliver the ions accelerated by means of a cyclotron or synchrotron. Nowadays, protons and carbon ions (heavy particles) are in clinical use.

For protons and heavy particles, unlike electrons or X-rays, the dose increases while the particle penetrates the tissue and loses energy continuously. Hence the dose increases with increasing thickness up to the Bragg peak that occurs near the end of the particle's range. Beyond the Bragg peak, the dose drops to zero (for protons) or almost zero (for heavy particles). The advantage of this energy deposition profile is that less energy is deposited into the healthy tissue surrounding the target tissue.

Although proton beams have approximately the same biological effectiveness as X-rays or electrons, carbon ions have 1.2 to 3.5 times as much effectiveness as X-rays. Carbon ions many other biological features, which X-rays don`t have, as follows; 1) having their reduced ability to repair damage DNA, 2) having smaller oxygen enhancement ratio, 3) effectiveness even against the hypoxic cancer cells, 4) effectiveness even against S-late phase cancer cells because of their being less of cell cycle dependence.

Investigators from National Institute of Radiological Sciences, Japan reported their experience in 927 patients treated with hypofractionated conformal carbon-ion radiation therapy between April 2000 and December 2010 [109]. Of 927 patients, 250, 216, and 461 patients were treated with 66 GyE (Gray equivalent (a measure of carbon-ion radiation dose base on an relative biological effectiveness (RBE) ratio of 3 with respect to photon radiation)) in 20 fractions (Fr), 63 GyE in 20 Fr, and 57.6 GyE in 16 Fr, respectively. Neoadjuvant ADT was given to the patients in the intermediate- and high-risk groups for 2 to 6 months. Adjuvant ADT was continued for a duration of 6 months for intermediate-risk patients and for 2 years for the high-risk patients. They reported the 5-year cause specific survival rates for the low-, intermediate-, and high-risk group patients as 100%, 100%, and 97.9%, respectively. The 5-year bRFS rates of the low-, intermediate-, and high-risk groups were 89.4%, 96.8%, and 88.4%, respectively. They reported that grade 2 rectal bleeding developed in 15 patients (1.6%), but no grade 3 or worse morbidities at the rectum were observed in all groups. They also reported that late grade 2 and grade 3 GU toxicities were observed in 57 (6.1%) and one (0.1%) of 927 patients, respectively. These incidences of late morbidities, especially of rectal bleeding are favorable compared with other RT methods (Table. 4).

| Authors | Method | Dose fractionation | No. patients | Morbidity rate | |
|---------|--------|--------------------|--------------|:----:|:----:|
|         |        | (Gy/Fr)            |              | GI | GU |
| Coote et al. [110] | IMRT | 60.0/20 | 60 | 9.5% | 4.0% |
| Martin et al. [111] | IMRT | 60.0/20 | 92 | 6.3% | 10.0% |
| Kupelian et al.[112] | IMRT | 70.0/28 | 770 | 4.4% | 5.2% |
| King et al. [113] | SRT | 36.25/5 | 41 | 15.0% | 29.0% |
| Madsen et al. [114] | SRT | 33.5/5 | 40 | 7.5% | 22.5% |
| Michalski JM et al. [115] | 3DCRT | 68.4-79.2/38-41 | 275 | 7-16% | 18-29% |
|  | 3DCRT | 78.0/39 | 118 | 25-26% | 23-28% |
| Schulte RW [116] | Proton | 75.0/39 | 901 | 3.5% | 5.4% |
| Ishikawa et al. [109] | Carbon-ion | 57.6-66.0/16-20 | 927 | 1.9% | 6.3% |

(Cited from Ishikawa et al [109])

**Table 4.** Comparison of Grade 2 or worse late morbidity rates according to RT method

# 6. Postoperative radiotherapy

## 6.1. Adjuvant radiotherapy (ART)

The results of three large phase III trials, which evaluated the merits of adjuvant versus expectant management in postoperative patients with positive surgical margins and/or pT3 disease, were reported.

EORTC 22911 confirmed the value of ART, which reduced the risk of biochemical failure and prolongs the time to clinical progression [117]. Patients eligible for this study had pT2-3N0M0 tumors and one or more pathologic risk factors (extracapsular extension (ECE), positive surgical margins (PSM), seminal vesicles invasion (SVI)). After a median follow-up of 5 years, biochemical and clinical progression-free survivals were significantly improved in the radiotherapy group (P < 0.0001 and P = 0.0009, respectively). The rate of local regional failure was also lower in the radiotherapy group (P = 0.07). Severe toxicity (grade 3 or higher) was similar, being 2.6% versus 4.2% at 5 years in the postoperative radiotherapy group (P = 0.07).

SWOG 8794 randomly assigned 473 node-negative patients initially treated with radical prostectomy, but found to have either PSM or pT3 (ECE and/or SVI) disease to ART or observation [118]. ART consisted of 60 to 64 Gy. ART resulted in an improvement in metastasis-free and overall survival compared with deferred therapy (HR 0.71; P = 0.016 and HR 0.72; P = 0.023, respectively). Although adverse effects were more common with radiotherapy versus observation, by 5 years there were no differences in health-related QOL, and a subset analysis suggests that earlier treatment is better than delayed treatment [119].

From the German Cancer Society, ARO 96-02/AUO AP 09/95 randomized 385 patients with pT3 or PSM to either ART (60Gy in 2 Gy fractions) or observation [120]. Although this study had the short median follow-up of 40 months, ART significantly improved progression-free survival (P < 0.0001) with a low incidence of late complications from radiotherapy.

### 6.2. Salvage radiotherapy (SRT)

A multi-institutional study suggests that early intervention with radiotherapy is better than delayed intervention for patients with biochemical failure [121, 122]. This analysis included patients with pT3-4N0 disease who received either SRT or early ART. Early ART for pT3-4N0 disease significantly reduces the risk of long-term biochemical progression after radical prostatectomy compared with SRT.

Stephenson et al. [123] reported on the outcomes and prognostic factors of 501 men who had salvage radiotherapy after a biochemical recurrence. In the entire cohort, the 4-year progression-free survival (PFS) was 45%, and 67% attained a PSA nadir of <0.1 ng/mL. Multivariate analyses demonstrated that Gleason score of 8 to 10, preradiotherapy PSA >2 ng/mL, negative margins, PSA-doubling time <10 months, and seminal vesicle invasion were associated with PSA progression. Supporting earlier intervention, preradiotherapy PSA <0.6 ng/mL had significantly improved PFS than a PSA of 0.61 to 2 ng/mL (P = 0.006) and >2 ng/mL (P = 0.001).

## Author details

Shinji Kariya*

Address all correspondence to: kariyas@kochi-u.ac.jp

Department of Diagnostic Radiology and Radiation Oncology, Kochi Medical School, Kohasu, Oko-town, Kochi, Japan

## References

[1] Bagshaw MA, Cox RS, Ray GR. Status of radiation treatment of prostate cancer at Stanford University. NCI Monogr 1988;( 7) 47-60.

[2] Pilepich MV, Krall JM, Sause WT, et al. Prognostic factors in carcinoma of the prostate —analysis of RTOG study 75-06. Int J Radiat Oncol Biol Phys 1987; 13(3) 339-349.

[3] Roach M 3rd, Pickett B, Weil M, et al. The "critical volume tolerance method" for estimating the limits of dose escalation during three-dimensional conformal radiotherapy for prostate cancer. Int J Radiat Oncol Biol Phys 1996; 35(5) 1019-1025.

[4]   Webb S. The physical basis of IMRT and inverse planning. Br J Radiol 2003; 76(910) 678-689.

[5]   Spirou SV, Chui CS. Generation of arbitrary intensity profiles by dynamic jaws or multileaf collimators. Med Phys 1994; 21(7) 1031-1041.

[6]   Kupelian PA, Elshaikh M, Reddy CA, et al. Comparison of the efficacy of local therapies for localized prostate cancer in the prostate-specific antigen era: a large single-institution experience with radical prostatectomy and external-beam radiotherapy. J Clin Oncol 2002; 20(16) 3376-3385.

[7]   D'Amico AV, Whittington R, Malkowicz SB, et al. Biochemical outcome after radical prostatectomy or external beam radiation therapy for patients with clinically localized prostate carcinoma in the prostate specific antigen era. Cancer 2002; 95(2) 281-286.

[8]   Roach M, Meehan S, Kroll S, et al. Radiotherapy for high grade clinically localized adenocarcinoma of the prostate. J Urol 1996; 156(5) 1719-1723.

[9]   Zelefsky MJ, Leibel SA, Gaudin PB et al. Dose escalation with three-dimensional conformal radiation therapy affects the outcome in prostate cancer. Int J Radiat Oncol Boil Phys 1998; 41(3) 491-500.

[10]  Fiveash JB, Hanks G, Roach M, et al: 3D conformal radiation therapy (3DCRT) for high grade prostate cancer: a multi-institutional review. Int J Radiat Oncol Biol Phys 2000; 47(2) 335-342.

[11]  Pollack A, Hanlon AL, Horwitz EM, et al. Prostate cancer radiotherapy dose response: an uptake of the fox chase experience. J Urol 2004; 171(3) 1132-1136.

[12]  Kupelian PA, Buchsbaum JC, Reddy CA, et al. Radiation dose response in patients with favorable localized prostate cancer (Stage T1-T2, biopsy Gleason < or = 6, and pretreatment prostate-specific antigen < or = 10). Int J Radiat Oncol Biol Phys 2001; 50(3) 621-625.

[13]  Spratt DE, Pei X, Yamada J, et al. Long-term survival and toxicity in patients treated with high-dose intensity modulated radiation therapy for localized prostate cancer. Int J Radiat Oncol Biol Phys 2012, in press.

[14]  Bolla M, Collette L, Blank L, et al. Long-term results with immediate androgen suppression and external irradiation in patients with locally advanced prostate cancer (an EORTC study): A phase III randomized trial. Lancet 2002; 360(9327) 103-106.

[15]  Pilepich MV, Winter K, Lawton CA, et al. Androgen suppression adjuvant to definitive radiotherapy in prostate carcinoma-long-term results of phase III RTOG 85-31. Int J Raiat Oncol Biol Phys 2005; 61(5) 1285-1290.

[16]  Pilepich MV, Winter K, John MJ, et al. Phase III radiation therapy oncology group (RTOG) trial 86-10 of androgen deprivation adjuvant to definitive radiotherapy in locally advanced carcinoma of the prostate. Int J Radiat Oncol Biol Phys 2001; 50(5) 1243-1252.

[17] Laverdiere J, Nabid A, De Bedoya LD, et al. The efficacy and sequencing of a short course of androgen suppression on freedom from biochemical failure when administered with radiation therapy for T2-T3 prostate cancer. J Urol 2004; 171(3) 1137-1140.

[18] Granfors T, Modig H, Damber JE, et al. Combined orchiectomy and external radiotherapy versus radiotherapy alone for nonmetastatic prostate cancer with or without pelvic lymph node involvement: A prospective randomized study. J Urol 1998; 159(6) 2030-2034.

[19] D'Amico AV, Manola J, Loffredo M, et al. 6-months androgen suppression plus radiation therapy vs radiation therapy alone for patients with clinically localized prostate cancer: A randomized controlled trial. JAMA 2004; 292(7) 821-827.

[20] Lawton CA, Won M, Pilepich M, et al. Long-term treatment sequelae following external beam irradiation of adenocarcinoma of the prostate: analysis of RTOG studies 7506 and 7706. Int J Radiat Oncol Biol Phys 1991; 21(4) 935-939.

[21] Michalski JM, Winter K, Purdy JA, et al. Toxicity after three-dimensional radiotherapy for prostate cancer on RTOG 9406 dose level V. Int J Radiat Oncol Biol Phys 2005; 62(3) 706-713.

[22] Zietman AL, DeSilvio ML, Slater JD, et al. Comparison of conventional-dose vs high-dose conformal radiation therapy in clinically localized adenocarcinoma of the prostate. JAMA 2005; 294: 1233-1239.

[23] Zelefsky MJ, Cowen D, Fuks Z, et al. Long-term tolerance of high dose three-dimensional radiotherapy in patients with localized prostate carcinoma. Cancer 1999; 85(11) 2460-2468.

[24] Peeters ST, Heemsbergen WD, Koper PC, et al. Acute and late complications after radiotherapy for localized prostate cancer: results of a multicenter randomized phase III trial comparing 68 Gy to 78 Gy. Int J Radiat Oncol Biol Phys 2005; 61(4) 1019-1034.

[25] Sandhu AS, Zelefsky MJ, Lee HJ, et al. Long-term urinary toxicity after 3-dimensional conformal radiotherapy for prostate cancer in patients with prior history of transurethral resection. Int J Radiat Oncol Biol Phys 2000; 48(3) 643-647.

[26] Lee WR, Schulthesis TE, Hanlon AL, et al. Urinary incontinence following external-beam radiotherapy for clinically localized prostate cancer. Urology 1996; 48(1) 95-99.

[27] Zelefsky MJ, Levin EJ, Hunt M, et al. Incidence of late rectal and urinary toxicities after three-dimensional conformal radiotherapy and intensity-modulated radiotherapy for localized prostate cancer. Int J Raiat Oncol Biol Phys 2008; 70(4) 1124-1129.

[28] Mamgani AA, Heemsbergen WD, Peeters STH, et al. Role of intensity-modulated radiotherapy in reducing toxicity in dose escalation for localized prostate cancer. Int J Radiat Oncol Biol Phys. 2009; 73(3) 685-691.

[29] Barringer BS. Radium in the treatment of prostatic carcinoma. Ann Surg 1924; 80(6) 881-884.

[30] Aronowitz JN. Benjamin Barringer: originator of the transperineal prostate implant. Urol 2002; 60(4) 731-734.

[31] Aronowitz JN. Dawn of prostate brachytherapy: 1915-1930. Int J Radiat Oncol Biol Phys 2002; 54(3) 712-718.

[32] Whitemore WF, Hilaris B, Grabstald H. Retropubic implantation of Iodine 125 in the treatment of prostatic cancer. J Urol 1972; 108(6) 918-920.

[33] Fuks Z, Leibel SA, Wallner KE, et al. The effect of local control on metastatic dissemination in carcinoma of the prostate: Long term results in patients treated with 125-I implantation. Int J Radiat Oncol Biol Phys 1991; 21(3) 337-347.

[34] Holm HH, Juul N, Pedersen JF, et al. Transperineal 125iodine seed implantation in prostatic cancer guided by transrectal ultrasonography. J Urol 1983; 130(2) 283-286.

[35] Charyulu KKN. Transperineal interstitial implantation of prostate cancer: a new method. Int J Radiat Oncol Biol Phys 1980; 6(9) 1261-1266.

[36] Orton CG, Webber BM. Time-dose factor (TDF) analysis of dose rate effects in permanent implant dosimetry. Int J Radiat Oncol Biol Phys 1977; 2(1-2) 55-60.

[37] Merrik G, Butler WM, Wallner KE, et al. Variability of prostate brachytherapy preimplant dosimetry: a multi-institutional analysis. Brachytherapy 2005; 4(4) 241-251.

[38] Kucway R, Vicini F, Huang R, et al. Prostate volume reduction with androgen deprivation therapy before interstitial brachytherapy. U Urol 2002; 167(6) 2443-2447.

[39] Solhjem MC, Davis BJ, Pisansky TM, et al. Prostate volume before and after permanent prostate brachytherapy in patients receiving neoadjuvant androgen suppression. Cancer J 2004; 10(6) 343-348.

[40] Crook J, McLean M, Gatton C, et al. Factors influencing risk of acute urinary retention after TRUS-guided permanent prostate seed implantation. Int J Radiat Oncol Phys 2002; 52(2) 453-460.

[41] Keyes M, Schellenberg D, Moravan V, et al. Decline in urinary retention incidence in 805 patients after prostate brachytherapy: The effect of learning curve? Int J Radiat Oncol Biol Phys 2006; 64(3) 825-834.

[42] Terk M, Stock R, Stone N. Identification of patients at increased risk for prolonged urinary retention following radioactive seed implantation of the prostate. J Urol 1998; 160(4)1379-1382.

[43] Lee N, Wuu CS, Rrody R, et al. Factors predicting for postimplantation urinary retention after permanent prostate brachytherapy. Int J Radiat Oncol Biol Phys 2000; 48(5) 1457-1460.

[44] Terk MD, Stock RG, Stone NN. Identification of patients at increased risk for prolonged urinary retention following radioactive seed implantation of the prostate. J Urol 1998; 160(4) 1379-1382.

[45]  Gutman S, Merrick GS, Butler WM, et al. Severity categories of the International Prostate Symptom Score before, and urinary morbidity after, permanent prostate brachytherapy. BJU Int 2006; 97(1) 62-68.

[46]  Zelefsky MJ, Yamada Y, Cohen GN, et al. Five-year outcome of intraoperative conformal permanent I-125 interstitial implantation for patients with clinically localized prostate cancer. Int J Radiat Oncol Biol Phys 2007; 67(1) 65-70.

[47]  Zelefsky MJ, Kuban DA, Levy LB, et al. Multi-institutional analysis of long-term outcome for stages T1-T2 prostate cancer treated with permanent seed implantation. Int J Radiat Oncol Biol Phys 2007; 67(2)327-333.

[48]  Henry AM, Al-Qaisieh B, Gould K, et al. Outcome following iodine-125 monotherapy for localized prostate cancer: The results of leeds 10-year single-center brachytherapy experience. Int J Radiat Oncol Biol Phys 2010; 76(1) 50-56.

[49]  Prada PJ, Juan G, Gonzalez-Suarez H, Fernandez J, et al. Prostate-specific antigen relapse-free survival and side-effects in 734 patients with up to 10 years of follow-up with localized prostate cancer treated by permanent $^{125}$iodine implants. BJU Int 2010; 106(1) 32-36.

[50]  Sylvester JE, Grimm PD, Wong J, et al. Fifteen-year biochemical relapse-free survival cause-specific survival, and overall survival following I125 prostate brachytherapy in clinically localized prostate cancer Seattle experience. Int J Radiat Oncol Boil Phys. 2011; 81(2) 376-381.

[51]  Kinnen KA, Batterman JJ, van Roermung JG, et al. Long-term biochemical and survival outcome of 921 patients treated with i-125 permanent prostate brachytherapy. Int J Radiat Oncol Biol Phys 2010; 76(5) 1433-1438.

[52]  Crook JM, Potters L, Stock RG, et al. Critical organ dosimetry in permanent seed prostate brachytherapy: Defining the organs at risk. Brachytherapy 2005; 4(3) 186-194.

[53]  Snyder KM, Stock RG, Hong SM, et al. Defining the risk of developing grade 2 proctitis following 125-I prostate brachytherapy using a rectal dose-volume histogram analysis. Int J Radiat Oncol Biol Phys 2001; 50(2) 335-341.

[54]  Papagikos MA, Deguzman AF, Rossi PJ, et al. Dosimetric quantifier for low-dose-rate prostate brachytherapy: Is V(100) superior to D(90)? Brachytherapy 2005; 4(4) 252-258.

[55]  Orio P, Wallner K, Merrick G, et al. Dosimetric parameters as predictive factors for biochemical control in patients with higher risk prostate cancer treated with Pd-103 and supplemental beam radiation. Int J Radiat Oncol Biol Phys 2007; 67(2) 342-346.

[56]  Morris WJ, Keyes M, Palma D, et al. Evaluation of dosimetric parameters and disease response after 125 iodine transperineal brachytherapy for low- and intermediate-risk prostate cancer. Int J Radiat Oncol Biol Phys 2009; 73(5) 1432-1438.

[57]  Merrick GS, Butler WM, Wallner KE, et al. Variability of prostate brachytherapy pre-implant dosimetry: A multi-institutional analysis. Brachytherapy 2005; 4(4) 241-251.

[58] Zelefsky MJ, Kuban DA, Levy BJ, et al. Multi-institutional analysis of long-term outcome for stage T1-T2 prostate cancer treated with permanent seed implantation. Int J Radiat Oncol Biol Phys 2007; 67(2) 327-333.

[59] Gomez-Iturriaga Pina A, Crook J, Borg J, et al. Biochemical disease-free rate and toxicity for men treated with iodine-125 prostate brachytherapy with d(90) > 180 Gy. Int J Radiat Oncol Biol Phys 2010; 78(2) 422-427.

[60] Sylvester JE, Grimm PD, Wong J, et al. Fifteen-year biochemical relapse-free survival, cause-specific survival, and overall survival following $I^{125}$ prostate brachytherapy in clinically localized prostate cancer: Seattle experience. Int J Radiat Oncol Biol Phys 2011; 81(2) 376-381.

[61] Prada PJ, Juan G, Gonzalez-Suarez H, et al. Prostate-specific antigen relapse-free survival and side-effects in 734 patients with up to 10 years of follow-up with localized prostate cancer treated by permanent $^{125}$iodine implants. BJU Int 2010; 106(1) 32-36.

[62] Henry AM, Al-Qaisieh B, Gould K, et al. Outcome following iodine-125 monotherapy for localized prostate cancer: the results of leeds 10-year single-center brachytherapy experience. Int J Radiat Oncol Biol Phys 2010; 76(1) 50-56.

[63] Zelefsky MJ, Kuban DA, Levy LB, et al. Multi-institutional analysis of long-term outcome for stages T1-T2 prostate cancer treated with permanent seed implantation. Int J Radiat Oncol Biol Phys 2007; 67(2) 327-333.

[64] Zelefsky MJ, Yamada Y, Cohen GN, et al. Five-year outcome of intraoperative conformal permanent I-125 interstitial implantation for patients with clinically localized prostate cancer. Int J Radiat Oncol Biol Phys 2007; 67(1) 65-70.

[65] D'Amico AV, Schultz D, Silver B, et al. The clinical utility of the percent of positive prostate biopsies in predicting biochemical outcome following external-beam radiation therapy for patients with clinically localized prostate cancer. Int J Radiat Oncol Biol Phys 2001; 49(3) 679-684.

[66] Critz FA, Levinson K. 10-year disease-free survival rates after simultaneous irradiation for prostate cancer with a focus on calculation methodology J Urol 2004; 172(6 Pt 1) 2232-2238.

[67] Merrick GS, Butler WM, Wallner KE, et al. Androgen deprivation therapy does not impact cause-specific or overall survival in high-risk prostate cancer managed with brachytherapy and supplemental external beam. Int J Radiat Oncol Biol Phys 2007; 68(1) 34-40.

[68] Sylvester JE, Grimm PD, Blasko JC, et al. 15-year biochemical relapse free survival in clinical stage T1-T3 prostate cancer following combined external beam radiotherapy and brachytherapy; Seattle experience. Int J Radiat Oncol Biol Phys 2007; 67(1):57-64.

[69] Stock RG, Cesaretti JA, Hall SJ, et al. Outcomes for patients with high-grade prostate cancer treated with a combination of brachytherapy, external beam radiotherapy and hormonal therapy. BJU Int 2009; 104(11) 1631-1636.

[70] Wernicke AG, Shamis M, Yan W, et al. Role of isotope selection in long-term outcomes in patients with intermediate-risk prostate cancer treated with a combination of external beam radiotherapy and low-dose-rate interstitial brachytherapy. Urol 2012; 79(5) 1098-1104.

[71] Brown D, Colonias A, Miller R, et al. Urinary morbidity with a modified peripheral loading technique of transperineal [125]I prostate implantation. Int J Radiat Oncol Biol Phys 2000; 47(2) 353-360.

[72] Crook J, McLean M, Catton C, et al. Factors influencing risk of acute urinary retention after TRUS-guided permanent prostate seed implantation. Int J Radiat Oncol Biol Phys 2002; 52(2) 453-460.

[73] Blasko JC, Ragde H, Grimm PD. Transperineal ultrasound-guided implantation of the prostate: Morbidity and complications. Scand J Urol Nephrol Suppl 1991; 137 113-118.

[74] Hu K, Wallner K. Urinary incontinence in patients who have a TURP/TUIP following prostate brachytherapy. Int J Radiat Oncol Biol Phys 1998; 40(4) 783-786.

[75] Kollmeier MA, Stock RG, Cesaretti J, et al. Urinary morbidity and incontinence following transurethral resection of the prostate after brachytherapy. J Urol 2005; 173(3) 808-812.

[76] Snyder KM, Stock RG, Hong SM, et al. Defining the risk of developing grade 2 proctitis following [125]I prostate brachytherapy using a rectal dose-volume histogram analysis. Int J Radiat Oncol Biol Phys 2001; 50(2) 335-341.

[77] Tran A, Wallner K, Merrick G, et al. Rectal fistulas after prostate brachytherapy. Int J Radiat Oncol Biol Phys 2005; 63(1) 150-154.

[78] Smith S, Wallner K, Han B, et al: Argon plasma coagulation for rectal bleeding following prostate brachytherapy. Int J Radiat Oncol Biol Phys 2001; 51(3) 636-642.

[79] Zelfsky MJ, Yamada Y, Cohen G, et al. Comparison of the 5-year outcome and morbidity of three dimensional conformal radiotherapy versus transperineal permanent iodine-125 implantation for early stage prostate cancer. J Clin Oncol 1999; 17(2) 517-522.

[80] Merrick GS, Butler WM, Wallner KE et al. The importance of radiation doses to the penile bulb vs. crura in the development of postbrachytherapy erectile dysfunction. Int J Radiat Oncol Biol Phys 2002; 54(4) 1055-1062.

[81] Merrck GS, Butler WM, Wallner KE, et al. Erectile function after prostate brachytherapy. Int J Radiat Oncol Biol Phys 2005; 62(2) 437-447.

[82] Raina R, Agarwal A, Goyal KK et al. Long-term potency after iodine-125 radiotherapy for prostate cancer and role of sildenafil citrate. Urology 2003; 62(6) 1103-1108.

[83] Potters L, Torre T, Fearn PA et al. Potency after permanent prostate brachytherapy for localized prostate cancer. Int J Radiat Oncol Biol Phys 2001; 50(5) 1235-1242.

[84] Chen YC, Chuang CK, Hsieh ML, et al. High-dose-rate brachytherapy plus external beam radiotherapy for T1 to T3 prostate cancer: An experience in Taiwan. Urology 2007; 70(1) 101-105.

[85] Demanes DJ, Brandt D, Schour L, et al. Excellent results from high dose rate brachytherapy and external beam for prostate cancer are not improved by androgen deprivation. Am J Clin Oncol 2009; 32(4) 342-347.

[86] Yamada Y, Bhatia S, Zaider M, et al. Favorable clinical outcome of three-dimensional computer-optimized high-dose-rate prostate brachytherapy in the management of localized prostate cancer. Brachytherapy 2006; 5(3) 157-164.

[87] Ducchesne GM, Williams SG, Das R, et al. Patterns of toxicity following high-dose-rate brachytherapy boost for prostate cancer: Mature prospective phase I/II study results. Radiother Oncol 2007; 84(2) 128-134.

[88] Hiratsuka J, Jo Y, Yoshida K, et al. Clinical results of combined treatment conformal high-dose-rate iridium-192 brachytherapy and external beam radiotherapy using staging lymphadenectomy for localized prostate cancer. Int J Radiat Oncol Biol Phys. 2004; 59(3) 684-690.

[89] Phan TP, Syed AM, Puthawala A, et al. High dose rate brachytherapy as a boost for the treatment of localized prostate cancer. J Urol 2007; 177(1) 123-127.

[90] Zwahlen DR, Andrianopoulos N, Matheson B, et al. High-dose-rate brachytherapy in combination with conformal external beam radiotherapy in the treatment of prostate cancer. Brachytherapy 2010; 9(1) 27-35.

[91] Martinez AA, Gonzalez J, Ye H. Dose escalation improves cancer-related events at 10 years for intermediate- and high-risk prostate cancer patients treated with hypofractionated high-dose-rate boost and external beam radiotherapy. Int J Radiat Oncol Biol Phys 2011; 79(2) 363-370.

[92] Morton G, Loblaw A, Cheung P, et al. Is single fraction 15 Gy the preferred high dose-rate brachytherapy boost dose for prostate cancer? Radiother Oncol 2011; 100(3) 463-467.

[93] Demanes DJ, Martinez AA, Ghilezan M, et al. High-dose-rate monotherapy: Safe and effective brachytherapy for patients with localized prostate cancer. Int J Radiat Oncol Biol Phys 2011; 81(5) 1286-1292.

[94] Ghilezan M, Martinez AA, Gustason G, et al. High dose rate brachytherapy as monotherapy delivered in two fractions within one day for favorable/intermediate risk prostate cancer: Preliminary toxicity data. Int J Radiat Oncol Biol Phys 2012; 83(3) 927-932.

[95] Jabbari S, Weinberg VK, Shinohara K, et al. Equivalent biochemical control and improved prostate-specific antigen nadir after permanent prostate seed implant brachytherapy versus high-dose three-dimensional conformal radiotherapy and high-

dose conformal proton beam radiotherapy boost. Int J Radiat Oncol Biol Phys 2010; 76(1) 36-42.

[96] Grills IS, Martinez AA, Hollander M, et al. High dose rate brachytherapy as prostate cancer monotherapy reduces toxicity compared to low dose rate palladium seed. J Urol 2004; 171(3) 1098-1104.

[97] Rogers CL, Alder AS, Rogers RL, et al. High dose rate brachytherapy as monotherapy for intermediate risk prostate cancer. J Urol 2012; 187(1) 109-116.

[98] Prada PJ, Jimenez I, Gonzalez-Suarez H, et al. High-dose-rate interstitial brachytherapy as monotherapy in one fraction and transperineal hyaluronic acid injection into the perirectal fat for the treatment of favorable stage prostate cancer: Treatment description and preliminary results. Brachytherapy 2012; 11(2) 105-110.

[99] Yoshioka K, Konishi K, Sumida I, et al. Monotherapeutic high-dose-rate brachytherapy for prostate cancer: Five-year results of an extreme hypofractionation regimen with 54 Gy in nine fractions. Int J Radiat Oncol Biol Phys 2011; 80(2) 469-475.

[100] Astrom L, Pedersen D, Mercke C, et al. Long-term outcome of high dose rate brachytherapy in radiotherapy of localized prostate cancer. Radiother Oncol 2005; 74(2) 157-161.

[101] Bachand F, Martin AG, Beaulieu L, et al. An eight-year experience of HDR brachytherapy boost for localized prostate cancer: Biopsy and PSA outcome. Int J Radiat Oncol Biol Phys 2009; 73(3) 679-684.

[102] Prada PJ, Gonzalez H, Fernandez J, et al. Biochemical outcome after high-dose-rate intensity modulated brachytherapy with external beam radiotherapy: 12 years of experience. BJU Int 2011; 109(12) 1787-1793.

[103] Rogers CL, Alder SC, Rogers RL, et al. High dose brachytherapy as monotherapy for intermediate risk prostate cancer. J Urol 2012; 187(1) 109-116.

[104] Demanes DJ, Rodriguez RR, Schour L, et al. High-dose-rate intensity-modulated brachytherapy with external beam radiotherapy for prostate cancer. Int J Radiat Oncol Biol Phys 2005; 61(5) 1306-1316.

[105] Deger S, Boehmer D, Roigas J, et al. High dose rate (HDR) brachytherapy with conformal radiation therapy for localized prostate cancer. Eur Urol 2005; 47(4) 441-448.

[106] Sullivan L, Williams SG, Tai KH, et al. Urethral stricture following high dose rate brachytherapy for prostate cancer. Radiother Oncol 2009; 91(2) 232-236.

[107] Pellizzon AC, Salvajoli JV, Maia MA, et al. Late urinary morbidity with high dose prostate brachytherapy as a boost to conventional external beam radiation therapy for local and locally advanced prostate cancer. J Urol 2004; 171(3) 1105-1108.

[108] Duchesne GM Williams SG, Das R, et al. Patterns of toxicity following high-dose-rate brachytherapy boost for prostate cancer: Mature prospective phase I/II study results. Radiother Oncol 2007; 84(2) 128-134.

[109] Ishikawa H, Tsuji H, Kamada T, et al. Carbon-ion radiation therapy for prostate cancer. Int J Urol 2012; 19(4) 296-305.

[110] Coote JH, Wylie JP, Cowan RA, et al. Hypofractionated intensity-modulated radiotherapy for carcinoma of the prostate: analysis of toxicity. Int J Radiat Oncol Biol Phys 2009; 74(4) 1121-1127.

[111] Martin JM, Rosewall T, Bayley, et al. Phase II trial of hypofractionated image-guided intensity-modulated radiotherapy for localized prostate adenocarcinoma. Int J Radiat Oncol Biol Phys 2007; 69(4) 1084-1089.

[112] Kupelian PA, Thakkar VV, Khuntia D, et al. Hypofractionated intensity-modulated radiotherapy (70 Gy at 2.5 Gy per fraction) for localized prostate cancer: long-term outcomes. Int J Radiat Oncol Biol Phys 2005; 63(5) 1463-1468.

[113] King CR, Brooks JD, Gill H, et al. Stereotactic body radiotherapy for localized prostate cancer: interim results of a prospective phase II clinical trial. Int J Radiat Oncol Biol Phys 2009; 73(4) 1043-1048.

[114] Madsen BL, His RA, Pham HT, et al. Stereotactic hypofractionated accurate radiotherapy of the prostate (SHARP), 33.5 Gy in five fractions for localized disease: first clinical trial results. Int J Radiat Oncol Biol Phy 2007; 67(4) 1099-1105.

[115] Michalski JM, Bae K, Roach M, et al. Long-term toxicity following 3D conformal radiation therapy for prostate cancer from the RTOG 9406 phase I/II dose escalation study. Int J Radiat Oncol Biol Phy 2010; 76(1) 14-22.

[116] Shulte RW, Slater JD, Rossi CJ Jr, et al. Value and perspectives of proton radiation therapy for limited stage prostate cancer. Strahlenther Onkol 2000; 176(1) 3-8.

[117] Bolla M, van Poppel H, Collette L, et al. Postoperative radiotherapy after radical prostatectomy: a randomized controlled trial (EORTC trial 22911). Lancet 2005; 366(9485) 572-578.

[118] Thompson IM, Tangen CM, Paradelo J, et al. Adjuvant radiotherapy for pathological T3N0M0 prostate cancer significantly reduces risk of metastases and improves survival: long-term followup of a randomized clinical trial. J Urol 2009; 181(3) 956-962.

[119] Swanson GP, Hussey MA, Tangen CM, et al. Predominant treatment failure in post-prostatectomy patients is local: analysis of patterns of treatment failure in SWOG 8794. J Clin Oncol 2007; 25(16) 2225-2229

[120] Wiegel T, Bottke D, Steiner U, et al. Phase III postoperative adjuvant radiotherapy after radical prostatectomy compared with radical prostatectomy alone in pT3 prostate cancer with postoperative undetectable prostate-specific antigen: ARO 96-02/AUO AP 09/95. J Clin Oncol 2009; 27(18) 2924-2930.

[121] Trabulsi EJ, Valicenti RK, Hanlon AL, et al. A multi-institutional matched-control analysis of adjuvant and salvage postoperative radiation therapy for pT3-4N0 prostate cancer. Urology 2008; 72(6) 1298-1302.

[122] Trock BJ, Han M, Freedland SJ, et al. Prostate cancer-specific survival following salvage radiotherapy vs observation in men with biochemical recurrence after radical prostatectomy. JAMA 2008; 299(23) 2760-2769.

[123] Stephenson AJ, Scardino PT, Kattan MW, et al. Predicting the outcome of salvage radiation therapy for recurrent prostate cancer after radical prostatectomy. J Clin Oncol 2007; 25(15) 2035-2041.

# Chapter 6

# Abdominoperineal Resection: Consideration and Limitations of Prostate Cancer Screening and Prostate Biopsy

Zachary Klaassen, Ray S. King, Kelvin A. Moses, Rabii Madi and Martha K. Terris

Additional information is available at the end of the chapter

## 1. Introduction

Prostate cancer and colorectal malignancies are the most common cancers in men, contributing to 15% and 9% of new cancer cases, respectively [1]. Furthermore, it is not uncommon to encounter patients with synchronous or metachronous colorectal and prostate cancers [2-3]. Abdominoperineal resection (APR) is often performed for surgical treatment of rectal cancer in addition to treatment of ulcerative colitis and familial polyposis coli. The technical aspects of an APR include a combined perineal and abdominal approach to resecting the rectum and mesorectum, in addition to the anus, perineal soft tissue and pelvic floor musculature [4].

The screening and treatment of patients with prostate cancer after an APR is challenging and unique. Enblad et al. [5] found a relative risk of 2.2 for the diagnosis of a second primary neoplasm in the prostate within 1 year after the diagnosis of rectal malignancy. After APR for colorectal pathologic features, however, there is no rectum for access to the prostate. This precludes the use of digital rectal examination (DRE) or transrectal ultrasound (TRUS)-guided prostate biopsies to diagnose primary tumors of the prostate [6-10].

Several methods have been described to evaluate the prostate in the patient with elevated prostate-specific antigen (PSA) levels who have undergone APR, including transperineal ultrasound (TPUS)-guided biopsy, transurethral ultrasounded guided perineal biopsy and computed tomography (CT)/magnetic resonance imaging (MRI) guided techniques. The aim of this chapter is to review the screening for prostate cancer in patients preparing for an APR and discuss post-APR screening and prostate biopsy techniques, limitations and practical considerations.

## 2. Abdominoperineal resection

Abdominoperineal resection is a surgery for carcinoma of the rectum and/or anus, performed through incisions in the abdomen and perineum. APR involves the removal of the anus, rectum, and the distal portion of the sigmoid colon along with regional lymph nodes. Without an anal opening, the patient has a permanent end-colostomy from the proximal sigmoid colon created through the anterior abdominal wall, typically placed in the left lower quadrant [11-12].

### 2.1. Diagnosis of rectal carcinoma

In patients with rectal cancer, the most common initial presenting symptom or complaint is bleeding, followed by changes in bowel habits, diarrhea, and lower abdominal pain. A DRE may detect rectal masses located within the distal 1/3 of the rectum. A potential source of confusion from a standard DRE may arise from carcinoma of the prostate encroaching on the nearby rectum, causing similar obstructive symptoms [11]. Flexible sigmoidoscopy or colonoscopy allow for a more thorough visual characterization, location, and size of the mass, and provides an opportunity for biopsy and histological examination. Endoluminal ultrasonography has recently been shown to be a diagnostic tool for characterizing the depth of invasion of the rectal mass. Pre-operative evaluation using colonoscopy and CT and/or MRI is indicated to rule-out synchronous lesions and/or metastatic disease [13].

### 2.2. Indications for treatment

Classic surgical dogma throughout the 20th century states that the standard treatment for rectal tumors located less than 8cm from the anal verge is to perform an APR. Careful surgical technique must be utilized to avoid complications such as recurrence of disease due to inadequate surgical margins, anastomotic breakdown, obstruction, and re-operation. Tumors located more proximally are generally treated successfully using the standard low anterior resection with restoration of bowel continuity. Absolute contraindications for anastomosis following resection of rectal cancer are invasion of the sphincter mechanism or the anal canal. The decision to preserve the anal sphincter can be affected by several factors including: level of the tumor, depth of invasion, extent of circumferential involvement, tumor fixation, local and metastatic invasion, age, and the ability to manage a colostomy. However, advances in instrumentation and techniques often allow for some tumors in the distal rectum to be resected and anastomosis performed [13-14].

### 2.3. Technique

APR can be performed by a single surgeon or with a two-surgeon (abdominal and perineal) team approach. Once the patient is prepped and draped, the anus is closed using a purse-string suture. A site for the colostomy should be selected prior to incision. The surgeon may consider preoperative ureteral stent placement to aid in identification of the ureters and to facilitate repair in case of inadvertent injury. A midline infra-umbilical incision is made, and the abdomen is explored for evidence of metastatic and/or synchronous disease. Once the tumor is deemed resectable, the surgeon on the perineal side can begin dissection simultaneously. In the abdominal compartment, the sigmoid colon and rectum is mobilized by incision of the left lateral mesentery, paying careful attention to avoid the left ureter as it courses over the bifurcation of the iliac vessels. Identification and control of the inferior mesenteric artery is followed by its ligation distal to the first branch to maintain adequate blood supply to the colon segment used for the stoma. The rectum is then bluntly dissected posterior along the presacral space and mobilized to the tip of the coccyx. Anteriorly, the rectum is retracted away from the bladder and Denonvillier's fascia is incised to free the rectum away from the prostate to its posterior margin. The lateral ligaments that contain the middle rectal arteries are controlled and ligated. At this point the proximal sigmoid colon is divided using a stapling device and brought through the anterior abdominal wall. The colostomy is then matured.

On the perineal side, an elliptical incision is made around the anus. Dissection is then made through the sphincters and the ischiorectal fossa is entered. The presacral space is entered from below and the rectum is mobilized circumferentially. Careful dissection is performed to avoid perforation of the rectum and compromise the containment of the malignancy. The perineal dissection is completed by dividing the levator muscle on each side. The distal sigmoid and rectum can be delivered through the perineal opening. The perineal wound is closed primarily, with a closed drain left in place. The peritoneum is repaired above and the floor of the pelvis is closed [12, 14-16].

## 3. Concomitant prostate cancer screening in the patient preparing for an APR

Patients scheduled to undergo APR represent a patient population in which prostate cancer screening may be indicated. Most cases of rectal cancer are diagnosed after 50 years of age [17], and are in the same age category of men at risk for prostate cancer diagnosis. However, the stage of rectal cancer should be taken into consideration when considering screening the same individual for prostate cancer: Stage T1 and T2 rectal tumors treated with APR have a ~90% 5-year survival, while stage T3 and T4 tumors are generally treated with neoadjuvant chemotherapy and/or radiation and generally have a 5-year survival of 50% and 25%, respectively [17]. Thus, prostate cancer screening in patients with advanced disease should be avoided.

Terris and Wren previously described a prostate cancer-screening program for 19 consecutive men scheduled for APR for colorectal carcinoma with no history of prostate cancer [18]. Screening included serum PSA and DRE and those with suspicious findings underwent TRUS-guided sextant biopsy. Six patients (31%) had a PSA >4.0 ng/mL (range 4.4 to 32.4 ng/mL, mean 9.3 ng/mL) of which two patients also had an abnormal DRE. TRUS-guided biopsy revealed prostate cancer in three individuals (50%). These patients included an individual with clinical stage T1c, Gleason 3+3=6 adenocarcinoma of the prostate treated with radiation, a second patient with clinical stage T2a, Gleason 3+4=7 adenocarcinoma of the prostate treated with radiation, and a third individual with a PSA of 32.4 ng/mL and DRE consistent with extracapsular extension of prostate cancer (clinical stage T3, Gleason 4+4=8 adenocarcinoma of the prostate) managed with androgen deprivation therapy. Concomitant prostate cancer screening for patients planning an APR should be a multi-disciplinary decision between the General Surgeons and Urologist in the male patient older than 50 years of age with clinical stage T1 or T2 rectal cancer and a life expectancy of more than 10 years.

## 4. Post-APR prostate cancer screening and modalities for prostate biopsy

The clinical scenario of a patient with an elevated PSA and no access to the rectum precludes the urologist from performing a DRE or a TRUS biopsy of the prostate. Other approaches to the prostate to allow a biopsy include CT and MRI guided techniques, transurethral ultrasound guided perineal biopsy and TPUS-guided biopsy.

### 4.1. CT and MRI-guided prostate biopsy

Transgluteal CT-guided prostate biopsy involves imaging the lower pelvis at 10-mm intervals and with a 10-mm slice thickness. The transgluteal approach allows sampling of both sides of the midline at the base, midgland and apical levels. When one entry site is used, the angle of the needle is projected to the contralateral side of the prostate; entry sites are chosen 3-4cm off the midline to avoid paraspinal ligaments and potential post-APR fibrosis around the tip of the coccyx (Figure 1) [19].

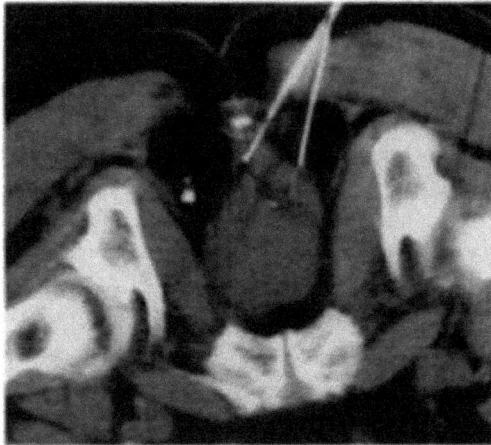

**Figure 1.** CT-guided percutaneous transgluteal biopsy of the prostate. Two needles are inserted at different angles to ensure adequate sampling of both sides of the prostate (Reprinted from American Journal of Roentgenology, Volume 166/Issue 6, Papanicolaou N, Eisenberg PJ, Silverman SG, McNicholas MM, Althausen AF. 1996, 1332-1334, with permission from The American Roentgen Ray Society).

Papanicolaou et al. [19] described this technique in 10 patients with a mean age of 67 years and mean PSA of 33.9 diagnosing prostate cancer in 6 patients (60%). While CT scan offers limited anatomical detail of the prostate, it does allow visualization of the peripheral zones to facilitate biopsy in patients without rectal access.

Limited experience with MRI-guided transperineal biopsy [20] and CT-MRI fusion to guide radiotherapy [21] has been described but is not widely available.

### 4.2. Transurethral ultrasound guided perineal prostate biopsy

The patient undergoing a transperineal biopsy guided by transurethral ultrasound is placed in the lithotomy position and a 26F resectoscope sheath is passed into the urethra. Subsequently, a 5.5 MHx transurethral ultrasound probe is passed through the sheath for visualization of the prostate. The width and height of the prostate are measured on the sagittal image and withdrawing the probe from the base to the apex of the prostate assesses length [22]. The advantage of this modality is that direct prostate imaging allows for precise guidance of transperineally placed biopsy needles. However, the major limitation is that one is only able to view the prostate in the sagittal plane. Seaman et al. [22] utilized this technique to perform 7 biopsies in 5 patients with a history of APR and elevated PSA (two patients had repeat biopsy secondary to increasing PSA), diagnosing prostate cancer in three patients (60%).

### 4.3. Transperineal Ultrasound (TPUS) guided prostate biopsy

The TPUS guided prostate biopsy is performed in the lithotomy position. A Foley catheter may be inserted to delineate the prostate anatomy and avoid the urethra with the biopsy needle [23]. The scrotum is then retracted anteriorly and the perineum is prepared in a sterile fashion. Then 1% Lidocaine is applied to the perineum for anesthesia. The transrectal ultrasound probe is adjusted to a frequency of 5-6 MHz and the prostate is visualized after traversing the course of the urethral catheter. The 18-guage biopsy needle is then directed at a 45-degree angle and biopsy specimens are obtained through the posterior aspect of the prostate. The needle forms an acute angle with the long axis of the prostate apex is nearly parallel with the long axis of the prostate base and mid-gland (Figure 2). Biopsy specimens are then obtained from the medial and lateral aspect of the prostate apex, mid-gland and base as is performed for TRUS biopsy. A "fan technique" for obtaining a six-core TPUS guided biopsy has also been described (Figure 3) [24].

A number of studies have compared the efficacy of TPUS-guided biopsies compared to TRUS-guided biopsies in patients with a rectum [8, 24]. Shinghal and Terris [8] prospectively identified 20 patients with prostate cancer diagnosed by TRUS-guided biopsies to evaluate the accuracy of TPUS prostate biopsies. Six TPUS-guided biopsies were obtained, followed by sextant TRUS-guided biopsies prior to radical prostatectomy. Final pathology demonstrated that all 20 patients had adenocarcinoma of the prostate. TPUS-guided biopsies identified cancer in only 2 of 20 patients (10%) compared to 13 of 20 patients (65%) for TRUS-guided biopsies. The positive TPUS-guided biopsy specimens were higher Gleason grade, and were found in patients with larger volume prostates and higher PSA. Emiliozzi et al. [24] performed a prospective study comparing TPUS versus TRUS-guided prostate biopsy in 107 patients with PSA > 4.0 ng/mL. The patients underwent TPUS-guided six core biopsy, followed by TRUS-guided six core biopsy. Prostate cancer was found in 43 of 107 patients (40%): 41 (95%) were found via the TPUS approach compared to 34 (79%) via the TRUS approach (p = 0.012).

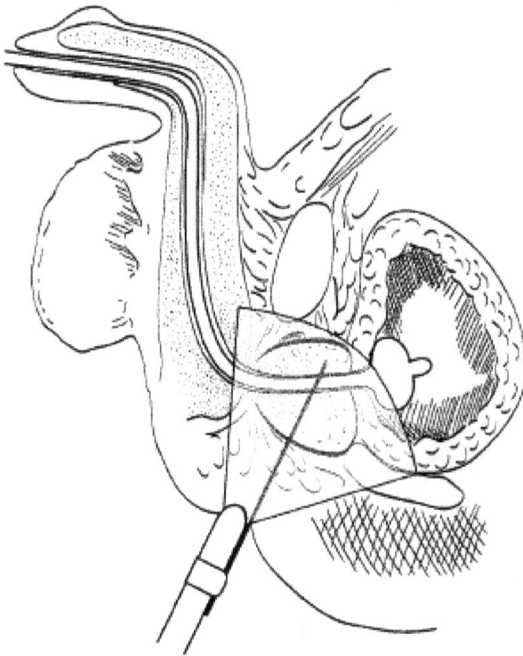

**Figure 2.** Transperineal prostate biopsy. There is a relatively acute angle of the needle in regard to the long axis of the prostate. The needle becomes almost parallel with the long axis of the prostate middle and base (Reprinted from The Journal of Urology, Volume 169/Issue 1, Shinohara K, Gulati M, Koppie TM, Terris MK. 2003, 141-144, with permission from American Urological Association).

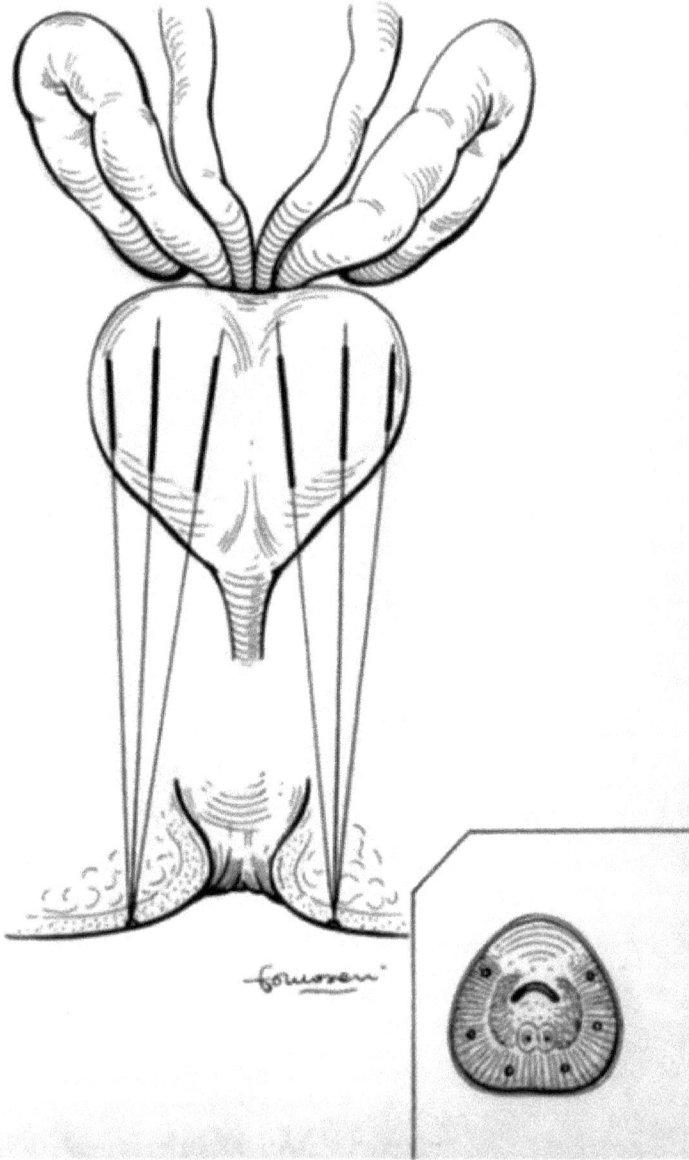

**Figure 3.** Scheme of the transperineal six-core fan biopsy. Cores are also taken from the far lateral aspect of the prostate (Reprinted from Urology, Volume 61/Issue 5, Emiliozzi P, Corsetti A, Tassi B, Federico G, Martini M, Pansadoro V. 2003, 961-966, with permission from Elsevier).

A number of studies have reported TPUS-guided biopsy in patients after APR [6, 9, 23] (Table). Shinohara et al. [23] reported the largest experience analyzing 28 patients with a history of APR who were referred for biopsy with a mean PSA of 22 ng/mL (median 9.5, range 4.1 to 237). The mean time from APR to referral was 14 years (range 1 to 33 years) and five patients had previously undergone radiation therapy as part of the treatment for colorectal cancer. Of the 28 patients, 23 were diagnosed with prostate cancer (82.1%), with a mean Gleason score of 6.6 (range 3 to 9). Twenty-two of the 23 patients (95.7%) elected for treatment, including prostatectomy (n=8), androgen deprivation therapy (n=7), external radiation therapy (n=6) and high dose radiation therapy (n=1).

| Study | Patients (N) | Median Age (Yrs) | Mean PSA (ng/mL) | Median PSA (ng/mL) | Mean Interval From APR to Biopsy (Yrs) | Biopsy Proven Prostate Cancer, N= (%) |
|---|---|---|---|---|---|---|
| Shinohara et al. [23] | 28 | 65 | 22 | 9.5 | 14 | 23 (82%) |
| Twidwell et al. [6] | 10 | 67 | NR | NR | 12 | 2 (20%) |
| Filderman et al. [99] | 5 | 62 | 16.5 | NR | NR | 2 (40%) |

**Table 1.** A comparison of studies analyzing transperineal ultrasound-guided prostate biopsy results in patients after abdominoperineal resection. (NR - not reported)

### 4.4. Practical considerations for TPUS-guided prostate biopsy

#### 4.4.1. Image quality

The image quality of TPUS of the prostate compared to TRUS has been previously described by Terris et al. [7]. In a prospective study of 50 patients who had not undergone APR, TPUS was performed with a 4-MHz abdominal probe at a frequency of 5 - 7 MHz and TRUS at 7 MHz (Figure 4). TPUS allowed good visualization of the prostate in 48 (96%) patients in the coronal plane and in 45 (90%) patients in the sagittal plane. Prostate volume, as calculated by the prolate spheroid method, correlated well with TRUS calculations (r = 0.876). Prostatic calcifications were seen in 12 patients (24%), identified by both TRUS and TPUS, however 29 patients (58%) with hypoechoic lesions identified by TRUS were not visualized by TPUS. Furthermore, six patients (12%) with cystic lesions visualized by TRUS were seen in half of the patients by TPUS (3/6). Image quality of TPUS is inadequate for staging purposes secondary to poor transverse and longitudinal visualization of the prostatic capsule. While the imaging quality of TPUS may be inferior to TRUS, it likely represents the most reliable modality in patients without access to the rectum and has been proposed as a diagnostic modality in patients at high risk for prostate cancer with previous negative TRUS-guided biopsies [25].

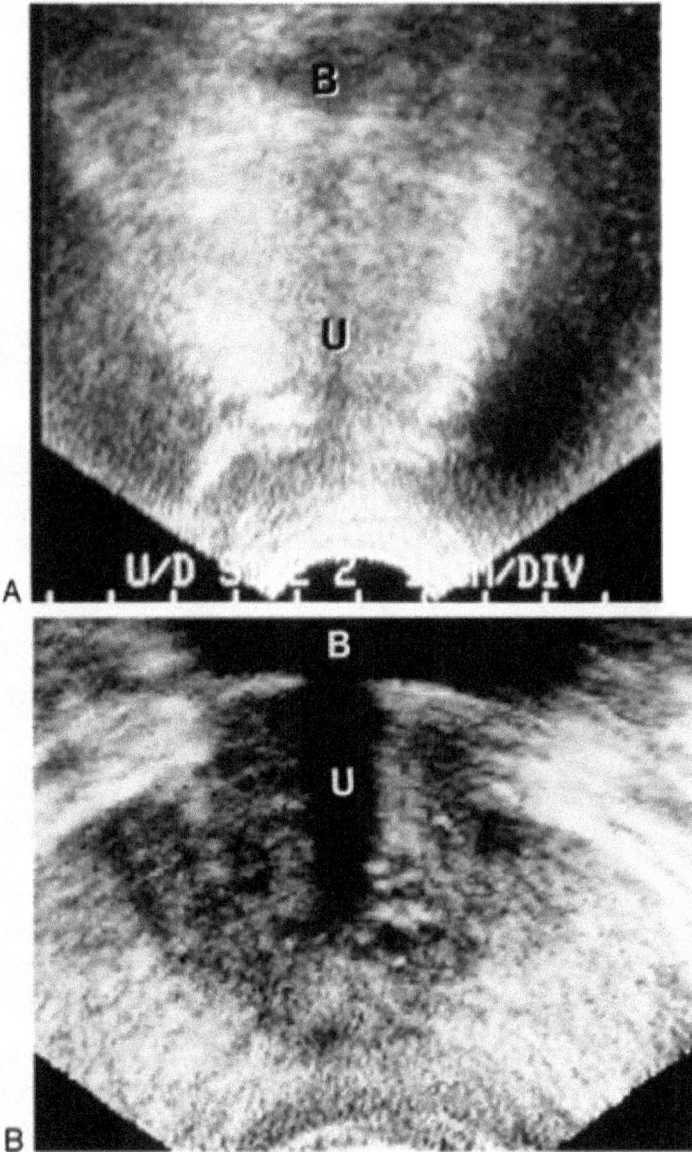

**Figure 4.** A) Transperineal image showing vague outline of the prostate in the coronal plane. (B) Transverse image of the prostate in the transverse plane. B = bladder; U = urethra (Reprinted from Urology, Volume 52/Issue 6, Terris MK, Hammerer PG, Nickas ME. 1998, 1070-1072, with permission from Elsevier).

*4.4.2. Improved sampling of the far lateral peripheral zone*

When performing TPUS-guided biopsy, the needle forms an acute angle with the long axis of the prostate apex before becoming nearly parallel with the long axis of the prostate base and mid-gland. Geometrically, this allows sampling of more peripheral zone tissue, notably the far lateral peripheral zone [23, 25]. Eskew et al. [26] performed sextant biopsies in addition to cores taken from the far lateral and mid regions of the prostate in 119 patients, diagnosing prostate cancer in 48 patients (40.3%). Among these 48 patients, 17 (35%) had carcinoma only in the far lateral and mid regions of the prostate.

# 5. Conclusions

Evaluation of the prostate in men with an elevated PSA who have undergone APR is challenging due to inability to perform DRE and TRUS-guided prostate biopsy. TPUS-guided prostate biopsy is the most cost effective and feasible modality for diagnosing prostate cancer in these patients. However, given that men aged 50-75 are at increased risk for both prostate cancer and colorectal cancer, preoperative prostate cancer screening in men who are planning APR allows for proper assessment of the prostate before access to the rectum is compromised, provides a baseline PSA to compare with further testing after the APR, and may detect synchronous malignancies. A multidisciplinary approach is ideal when considering prostate cancer screening in men 50 years of age or older with reasonable life expectancy who are planning APR.

# Author details

Zachary Klaassen[1], Ray S. King[2], Kelvin A. Moses[1], Rabii Madi[1] and Martha K. Terris[1*]

1 Department of Surgery, Section of Urology, Georgia Health Sciences University, Augusta, Georgia

2 Department of Surgery, Georgia Health Sciences University, Augusta, Georgia

# References

[1]  Siegel R, Naishadham D, Jemal A. Cancer Statistics, 2012. CA – A Cancer Journal for Clinicians 2012;62(1) 10-29.

[2]  Lee T, Barringer M, Myers RT, Sterchi JM. Multiple primary carcinomas of the colon and associated extracolonic primary malignant tumors. Annals of Surgery 1982;195(4) 501-507.

[3]   Weir JA. Colorectal cancer: metachronous and other associated neoplasm. Diseases of the Colon and Rectum 1975;18(1) 4-5.

[4]   Park J, Guillem JG. Chapter 47 – Rectal Cancer. In: Cameron JL, Cameron AM (eds). Current Surgical Therapy, 10th ed. Philadelphia, PA: Elsevier Health Sciences; 2011.

[5]   Enblad P, Adami H, Glimerlius B, Krusemo U, Pahlman L. The risk of subsequent primary malignant diseases after cancers of the colon and rectum. Cancer 1990;65(9) 2091-2100.

[6]   Twidwell JJ, Matthews RD, Huisam TK, Sands JP. Ultrasound evaluation of the prostate after abdominoperineal resection. The Journal of Urology 1993;150(3) 902-904.

[7]   Terris MK, Hammerer PG, Nickas ME. Comparison of ultrasound imaging in patients undergoing transperineal and transrectal prostate ultrasound. Urology 1998;52(6) 1070-1072.

[8]   Shinghal R, Terris MK. Limitations of transperineal ultrasound-guided prostate biopsies. Urology 1999;54(4) 706-708.

[9]   Filderman PS, Jacobs SC. Prostatic ultrasound in the patient without a rectum. Urology 1994;43(5) 722-724.

[10]  Koppie TM, Presti JC, Shinohara K, Terris MK, Carroll PR. Transperineal biopsy after abdominoperineal resection: A two center experience. J Urol 2000;163(1) 260.

[11]  Corman ML. Colon and Rectal Surgery, 5th Ed. Philadelphia: Lippincott Williams & Wilkins; 2005.

[12]  Perry WB, Connaughton JC. Abdominoperineal resection: how is it done and what are the results? Clinics in Colon and Rectal Surgery 2007;20(3) 213-220.

[13]  Murrell ZA, Dixon MR, Vargas H, Arneel TD, Kumar R, Stamos MJ. Contemporary indications for and early outcomes of abdominoperineal resection. American Surgeon 2005;71(10) 837-840.

[14]  Reshef A, Lavery I, Kiran R. Factors associated with onocologic outcomes after abdominoperineal resection compared with restorative resection for low rectal cancer: patient and tumor related or technical factors only? Diseases of the Colon and Rectum 2012;55(1) 51-58.

[15]  Simorov A, Reynoso J, Dolghi O, Thompson J, Oleynikov D. Comparison of perioperative outcomes in patients undergoing laparoscopic versus open abdominoperineal resection. The American Journal of Surgery 2011;202(6) 666-672.

[16]  Marr R, Birbeck K, Garvican J, Macklin CP, Tiffin NJ, Parsons WJ, Dixon MF, Mapstone NP, Sebag-Montefiore D, Scott N, Johnston D, Sagar P, Finan P, Quirke P. The modern abdominoperineal excision: the next challenge after total mesorectal excision. Annals of Surgery 2005;242(1) 74-82.

[17]  Surveillance, Epidemiology, and End Results (SEER) Program (www.seer.cancer.gov). Research Data (1973-2009), National Cancer Institute, DCCPS, Surveillance

Research Program, Surveillance Systems Branch, released April 2012, based on the November 2011 submission.

[18] Terris MK, Wren SM. Results of a Screening Program for Prostate Cancer in Patients Scheduled for Abdominoperineal Resection for Colorectal Pathologic Findings. Urology 2001;57(5) 943-945.

[19] Papanicolaou N, Eisenberg PJ, Silverman SG, McNicholas MM, Althausen AF. Prostatic biopsy after proctocolectomy: a transgluteal, CT-guided approach. AJR American Journal of Roentgenology 1996;166(6) 1332-1334.

[20] D'Amico AV, Tempany CM, Cormack R, Hata N, Jinzaki M, Tuncali K, Weinstein M, Richie JP. Transperineal magnetic resonance image guided prostate biopsy. The Journal of Urology 2000;164(2) 385-387.

[21] Lau HY, Kagawa K, Lee WR, Hunt MA, Shaer AH, Hanks GE. Short communication: CT-MRI image fusion for 3D conformal prostate radiotherapy: use in patients with altered pelvic anatomy. The British Journal of Radiology 1996;69(828) 1165-1170.

[22] Seaman EK, Sawczuk IS, Fatal M, Olsson CA, Shabsigh R. Transperineal prostate needle biopsy guided by transurethral ultrasound in patients without a rectum. Urology 1996;47(3) 353-355.

[23] Shinohara K, Gulati M, Koppie TM, Terris MK. Transperineal prostate biopsy after abdominoperineal resection. The Journal of Urology 2003;169(1) 141-144.

[24] Emiliozzi P, Corsetti A, Tassi B, Federico G, Martini M, Pansadoro V. Best approach for prostate cancer detection: A prospective study on transperineal versus transrectal six-core prostate biopsy. Urology 2003;61(5) 961-966.

[25] Igel TC, Knight MK, Young PR, Wehle MJ, Petrou SP, Broderick GA, Marino R, Parra RO. Systematic transperineal ulatrasound guided template biopsy of the prostate in patients at high risk. The Journal of Urology 2001;165(5) 1575-1579.

[26] Eskew LA, Bare RL, McCullough DL. Systematic 5 region prostate biopsy is superior to sextant method for diagosing carcinoma of the prostate. The Journal of Urology 1997;157(1) 199-202.

# High-Dose-Rate Interstitial Brachytherapy as Monotherapy in One Fraction for the Treatment of Favorable Stage Prostate Cancer

Pedro J. Prada

Additional information is available at the end of the chapter

## 1. Introduction

Low dose rate (LDR) brachytherapy has rapidly gained popularity in the USA [1, 2] and Europe [3, 4] as an accepted, effective and safe therapy for localized prostate cancer. Many reports are now available which confirm good outcomes in selected patients with PSA relapse-free survivals that are equivalent to those achieved by surgery.

The potential for a therapy that is equally efficient but less harmful than other interventions is especially attractive for patients with early prostate cancer.

On the other hand, treatment with temporary high dose rate (HDR) brachytherapy with 192-Ir as monotherapy has a number of advantages compared to LDR. The overall treatment time is decreased from many months with LDR to several minutes with HDR. Besides, HDR improves the dose distribution because of the possibility of accurately controlling the source and vary the source dwell time during treatment. The intraoperative optimization used with HDR allows better source position targeting with the potential for limiting toxicity. There are also advantages in radiation safety for both staff and patient who leave the treatment room without any radioactive implants.

The purpose of this chapter was to determine the possibility to treat patients with favorable stage prostate cancer (5, 6) with HDR monotherapy in one fraction and transperineal hyaluronic acid injection into the perirectal fat.

High-Dose-Rate Interstitial Brachytherapy as Monotherapy in One Fraction for the Treatment of Favorable Stage Prostate Cancer

143

## 2. Brachytherapy implant characteristics

Patients received one implant and one fraction of HDR. Fraction dose is 20.5 Gy because it is considered to correspond biologically (biologic effective dose) to > 90 Gy administered at 2 Gy/fraction according to the linear quadratic model, assuming an $\alpha/\beta$ of 1.2 Gy (7, 8, 9, 10).

Brachytherapy procedure is done under spinal anesthesia with the patient in the lithotomy position (Fig. 1). A Foley catheter is placed, and the bladder is partially filled with 100 cm$^3$ of sterile water. The needles are positioned (Fig. 2) by transperineal placement under real time TRUS guidance using a template. Axial cross-sections is captured in 5mm steps and transferred to the Treatment Planning Software. Prostate gland, normal structures (urethra and rectum) and needle positions are identified and mapped based on the ultrasound image. Dose optimization is done on the reconstructed applicator geometry using dose point and manual optimization algorithms to determine dwell positions and times (Fig. 3).

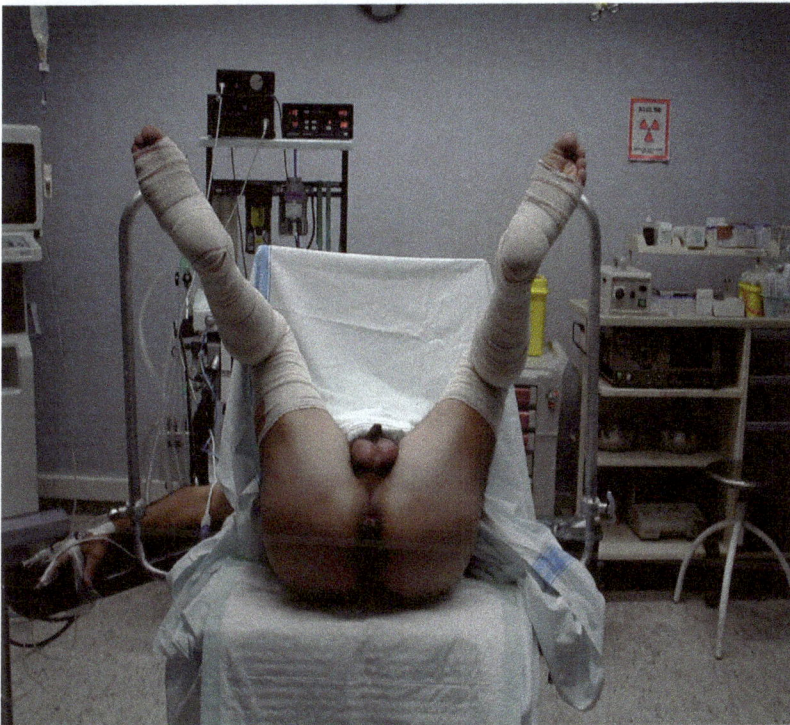

**Figure 1.** Lithotomy position

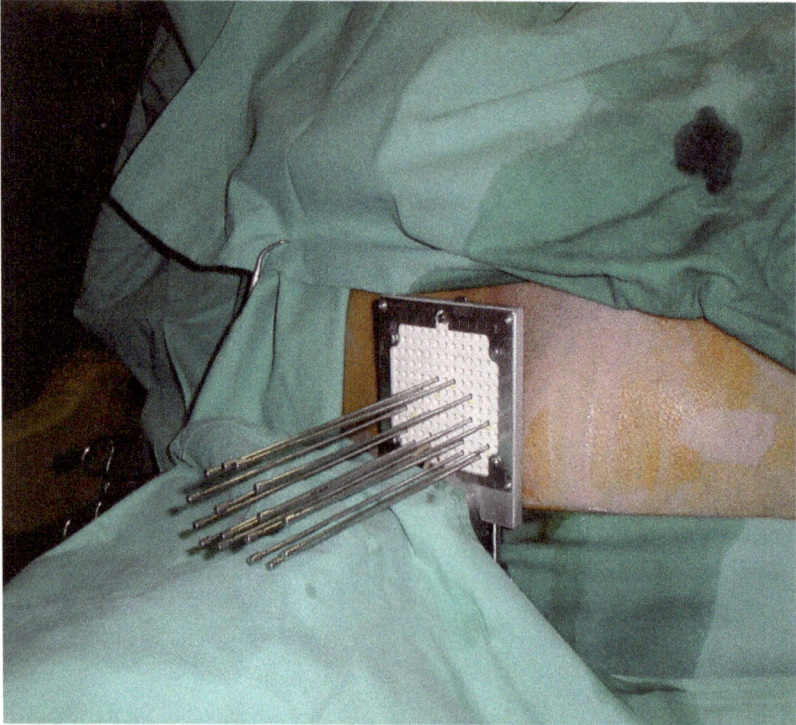

**Figure 2.** The needles are positioned

High-Dose-Rate Interstitial Brachytherapy as Monotherapy in One Fraction for the Treatment
of Favorable Stage Prostate Cancer

145

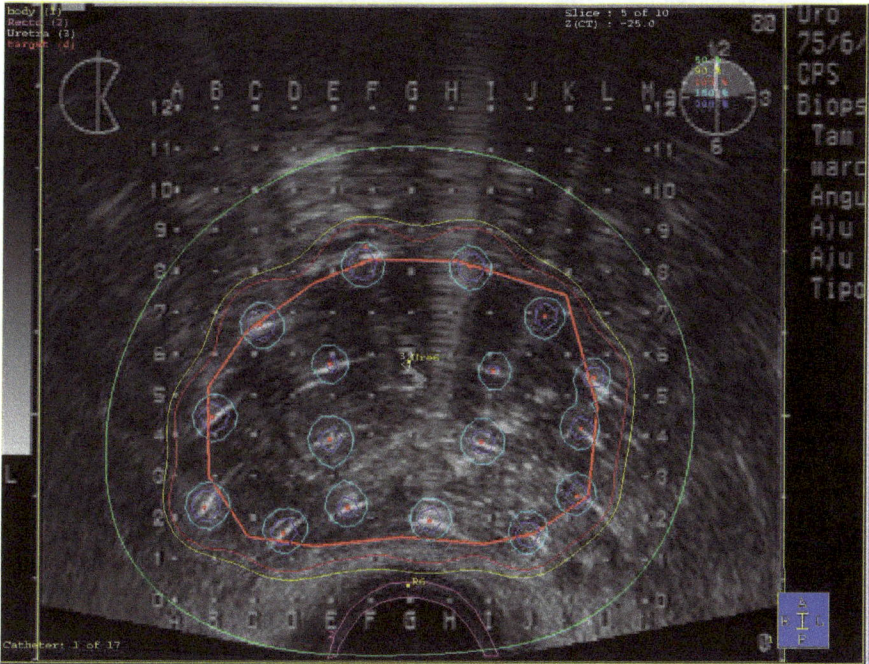

**Figure 3.** Dose optimization

The prostate without safety margins is then defined as the planning target volume (PTV) to
be treated (Fig. 4) with the prescribed dose (PD).

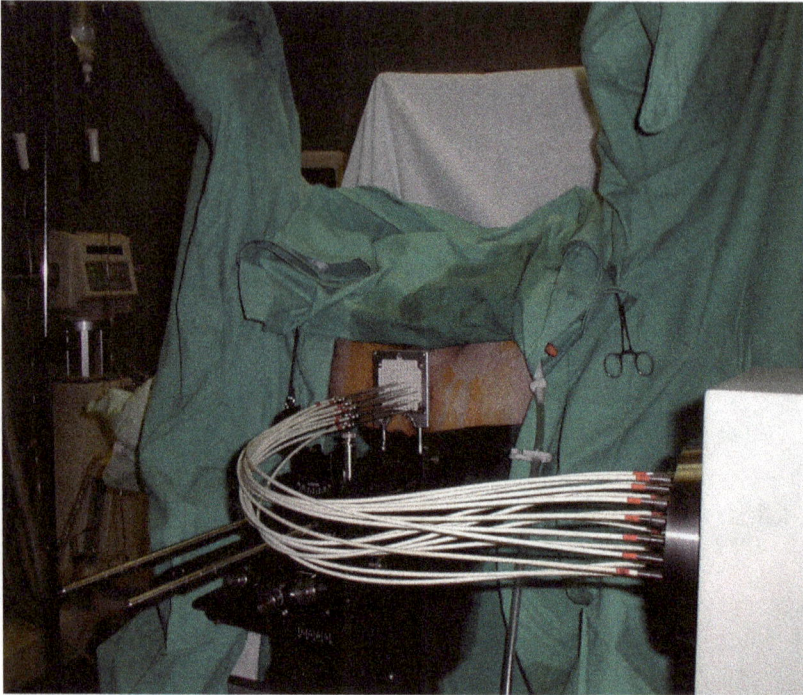

**Figure 4.** Treatment

Based on the dose volume histograms (DVH) data, the quality of plans and implants is evaluated using following indicators:

- The rectal dose is calculated at the anterior edge of the TRUS probe and is limited to ≤ 75% of the prescription dose.

- The dose to any segment of the urethra is limited to ≤ 110% of the prescription dose. V120 and D100 of the prostatic urethra are determined (volume that received a dose of 120% and dose delivered to 100% of the urethra).

- The PTV V90, V100, V150 and V200 (% of PTV receiving 90%, 100%, 150% and 200% of the PD) are recorded.

- D90 (dose delivered to 90% of the PTV) is calculated.

All patients are discharged from the center on the same day of the procedure between 6-8 hours of implantation.

To decrease rectal toxicity, transperineal hyaluronic acid (HA) injection into the peri-rectal fat is used to consistently displace the rectal wall away from the radiation sources in all patients. We believe that the increase in distance (mean 2 cm along the length of the

 ⌐ enough to provide a significant radiation dose reduction from HDR bra-
⌐apy [11, 12].

## 3. Hyaluronic acid

The Hyaluronic acid (HA) is a polysaccharide normally found in human tissues as a component of the connective tissue. Normally, it plays a vital role on the skin and in the synovial
fluid of the joints. It is normally degradable by the normal enzymatic system in relative
short time. However, to make it last for months when used for the treatment of skin wrin-
kles and osteoarthritis, the compound is modified making it stable for duration close to 1
year before it is reabsorbed by the body. Only one type of HA is used in our Department
(Restylane sub-Q).

The total injected amount is related to the need for systematically creating a minimum of a 2
cm space between the prostate and rectum throughout this length. Usually, we use between
6 and 8 cc per patient

## 4. Technique of hyaluronic
## acid injection

The injection technique of HA in the perirectal fat occurs before all needles are in treatment
position according to the following procedure.

- Step 1. The transrectal ultrasound (TRUS) probe with the transperineal template is placed
  and fixed in the standard fashion.

- Step 2. Using TRUS guidance, the needle tip is placed in the perirectal fat (Fig. 5), between
  the posterior prostate capsule and the anterior rectal wall, at the level of the maximum
  transverse diameter of the prostate (reference level). Then under direct TRUS guidance,
  the needle tip is advanced to the level of the seminal vesicles.

- Step 3. The needle is connected to the syringe containing of HA. After aspirating to be certain that we are not in a vessel, we proceed to inject between 6 and 8 cc within the space
  between the seminal vesicles and the apex of the prostate. This is performed under TRUS
  guidance to see and verify the new space created by the injection of HA (Fig. 6). The total
  injected amount allows us to create the new space >2 cm.

- Step 4. The needle is removed and all needles treatment is placed under TRUS Guidance.
  It can be performed as an outpatient. After the discharge from the theater clinic, the patient continues normal-life activities

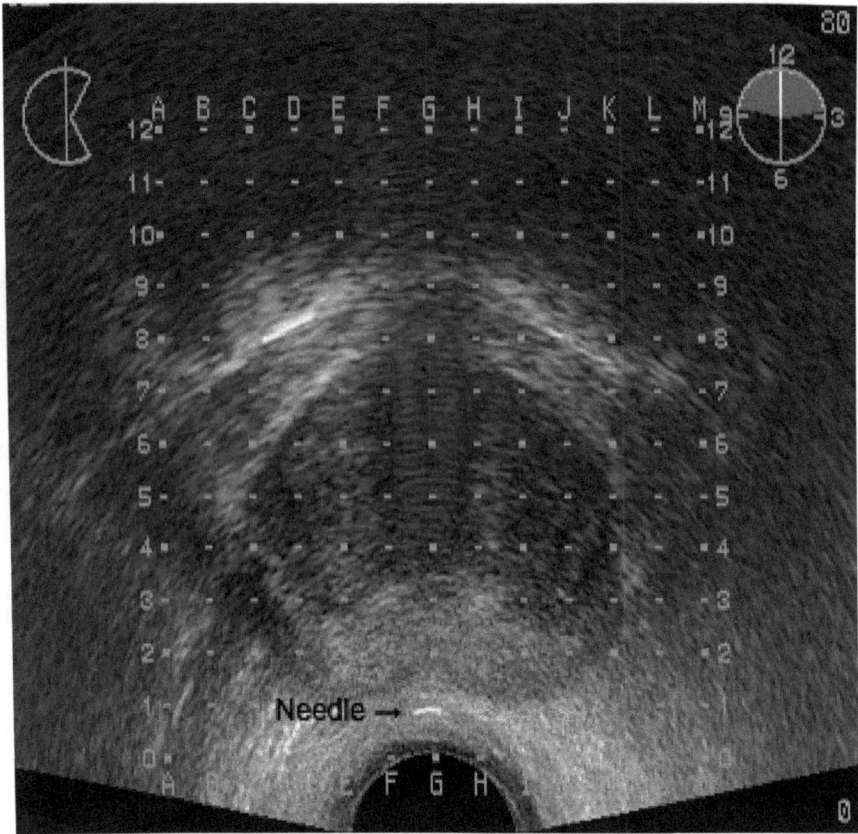

**Figure 5.** The needle tip is placed in the perirectal fat

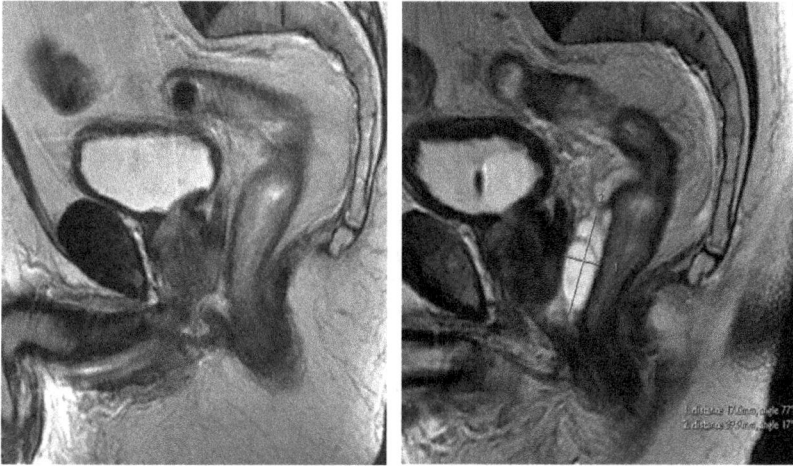

**Figure 6.** Magnetic resonance image demonstrating the additional perirectal space created by the hyaluronic acid injection

## 5. Results

In our Centre a total of 70 patients have been treated with this technique and is the first in the medical literature using in patients with favorable risk prostate cancer. Our technique has the great advantage of being practically a one-time procedure which prevents any movement of the needles.

In our series acute and late genitourinary toxicity grade 2 or more was not observed in any patient. The median of flow rate test pretreatment in our study was 12.5 ml/s (3-30 ml/s) but acute urinary retention was seen in only 1 patient, requiring a temporary postimplant bladder catheter during seven days, this results are better than other investigators [13-16].

The lasted follow-up visit the sexual preservation rate was 89% in patients who were potent preoperatively and not receiving hormonal therapy, this result is similar to that other investigators.

The late grade I genitourinary toxicity caused by our treatment was significantly associated with the dose administered to the PTV represented by D90 (p=0.050).

In our study no gastrointestinal toxicity, such as anal pain, rectal bleeding, diarrhea, anal ulcer and/or rectourethral fistula has been observed after treatment. We believe that the increase in distance between rectum and posterior prostatic capsule created by the peri-rectal injection of hyaluronic acid is enough to provide a significant radiation dose reduction from HDR brachytherapy and have significantly smaller incidence of mucosal damage [11, 12].

The actuarial biochemical control in our series was 100% and 88% respectively for low and intermediate risk groups at 32 months, but is too early to draw final conclusion respect to biochemical control.

## 6. Conclusions

High dose rate brachytherapy as monotherapy in one fraction with a transperineal hyaluronic acid injection into the peri-rectal fat to decrease rectal toxicity for patients with favorable risk prostate cancer is feasible and very well tolerated with advantages compared to LDR and HDR brachytherapy as monotherapy using the fractionation schema of 4 fractions administered 2 times daily during two days.

HDR monotherapy in one fraction resulted in a low genitourinary morbidity and no gastrointestinal toxicity but clinical and biochemical control rates will be reported as longer follow-up.

## Author details

Pedro J. Prada

Address all correspondence to: pprada@telecable.es

Department of Radiation Oncology, Hospital Universitario Marques de Valdecilla, Santander, Spain

## References

[1] Mettlin CJ, Murphy GP, McDonald CJ, et al. The National cancer data base report on increase use of brachytherapy for the treatment of patients with prostate carcinoma in the USA. Cancer 1999; 86: 1877-1882.

[2] Lee RW, Moughan J, Owen J, et al. The 1999 Patterns of care Study of radiotherapy in localized prostatic carcinoma. A comprehensive survey of prostate brachytherapy in the United States. Cancer 2003; 98 (9): 1987-1994.

[3] Ash D, Flynn A, Battermann J, Reijke T, et al. ESTRO/EAU/EORTC recomendations on permanent seed implantation for localizad prostate cancer. Radiotherapy and Oncology. 2000, 57:315-321.

[4] Battermann JJ, Boon TA, Moerland A et al. Results of permanent prostate brachytherapy, 13 years of experience at a single institution. Radiotherapy and Oncology 2004; 71:23-28.

[5]  Fleming I, Cooper JS, Henson DE, et al. AJCC Cancer staging Manual, 5th edn. Philadelphia, Pennsylvania; Lippincitt-Raven, 1997.

[6]  Zelefsky MJ, Leibel SA, Gaudin PB, et al. Dose escalation with three-dimensional
conformal radiation therapy affects the outcome in prostate cancer. Int J Radiat Oncol
Biol Phys 1998; 41:491-500.

[7]  Brenner DJ, Martinez AA, Edmundson GK, et al. Direct evidence that prostate tumors show high sensitivity to fractionation (low alpha/beta ratio), similar to late-re-
sponding normal tissue. Int J Radiat Oncol Biol Phys 2002;52:6-13.

[8]  Duchesne GM, Peters LJ. What is the alpha/beta ratio for prostate cancer? Rationale
for hypofractionated high-dose-rate brachytherapy.[editorial]. Int J Radiat Oncol Biol
Phys 1999;44:747-748.

[9]  Fowler JF. The radiobiology of prostate cancer including new aspects of fractionated
radiotherapy. Acta Oncol 2005;44:265-276.

[10]  Fowler JF. The linear-quadratic formula and progress in fractionated radiotherapy.
Br J Radiol 1989;62:679-694.

[11]  Prada PJ, Fernandez J, Martinez A, et al. Transperineal injection of hyaluronic acid in
the anterior peri-rectal fat to decease rectal toxicity from radiation delivered with intensity modulated brachytherapy or EBRT for prostate cancer patients. Int J Oncol Biol Phys. 2007; 69 (1):95-102.

[12]  Prada PJ, González H, Menéndez C, et al. Transperineal Injection of Hyaluronic Acid
in the Anterior Peri-rectal Fat to Decrease Rectal Toxicity from Radiation Delivered
with Low Dose Rate Brachytherapy for Prostate Cancer Patients. Brachytherapy. 8(2):
210-217, 2009.

[13]  Ghadjar P, Keller T, Rentsch C A, et al. Toxicity and early treatment outcomes in low
and intermediate-risk prostate cancer managed by high-dose-rate brachytherapy as a
monotherapy. Brachytherapy 2009; 8:45-51.

[14]  Martin T, Baltas D, Kurek R, et al. 3-D conformal HDR brachytherapy as monotherapy for localized prostate cancer. A pilot study. Strahlenther Onkol 2004; 180:225-232.

[15]  Yoshioka Y, Takayuki N, Yoshida K, et al. High-dose-rate interstitial brachytherapy
as a monotherapy for localized próstata cáncer: treatment description and preliminary results of a phase I/II clinical trial.. Int J Oncol Biol Phys 2000; 48(3):675-681.

[16]  Konishi K, Yoshioka Y, Isohashi F, et al. Correlation between dosimetric parameters
and late rectal and urinary toxicities in patients treated with high-dose-rate brachytherapy used as monotherapy for prostate cancer. Int J Oncol Biol Phys 2009; 75(4):
1003-1007.

# Prostate Cancer Markers

# Chapter 8

# Testosterone Measurement and Prostate Cancer

Tine Hajdinjak

Additional information is available at the end of the chapter

## 1. Introduction

Testosterone is important growth factor for prostate cells. If testosterone availability drops, prostate cells stop thriving. Benign prostate shrinks and the same happens with prostate cancer cells. Larger decrease in testosterone availability means larger reduction in prostate cells mass. Although only reduction in testosterone levels will not, in most occasions, permanently heal prostate cancer, it causes its regression and significantly delays further progression of prostate cancer. Therefore, reduction of body's testosterone level is important prostate cancer treatment modality. When surgical removal of prostate due to cancer is not an opinion (for example because of advanced age, significant comorbidity or because cancer has already spread beyond prostate) or was unsuccessful as noted by rising PSA, which indicates cancer growth, serum testosterone value becomes very important factor in treatment related decisions. If testosterone values are high, reduction of testosterone level will be helpful – it is expected prostate cells will react, shrink, PSA will fall. If testosterone values are already low, their further reduction with different agent may be possible. If testosterone values are already at the lowest reachable levels, other ways of treatment should be sought. After reduction of testosterone levels in the body (castration), prostate cancer cells with time (sometimes months, sometimes years, sometimes decades) develop alternative signaling mechanisms and ways of paracrine androgens supply. It is estimated this happens in a third of all prostate cancer patients [1].

As this chapter focuses primarily on prostate cancer, some topics, like free-testosterone or salivary testosterone measurements are not included, because although they are related to testosterone measurement in general, they are, at least at present (things may change in the future), not used in day-to-day care of prostate cancer patients. All testosterone values mentioned relate to serum testosterone measurements.

## 2. Some characteristics of testosterone

Testosterone is principal male androgen, sex hormone and anabolic steroid. It is found not only in humans, but also in many other vertebrates. In males, testosterone is secreted by Leydig cells in testicles, in females by theca cells in ovaries. Small amount is produced also in zona reticularis of adrenal cortex in both genders and in placenta. Chemically (figure 1), it is white powder, soluble in methanol, name is17beta-Hydroxyandrost-4-en-3-on or 4-Androsten-17beta-ol-3-on, Chemical Abstracts Service number 58-22-0, ATC code G03BA03. It is a controlled substance, in US by Drug Enforcement Administration (DEA). It's inactive epimer – difference in configuration of OH at C17 - is called epitestosterone. Testosterone's biosynthesis starts from cholesterol. Metabolism: up to one tenth of testosterone is converted by 5-alpha reductase to dihydrotestosterone, less than 0.5% by aromatase to estradiol. Most of testosterone is deactivated and excreted as glucoronides.

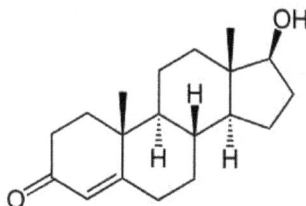

**Figure 1.** Testosterone structure (Picture in public domain – Wikimedia: NEUROtiker)

## 3. Reasons for testosterone measurement in prostate cancer

Testosterone measurement in prostate cancer patients has more than 40 years history [2]. Confirmation of castrate testosterone level is necessary before identifying prostate cancer as castration resistant. Castrate states are at present defined as serum testosterone level below 20 ng/dl (=0.69 nmol/l) or below 50 ng/dl (=1.73 nmol/l) [3], but it was not always this way and different testosterone measurement methods have important implications.

Need for controlling quality of chemical castration treatment of prostate cancer steams from reports of up to 15% castration failures [4,5]. This means LHRH treated patients may not reach castration levels of testosterone due to different reasons [6], not only non-compliance, application failures, but also other reasons, for example problems with depot formulation resorption due to granuloma formation on injection site [7] or may simply need more frequent dosages [8].

Further reason for testosterone measurements in prostate cancer patients lies in reports of correlation between success of castration and time to PSA progression: better castration (lower testosterone value) gives longer time to progression [9,10]. Therefore hormonal treatment of prostate cancer should not be followed with PSA measurement only (as indirect indication of treatment success), but also with testosterone measurement [11].

Before any treatment, at diagnosis, serum testosterone value is predictor of disease aggressiveness – lower testosterone values are related to less differentiated cancer and worse prognosis [12]. For all stated reasons, measurement of serum testosterone is important for clinicians who treat prostate cancer patients.

After long term of androgen suppression with LHRH (GnRH) analogues, sometimes testosterone levels do not recover after stopping treatment (which may be due to permanent dysfunction of Lydig cells), therefore application of LHRH drugs may be stopped in selected patients [13]. However, this should be confirmed and followed with testosterone measurement.

But testosterone measurements are not important only for urologists, who, apart from main reason – decisions related to prostate cancer management, use it for example also for aging male symptomatology and evaluation of patients with erectile dysfunction. Also other medical specialties, like endocrinology, pediatrics, gynecology or oncology use testosterone measurements for their conditions, like diagnosing and monitoring hyper- or hypo- androgenic disorders in women, like polycystic ovary syndrome, alopecia, acne, hirsutism or hypoactive sexual desire disorder; androgen secreting neoplasms; congenital syndromes with ambiguous genitalia... Pediatrics and endocrinology were in the past probably most frequent users of testosterone assays, but nowadays most laboratories receive most testosterone requests from urologists.

## 4. Prostate cancer incidence will increase in future

Prostate cancer is already most frequently diagnosed cancer among men in the developed world. As a cause of death among males, it is second in the USA and third in Europe. Large increase in prostate cancer incidence in recent years is not only due to availability of PSA (biochemical marker, which is useful for screening purposes) and due to better awareness of doctors and population at large, but in large part also due to changes in population pyramid and increased life expectancy. As breast cancer, which is most common in females over 60 years of age, also prostate cancer is cancer of older people. For example, in Slovenia (which may be in health related issues regarded somewhere in-between developed western and less advanced other parts of the world), incidence of prostate cancer increased 50% from 2000 to 2011 [14]. At the same time, population at main risk (males above age 60) increased 28%. Therefore more than half of increase of prostate cancer incidence can not be attributed to, as some people, even health care professionals, claim, "artificial" increase of incidence due to "over-screening", but simply to the fact that population at risk has significantly increased. And among those (males between 55 and 70), screening is most appropriate because life expectancy also increases (at present, for 75 year old man in Slovenia it is on average more than 10 years) and therefore cancer control is worthwhile.

In our country, recently prostate cancer incidence has been higher compared to breast cancer. Cause for this is not better prostate cancer "screening", but simple fact of changes in population pyramid, in numbers of populations at risk: relation between males and females in most important age range for prostate and breast cancer detection has changed – number of males grows significantly faster than number of females. In year 2000, 700 more females reached age of 60 compared to males, in 2011, 500 more males reached age 60 compared to females [15]. Although among oldest old, number of females will remain higher compared to men, present big gap in number of men compared to women in age group 50-70 is getting smaller and smaller and this also contributes to further increase of significance of prostate compared to breast cancer.

According to population pyramid, further increase of burden due to prostate cancer is expected, for example in our country, until year 2050, when overall population in Slovenia will, according to present trends, decrease from current 2 to 1.9 million, but number of males, age 60 or more, will peak at 1.8 times the number in 2011. Similar trend is expected to happen in most countries in the world sooner or later and therefore prostate cancer will remain important health problem in future.

## 5. Need for hormonal treatment of prostate cancer may not decrease in future

Despite facts about prostate cancer incidence, presented in section 4 and despite undeniable proof that population based PSA prostate cancer screening reduces mortality due to prostate cancer [16], it seems some professional bodies, like U.S. preventive services task force [17,18] recently advised against screening.

Further, among young UK general practitioners, during non-formal conversation, in year 2012, one can easily hear claims like "PSA – oh I thought it is NOT for screening, it is only for follow up purposes, only for patients, who have diagnosis of prostate cancer already" (personal experience).

With this recent trend by policy-makers, it seems hopes of urologists, who treat prostate cancer patients, that we will in the future find only very few patients, who will present with stage of disease, where nothing else but hormonal treatment would be possible or hormonal treatment will become necessary during the course of their disease, are dispelled. As it seems focus of attention is turned away from early detection and managing (watchful waiting, not necessary treating patients with prostate cancer), towards second and third line treatments for advanced disease, testosterone measurement in patients with prostate cancer will become even more important in the future.

## 6. Different hormonal treatments influence testosterone differently

Different drugs for hormonal treatment of prostate cancer have different effects on serum testosterone. Non-steroidal antiandrogens increase overall serum testosterone levels. Steroidal antiandrogen (cyproterone) reduces testosterone levels, but not to castrate values. Often old patients take two 100 mg tablets daily and testosterone values are than commonly around 7 nmol/l. With proper dosing (3 times 100 mg daily), values nearing castration levels have been reported (mean 2.5 nmol/l, [19]), on the other side, with dose 200 mg daily, relatively small decrease only to low-normal levels has been reported for healthy young to middle-aged men (mean 11.4 nmol/l [20]).

LHRH agonists injections are supposed to universally reduce testosterone levels to castration values, but sometimes this is not the case. LHRH antagonists are gaining popularity very slowly with similar effect on testosterone. They may reduce testosterone levels in a proportion of patients a bit further compared to LHRH agonists [21] and they do not cause microsurges of testosterone, which are often present with every re-dosing of LHRH agonists.

Surgical castration remains a viable opinion in many countries and for many patients. Steroids are available to further reduce serum androgen levels in castrate resistant disease states by blocking adrenal production. 5 alpha reductase inhibitors may, according to some theories, play a role in combination treatment.

In the past, castrate values of testosterone were achieved with estrogens, like stilbestrol. Due to side effects (blood cloths), this is not used any more. Ketoconazole, inhibitor of steroid synthesis, is still available for fast testosterone levels reduction, but in practice is is used mainly in experimental settings after chemotherapy failure in castration resistant states [22].

Typical testosterone responses to some hormonal agents are summarized in Table 1.

| Agent | Typical testosterone response |
|---|---|
| non-steroidal antiandrogen (bicalutamide, flutamide) | increase (may go above 30 nmol/l) |
| steroidal antiandrogen (cyproterone acetate) | decrease, very dependent on dosage regimen, with 3x100 mg it may approach, but not reach castrate values, in a few days |
| GnRH (LHRH) agonists (triptorelin, goserelin, leuporolide) | designed to decrease levels below castrate values (below 1.73 nmol/l), may take a month after first application to reach castrate level |
| GnRH antagonists (degarelix) | designed to decrease levels below castrate values without surges |
| surgical castration (bilateral orchiectomy) | gold standard, decrease below castration level in few hours, however, adrenal androgens remain |
| ketoconazole | decrease below castration levels if dose is high enough in 2-4 days, but sometimes variable response, corticosteroids should be supplemented simultaneously |
| estrogens (stilbestrol – of historical interest only) | decrease below castration levels after approx. 5 days, later surges may appear |

**Table 1.** Typical serum testosterone responses to different hormonal agents. In practice, individual responses may vary significantly, therefore confirmation with individual measurement is important.

# 7. Methods for serum testosterone measurement

With introduction of indirect RIA techniques (double isotope derivative dilution technique) to measure serum testosterone in 1970ties and later automated chemiluminescent assays, serum testosterone values became widely available to practicing urologists.

Manufacturers mainly use similar principles of assays. As an example of principle, Abbott's chemiluminescent assay is described [23]. It is "delayed one step", competitive heterogeneous assay. First, testosterone in serum sample is displaced from sex binding globulin (SHBG) with low-pH buffer. Sample is mixed with microparticles, coated with mouse monoclonal anti-testosterone antibody. After incubation, addition of labeled testosterone (in this case, conjugated with alkaline phosphatase), follows. Labeled testosterone binds to unoccupied sites on microparticles, coated with the antibodies against testosterone. More testosterone in the sample – less sites are free for labeled testosterone to bind. After another incubation, reaction mixture is transferred to cells, where microparticles fix and bind. Wash step follows – it removes unbound conjugate (labeled testosterone and other substances which may interfere with next step). Then, labeled antigen is visualized and measured. Signal is inversely proportional to amount of testosterone in the sample – as according to principle of competitive assay – stronger signal indicates more added, with marker conjugated testosterone present, therefore less "original" testosterone in the sample. In Abbott's example, 4-methylumbelliferyl phosphate is added and alkaline phosphatase, conjugated to added testosterone, hydrolyzes phosphate from 4-methylumbelliferryl phosphate to 4-methylumbelliferone, which fluorescence is measured [23].

In direct RIA methods, principle is the same, only marking of competing antigen is performed with radioactive substance instead of alkaline phosphatase or other enzymatic, fluorescence-based technique. Large variability was observed for direct RIA methods [24]. In indirect RIA methods, quantification follows organic solvent extraction and purification steps with monitoring of procedural losses. Although correlations between indirect RIA and mass spectrometry methods are good (above 0.9), absolute concentrations were reported to be significantly higher, probably (as in direct assays), due to cross-reaction of immunoreactive material [25].

Indirect assays (extraction and chromatography followed by RIA) are not available any more in our practice. Main method for serum testosterone determination in most present day clinical laboratories around the world (perhaps it is different in parts of US) is still direct automated chemiluminescent assay [26]. This assay mixes antibodies directly with serum and skips extraction step. This holds true for all direct assays, not only chemiluminescent but also radio-immuno (RIA) based.

Mass spectrometry (MS) of steroid compounds, which includes testosterone, has a long history of research and development [27]. It is coupled to liquid chromatography (LC, a separation technique in which the mobile phase is liquid) or gas chromatography (GC, a separation technique where the mobile phase is gas). After first separation and before ionization, in the past, derivatization (conversion of chemical compound into derivative) was often used to improve, for example, ionization efficiency and other characteristics of analyte[28]. With development of more sensitive techniques, today derivatization seem not included any more in a typical setting for testosterone determination with HPLC-tandem mass spectrometry. Sample must be ionized before ions are separated according to mass and charge in the spectrometer. Among methods of ionization are for example atmospheric pressure photoionization (suggested to be most optimal for testosterone analysis) or (less optimal for testosterone) electrospray ionization. Tandem mass spectrometry (MS/MS) means that spectrometry is performed in an arrangement in which ions are subjected to two or more sequential stages of analysis (which may be separated spatially or temporally).

High throughput LC/MS/MS has become gold standard for measurement of testosterone and other well defined steroid substances in biological fluids. GC/MS can also be used to quantify testosterone, but represents today mainly a "discovery tool" which provides "integrated picture of individual's metabolome" [29].

Some characteristics of testosterone assays are summarized in Table 2.

| Type | Characteristics |
|---|---|
| chemiluminescet | uses antibodies, direct, most laboratory platforms (Abbott, Siemens, Roche) have their own antibodies, which all cross react to some extent to other substances and give consistent, but different results, typically higher than reference methods in/near castrate range |
| RIA – radio -immuno assay | uses antibodies, rarely in use those days, typically good results if indirect – radio- immuno - detection after chromatography step, for direct RIA's, same as for chemiluminescence – problems with antibody selectivity |
| LC-MS/MS: liquid chromatography – tandem mass spectrometry | uses molecular mass based identification, indirect, uses different liquid chromatography methods to extract testosterone from sample (for example "high turbulent flow") and tandem mass spectrometry to confirm and quantify sample, gold standard |
| GC-MS: gas chromatography – mass spectrometry | uses molecular mass based identification, indirect, research mainly, useful for profiling different steroids in the sample, reference method, issues with "in-house" development, sample preparation, most labor and resource intensive |

**Table 2.** Most prevalent types of testosterone assays.

## 8. Units for testosterone measurement

Guidelines [3] state testosterone values in ng/dl only and some countries still use old values (for example US, Germany, Belgium), but in many countries laboratory results only in SI units - International System of Units - (nmol/l) - are available (for example Slovenia). Some articles, to further confusion, use other combinations, like ng/ml or mg/dl. To allow easier reference to practicing physicians, in Table 3, some typical serum testosterone values are presented in different units.

Conversion factors: as molecular formula of testosterone is $C_{19}H_{28}O_2$, molecular mass of testosterone is 288.42 g/mol. Therefore, if value in ng/dl is available, multiply it with 0.0347 nmol/l / ng/dl to get value in nmol/l. If value in nmol/l is available and one needs ng/dl, value in nmol/l should be multiplied by 28.8 ng/dl / nmol/l to get ng/dl. 1 ng/ml (or microg/l) = 100 ng/dl.

| Clinical meaning | value |
|---|---|
| normal morning value for males, above | 12 nmol/l (= 346 ng/dl = 3.46 ng/ml) |
| advised supplementation for healthy males, regardless of symptoms, below | 8 nmol/l (= 231 ng/dl = 2.31 ng/ml) |
| "old" castration value | 1.73 nmol/l (= 50 ng/dl = 0.5 ng/ml) |
| median value for premenopausal females | 1.39 nmol/l (= 40 ng/dl = 0.4 ng/ml) |
| "Morote's" value | 1.11 nmol/l (= 32 ng/dl = 0.32 ng/ml) |
| "new" castration value | 0.69 nmol/l (= 20 ng/dl = 0.2 ng/ml) |

**Table 3.** Typical serum testosterone values in different units. "Morote's" value represents level of serum testosterone, determined with direct chemiluminescent immuno assay in prostate cancer patients on hormonal treatment, above which shorter time to progression was observed compared to patients with testosterone values below this level [9]. For curiosity, median value for premenopausal females can also be used as guideline for supplementation in hypoactive sexual desire disorder [30].

## 9. Daily rhythm of testosterone

Circadian and "ultradian" mean testosterone level fluctuations peak is around 8 AM and through level around 8 PM. Over this, there is a 90 min oscillation in testosterone values as reflection of pulsatile secretory pattern.

Sleeping increases testosterone values [31]. Some even claim sleep, not circadian rhythm to be more important for regulation of testosterone [31]. Pattern of physical activity (physical work or training in the morning versus evening) does not influence testosterone concentrations or testosterone diurnal pattern [32]. Food (mixed meal) decreases testosterone value, if blood is taken 1-2 hours after, by 30% in comparison to overnight fast [33]. Better sleep increases testosterone value [34]. Anxiety may increase testosterone levels, it was even suggested, patient's samples on the day of admission to hospital should not be used because anxiety may be associated with increased testosterone level [35]. On LHRH agonists, diurnal pattern is expected to be abolished [36]. Age reduces circadian fluctuations [37].

Due to stated variations in testosterone levels during the day, morning fasting blood samples are standard.

## 10. What can one expect from direct chemiluminescent assays –Example

Wide availability of automated testosterone assays should make easy for clinicians to follow prostate cancer patients testosterone levels, as at present almost every clinical laboratory offers testosterone measurement with one of direct chemiluminescent assays methods.

Aim was to evaluate use of such a testosterone measurement tool in every-day clinical practice and consequences that might follow. Claims from some pharmaceutical company representatives on their LHRH agonist formulations to be better than others were also addressed.

### 10.1. Materials and methods

In a cross-sectional audit study, serum testosterone level was determined in all patients on 3-month LHRH formulations, treated in out-patient clinic in two months period. Blood samples were taken immediately before the next injection. Only patients, who previously received more than one injection and with previous injection exactly 3 months or less before examination were eligible.

Three preparations were found to be used: Diphereline (triptorelin 11.25 mg), Eligard (modern leuprolide formulation, 22.5 mg) and Zoladex (goserelin 10.8 mg).

Further 10 samples were taken from patients with surgical castration performed more than 6 months ago, who appeared on regular follow up out-patient visit during the study period.

Testosterone measurement was performed with direct chemiluminescent microparticle immunoassay Architect from Abbott Laboratories. According to procedural leaflet, functional sensitivity of this assay was 0.49 nmol/l (95% confidence interval 0.38 – 0.59) and analytical sensitivity 0.28 nmol/l.

As SI units (nmol/L) are obligatory in our country, all testosterone measurements were originally reported in SI units and conversion to US units (ng/dl) was performed for the purpose of this report using conversion factor of 0.0347.

For statistical evaluation of differences between groups of patients on different LHRH agonist formulations, analysis of variance between groups was calculated using open source statistical software R [38].

### 10.2. Results

125 patients aged 50 to 92 (median 74 years, lower quartile 70, upper quartile 78 years) were included.

For the whole group, serum testosterone values ranged from 14 ng/dl (0.5 nmol/l, lowest reportable result) to 107 ng/dl (3.7 nmol/l), median 37 ng/dl (1.3 nmol/l), lower quartile 32 ng/dl (1.1 nmol/l), upper quartile 58 ng/dl (2.0 nmol/l).

According to those results, considering castrate level of 20 ng/dl (=0.694 nmol/l), only 7% of patients on LHRH treatment and 2/10 patients after surgical castration could be classified to castrate state of disease. Considering castrate level of 50 ng/dl (1.735 nmol/l), 66% of patients on chemical castration and 8/10 patients after surgical castration would comply.

Testosterone measurement results, according to LHRH agonist, are presented in Table 4. According to analysis of variance, differences between groups of patients, treated with different LHRH agonists, were not significantly different (F=0.69, p=0.5).

| LHRH formulation | N | TST:min-max | TST-median | TST-75% | TST-90% |
|---|---|---|---|---|---|
| triptorelin 11.25 mg | 53 | 20-98 | 37 | 58 | 72 |
| goserelin 10.8 mg | 41 | 14-107 | 37 | 52 | 69 |
| leuprolide 22.5 mg | 21 | 14-84 | 49 | 63 | 72 |

**Table 4.** Testosterone measurement results with Abbot Architect assay in patients on different 3-month LHRH agonists. Samples were taken immediately before next injection. TST – testosterone. Units: ng/dl (1,73nmol/L=50 ng/dl). Differences between different LHRH formulations were not statistically significant.

## 11. Problems with direct testosterone immunoassays

Large differences were reported from measurements of the same serum sample with chemiluminescent assays from different manufacturers [39,40]. Direct RIA techniques were not better [41]. In the low range (values of interest for castration control in patients with prostate cancer), which was close to range of female testosterone levels, direct assays gave results more than 20% different from the gold standard [41]. Abbot Architect assay was also reported to give consistently up to 20% higher results compared to standard in this range of values [39].

One of the reasons for variability is in the fact that antibodies are different among manufacturers, with different cross-reactivity profiles. All present direct chemiluminescent assays are matrix dependent, which was extensively studied by the British group [42]. It was confirmed there was significant cross-reactivity for example with dehydroepiandrosteronesulphate (DHEA-S) [43]. The described issue is not only in urology regarding testosterone – also other areas of endocrinology where steroid hormones measurements are important, have reported and discussed similar issues [44,45]. College of American Pathologists proficiency testing revealed in 2008, highest mean compared to lowest mean for testosterone, to differ by factor 2.8 [46]. Differences for mass spectrometry assays were much lower, by factor 1.4.

## 12. Problems with mass spectrometry testosterone assays

Mass spectrometry (MS) assays are not commercially available in classical sense, but are to much larger extent dependent on each laboratory's own development. As mass spectrometry technology is capable of very high sensitivity and specificity, those assay are accepted as gold standard. But, they are more than direct commercial assays dependent on proper calibration and sample preparation[47]. Research has shown biases as high as 25.3% for testosterone values near castrate ranges [47]. Others reported up to 26% of results outside total error limit of 14% due to improper calibration and between-run calibration [48]. Although MS techniques are becoming standard assays for steroid hormones, this presents several challenges, for example affordability for smaller laboratories, high operating costs of equipment, need for standardization of MS assays and in many occasions, actually setting new reference ranges [49] and relating them to physiological and pathological conditions, as happens with testosterone, where castrate values have been moved from 50 ng/dl to 20 ng/dl.

## 13. Castrate testosterone values in different prostate cancer studies

Serum testosterone value around 1.735 nmol/l or 50 ng/dl as castrate level for the purpose of hormonal treatment of prostate cancer was used already in 1970'ties [2]. Later, some LHRH formulations were designed to achieve serum testosterone below this value in 95% of treated patients. It was accepted as standard value in guidelines [50]. Guidelines have at present gone even a step further and stated testosterone levels above 50 ng/dl to be in-sufficient and additional hormonal manipulation to be warranted in such patients [3]. It is further generally accepted patients with surgical castration to have lower levels of testosterone – around 15 ng/dl and certainly below 30 ng/dl [51]. As surgical castration provides lower testosterone levels, there were always claims one should aim as low as possible with testosterone levels and should try to reach below 20 ng/dl – for example in a small study of 38 patients, treated with LHRH agonists, Oefelein found 5% did not reach values below 50 ng/dl and 13% did not reach values below 20 ng/dl [52]. This movement, which aims to decrease castrate testosterone level, was further supported by publication which claims patients with castrate testosterone levels below 32 ng/dl (1.1 nmol/l) – Morote's value - to have longer time to biochemical progression [9]. In their study, which also used chemiluminescent antibody testosterone assay, in 25% of patients testosterone levels above 50 ng/dl were identified. Further, with serial measurements, 55% of patients on chemical castration had testosterone values found above 20 ng/dl [8]. Studies which use HPLC/MS/MS for determination of testosterone levels do see lower values [53].

Some studies seem to oversee guidelines and post their own castrate testosterone levels, which are significantly higher and set to a value which offers approximately 95% successful castration. In their article on testosterone escape, group from Norway claims their castration level is 2.8 nmol/l which equals 81 ng/dl [6]. This value was selected as their laboratory's upper normal limit for women. And with this value, they identified 10% of patients who failed to reach this castration level. The present study was similar to this in testing patient's serum for testosterone at the end of 3 month dosing interval, which may also influence results.

Another group from Turkey, which evaluated influence of androgen deprivation therapy on hand function in 2008 article used radioimmunoassay for testosterone measurement and in a castrate group mean value of testosterone was 52 ng/dl +- 35 ng/dl [54]. One can assume for approximately half of their patients testosterone levels were not in castrate area according to guidelines. Surgical castration study, using chemiluminescent assay, found values up to or above 50 ng/dl for surgically castrated patients [55]. Further surgical castration study found patients on LHRH treatment before surgical castration to have values above 50 ng/dl in 28% of patients and after surgical castration in up to 8% [56]. Unfortunately method of testosterone measurement is not stated in this article, but it correlates perfectly with data presented here, where chemiluminescent method was used. Further, recent LHRH agonists report from Canada, which also used "competitive immunoassay using direct chemiluminescent technology" [57], found median testosterone values for different LHRH agonists to be (in nmol/l) 1.2, 1.3, 1.1 and 1.3 and in two of five formulations, upper quartal value was 1.8, indicating 25% of patients on particular formulation to be even above "old" castration value of 1.72 nmol/l (50 ng/dl). Another study from Canada, also using chemiluminescent immunoassays, although claiming they were "newer technology", indicates risk for breakthrough levels of serum testosterone (value measured higher than castrate value) in patients on LHRH agonist injections to be 5.4% and 2.2% (for castration values 1.1 nmol/l and 1.7 nmol/l, respectively) per each LHRH injection [58]! Cancer control was claimed to be inferior in patients with breakthroughs of serum testosterone measured [58].

## 14. Direct testosterone assays and prostate cancer – The verdict

Probably one of most important reasons for observed discrepancies in testosterone measurements lies in "matrix" issue, in cross-reactivity. Immunolite assay and Abbot Architect both cross-react with DHEA and give consistently higher values for serum testosterone in range of castration male values [39,42]. Therefore results of studies, which use direct chemiluminescent testosterone assays in clinical setting cannot be compared to studies, which use chromatography followed by mass spectrometry techniques, because they do not measure the same things.

Inaccuracy of present day direct testosterone assays is already recognized in the field of female and male testosterone replacement, in pediatrics [59] and should be recognized also in the field of prostate cancer. Until indirect testosterone assays applying mass spectroscopy become widely available, publications should set realistic values of castrate levels and precisely state measurement methods used. They may be universally available in the USA, but in Europe, even western university hospitals are not quick in replacing direct immuno-assays with gas chromatography methods – for example in Ghent they changed only recently, also for reasons like "one can not publish any more anything about testosterone without this method". And even mass spectrometry methods show significant errors and inconsistencies.

On the downside, it becomes clear using direct present day techniques to control castration methods (either chemical or surgical) is not appropriate and invariably leads to disputable results. Above findings also in part explain long term debate about subcapsular or classical simple orchiectomy and part of an occasional finding of non-castrate testosterone level after orchiectomy [56]. Also our own impulse for studying the field come from initial observations that patients after surgical castration have higher testosterone values compared to guideline's requests.

On the upside, direct chemiluminescent assays do measure something. They can unmask occasional testosterone outlier (skipped dose of drug, granuloma formation or an individual in need for more frequent dose of a drug – reduced dose interval, as explained for example in dr. Garnick's editorial comment [8]). They can identify hypogonadal men with prostate cancer before starting androgen deprivation therapy, who have very bad prognosis or may in the future benefit from modified treatments, like incorporating early use of new antiandrogens (for example MDV3100 [60]). They are necessary if one embarks on "on demand" redosing of LHRH agonists [61].

It is obvious chemiluminescent direct testosterone measurements do not show only testosterone values and as such can not serve as a tool to decide which LHRH agonist reduces testosterone more compared to other drugs. But results of such assays, as for example Abbot Architect testosterone assay, are consistent [39] and according to published and our results, there are great differences in measured levels of androgens in patients on LHRH agonist therapy (740%, from 0.5 to 3.7 nmol/L, 14 – 107 ng/dL). Perhaps, at present a pure speculation, chemiluminescent assays, which give consistent results, only with some cross-reactivity and therefore systematic overestimation of testosterone values in the low range, like Architect and Immunolite, can give estimation of overall serum androgen levels. Importance of extratesticular androgens is becoming more and more evident [62,63]. This may explain findings from Morote et al, who used same technically problematic direct chemiluminiscent assay and found correlation between assay results and time to biochemical progression [9] or from Perachino et al, who found even correlation between assay results and survival [10]. Also Hashimoto et al [64], although failing to provide details about their testosterone assay and reporting questionably low testosterone values, report usefulness of testosterone measurement for prediction of antiandrogen treatment results – when testosterone levels were low, no additional clinical benefit of antiandrogen treatment was observed, when testosterone was higher, antiandrogens were useful. If future can confirm those propositions, direct testosterone tests, despite their imprecision for their original purpose, may well serve us in selecting patients for antiandrogen addition to castration or for secondary hormonal treatment, especially in perspective of new androgen manipulating drugs, like abiraterone acetate (Zytiga) and MDV3100 [60].

## 15. Conclusions

Serum testosterone levels provide objectivity for proper prostate cancer disease states characterization. Testosterone level before treatment may add to prognosis. More importantly, testosterone levels during treatment become main issue in individual's prostate cancer treatment decisions, as soon as increasing PSA levels indicate failure of primary local treatment.

Apparent difference between guidelines (which ask for 20ng/dl) and practice in serum tes-tosterone values of hormonally treated prostate cancer patients was investigated and could be explained in methodologies of testosterone determination. Most present day available testosterone assays in hospitals are direct assays, which overestimate testosterone values in the castrate range. Antibodies cross-react with other androgens in serum (which prevail in low testosterone range) and result is overall androgen estimation, not pure testosterone val-ue. Studies should recognize this and find use for this "overall androgen" value, which is, contrary to indirect mass spectroscopy assays, universally available and was found to be re-lated to disease progression and treatment results. Further, it is useful for identification of high risk patients with low testosterone values at diagnosis and identification of patients with poor response to LHRH agonists. Testosteron results are necessary for prolongation of interval between injections, which may be possible in approximately half of patients on LHRH agonists treatment where values are well below castration levels and at the same time, some patients may need injections of LHRH agonists in shorter intervals. In the future, tests which estimate not only pure testosterone, but overall androgen level, may become clinically relevant with awareness of prostate cancer cell's ability to use different androgen molecules and as a consequence patient tailored use of new androgen manipulating drugs.

## Acknowledgements

Study was strongly supported by Prim. KarelKisner, Former Head of Department of Urolo-gy in UKC Maribor, Slovenia and Mag. MaksimiljanGorenjak, Head of Department of Labo-ratory Medicine at the same institution.

## Author details

Tine Hajdinjak[1,2,3]

Address all correspondence to: tine.hajdinjak@gmail.com

1 Center UROL Maribor, Slovenia

2 Medical Faculty, University of Maribor, Maribor, Slovenia

3 Division of Urology, Department of Surgery, General Hospital Murska Sobota, Slovenia

## References

[1] Bianco FJ Jr. Paradigms in androgen/castrate resistant states of prostate cancer in a biomarker era. Urol. Oncol. 2008;26(4):408–14.

[2]  Shearer RJ, Hendry WF, Sommerville IF, Fergusson JD. Plasma testosterone: an accurate monitor of hormone treatment in prostatic cancer. Br J Urol. 1973;45(6):668–77.

[3]  Mottet N, Bellmunt J, Bolla M, Joniau S, Mason M, Matveev V, idr. EAU guidelines on prostate cancer. Part II: Treatment of advanced, relapsing, and castration-resistant prostate cancer. Eur. Urol. 2011;59(4):572–83.

[4]  Peyromaure M, Rebillard X, Ruffion A, Salomon L, Villers A, Soulie M. Time-course of plasma testosterone in patients with prostate cancer treated by endocrine therapy. Prog. Urol. 2008;18(1):2–8.

[5]  Morote J, Esquena S, Abascal JM, Trilla E, Cecchini L, Raventós CX, et al. Failure to maintain a suppressed level of serum testosterone during long-acting depot luteinizing hormone-releasing hormone agonist therapy in patients with advanced prostate cancer. Urol. Int. 2006;77(2):135–8.

[6]  Yri OE, Bjoro T, Fossa SD. Failure to achieve castration levels in patients using leuprolide acetate in locally advanced prostate cancer. Eur. Urol. 2006;49(1):54–58; discussion 58.

[7]  Shiota M, Tokuda N, Kanou T, Yamasaki H. Incidence rate of injection-site granulomas resulting from the administration of luteinizing hormone-releasing hormone analogues for the treatment of prostatic cancer. Yonsei Med. J. 2007;48(3):421–4.

[8]  Morote J, Planas J, Salvador C, Raventós CX, Catalán R, Reventós J. Individual variations of serum testosterone in patients with prostate cancer receiving androgen deprivation therapy. BJU Int. 2009;103(3):332–335; discussion 335.

[9]  Morote J, Orsola A, Planas J, Trilla E, Raventós CX, Cecchini L, et al. Redefining clinically significant castration levels in patients with prostate cancer receiving continuous androgen deprivation therapy. J. Urol. 2007;178(4 Pt 1):1290–5.

[10] Perachino M, Cavalli V, Bravi F. Testosterone levels in patients with metastatic prostate cancer treated with luteinizing hormone-releasing hormone therapy: prognostic significance? BJU Int. 2010;105(5):648–51.

[11] Schulman CC, Irani J, Morote J, Schalken JA, Montorsi F, Chlosta PL, et al. Testosterone measurement in patients with prostate cancer. Eur. Urol. 2010;58(1):65–74.

[12] Schatzl G, Madersbacher S, Thurridl T, Waldmüller J, Kramer G, Haitel A, et al. High-grade prostate cancer is associated with low serum testosterone levels. Prostate. 2001;47(1):52–8.

[13] Pedraza R, KwartAM. Hormonal therapy for patients with advanced adenocarcinoma of the prostate: is there a role for discontinuing treatment after prolonged androgen suppression? Urology. 2003;61(4):770–3.

[14] Slora: Slovenija in rak (Slovenian cancer registry) [Internet]. [accessed 2012 aug 8]. Available from: http://www.slora.si/

[15]  Prebivalstvenapiramida (Statistical office of the Republic of Slovenia) [Internet]. [accessed 2012 aug 8]. Available from: http://www.stat.si/Piramida.asp

[16]  Schröder FH, Hugosson J, Roobol MJ, Tammela TLJ, Ciatto S, Nelen V, et. al. Prostate-cancer mortality at 11 years of follow-up. N. Engl. J. Med. 2012 15;366(11):981–90.

[17]  Chou R, Croswell JM, Dana T, Bougatsos C, Blazina I, Fu R, et al. Screening for prostate cancer: a review of the evidence for the U.S. Preventive Services Task Force. Ann. Intern. Med. 2011;155(11):762–71.

[18]  Prostate Cancer: We Can Do Better: Editorial on Screening for Prostate Cancer from USPSTF Chair Dr. Virginia Moyer [Internet]. [accessed 2012 aug 8]. Available from: http://www.uspreventiveservicestaskforce.org/prostatecancerscreening/prostatecanoped.htm

[19]  Appu S, Lawrentschuk N, Grills RJ, Neerhut G. Effectiveness of cyproterone acetate in achieving castration and preventing luteinizing hormone releasing hormone analogue induced testosterone surge in patients with prostate cancer. J. Urol. 2005;174(1):140–2.

[20]  Morse HC, Leach DR, Rowley MJ, Heller CG. Effect of cyproterone acetate on sperm concentration, seminal fluid volume, testicular cytology and levels of plasma and urinary ICSH, FSH and testosterone in normal men. J. Reprod. Fertil. 1973;32(3):365–78.

[21]  Masson-Lecomte A, Guy L, Pedron P, Bruyere F, Rouprêt M, Nsabimbona B, et al. A switch from GnRH agonist to GnRH antagonist in castration-resistant prostate cancer patients leads to a low response rate on PSA. World journal of urology. 2012. DOI: 10.1007/s00345-012-0841-1.

[22]  Heyns W, Drochmans A, van der Schueren E, Verhoeven G. Endocrine effects of high-dose ketoconazole therapy in advanced prostatic cancer. ActaEndocrinol. 1985;110(2):276–83.

[23]  Novotny M, Wilson HD. Testosterone testing: an immunoassay with improved accuracy in samples from both males and females. CLI [Internet]. 2005; Accessed 2012 Aug 8. Available from: http://www.cli-online.com/fileadmin/pdf/pdf_general/testosterone-testing-an-immunoassay-with-improved-accuracy-in-samples-from-both-males-and-females.pdf

[24]  Stanczyk FZ, Cho MM, Endres DB, Morrison JL, Patel S, Paulson RJ. Limitations of direct estradiol and testosterone immunoassay kits. Steroids. 2003;68(14):1173–8.

[25]  Hsing AW, Stanczyk FZ, Bélanger A, Schroeder P, Chang L, Falk RT, idr. Reproducibility of serum sex steroid assays in men by RIA and mass spectrometry. Cancer Epidemiol. Biomarkers Prev. 2007;16(5):1004–8.

[26]  Newman JD, Doery JCG. Assessing hypogonadism in men - how helpful are current testosterone assays? AustFam Physician. 2008;37(8):670–1.

[27]  Friedland SS, Lane GH, Longman RT, Train KE, O'Neal MJ. Mass Spectra of Steroids. Anal. Chem. 1959;31(2):169–74.

[28]  Santa T, Al-Dirbashi OY, Fukushima T. Derivatization reagents in liquid chromatography/electrospray ionization tandem mass spectrometry for biomedical analysis. Drug DiscovTher. 2007;1(2):108–18.

[29]  Krone N, Hughes BA, Lavery GG, Stewart PM, Arlt W, Shackleton CHL. Gas chromatography/mass spectrometry (GC/MS) remains a pre-eminent discovery tool in clinical steroid investigations even in the era of fast liquid chromatography tandem mass spectrometry (LC/MS/MS). J Steroid BiochemMol Biol. 2010;121(3-5):496–504.

[30]  Palacios S. Hypoactive Sexual Desire Disorder and current pharmacotherapeutic options in women. Womens Health (LondEngl). 2011;7(1):95–107.

[31]  Andersen ML, Alvarenga TF, Mazaro-Costa R, Hachul HC, Tufik S. The association of testosterone, sleep, and sexual function in men and women. Brain Res. 2011;1416:80–104.

[32]  Sedliak M, Finni T, Cheng S, Kraemer WJ, Häkkinen K. Effect of time-of-day-specific strength training on serum hormone concentrations and isometric strength in men. Chronobiol. Int. 2007;24(6):1159–77.

[33]  Lehtihet M, Arver S, Bartuseviciene I, Pousette A. S-testosterone decrease after a mixed meal in healthy men independent of SHBG and gonadotrophin levels. Andrologia. 2012. doi: 10.1111/j.1439-0272.2012.01296.x.

[34]  Penev PD. Association between sleep and morning testosterone levels in older men. Sleep. 2007;30(4):427–32.

[35]  Robinson MR, Thomas BS. Effect of hormonal therapy on plasma testosterone levels in prostatic carcinoma. Br Med J. 1971;4(5784):391–4.

[36]  Grant JB, Ahmed SR, Shalet SM, Costello CB, Howell A, Blacklock NJ. Testosterone and gonadotrophin profiles in patients on daily or monthly LHRH analogue ICI 118630 (Zoladex) compared with orchiectomy. Br J Urol. 1986;58(5):539–44.

[37]  Copinschi G, Van Cauter E. Effects of ageing on modulation of hormonal secretions by sleep and circadian rhythmicity. Horm. Res. 1995;43(1-3):20–4.

[38]  R Core Team. R: A Language and Environment for Statistical Computing. Vienna, Austria; Available from: www.R-project.org

[39]  Taieb J, Mathian B, Millot F, Patricot M-C, Mathieu E, Queyrel N, et al. Testosterone measured by 10 immunoassays and by isotope-dilution gas chromatography-mass spectrometry in sera from 116 men, women, and children. Clin. Chem. 2003;49(8):1381–95.

[40]  Moal V, Mathieu E, Reynier P, Malthièry Y, Gallois Y. Low serum testosterone assayed by liquid chromatography-tandem mass spectrometry. Comparison with five immunoassay techniques. Clin. Chim. Acta. 2007;386(1-2):12–9.

[41] Sacks SS. Are routine testosterone assays good enough? ClinBiochem Rev. 2005;26(1): 43–5.

[42] Middle JG. Dehydroepiandrostenedionesulphate interferes in many direct immuno-assays for testosterone. Ann. Clin. Biochem. 2007;44(Pt 2):173–7.

[43] Warner MH, Kane JW, Atkin SL, Kilpatrick ES. Dehydroepiandrosteronesulphate in-terferes with the Abbott Architect direct immunoassay for testosterone. Ann. Clin. Biochem. 2006;43(Pt 3):196–9.

[44] Pearson Murphy BE. Lack of specificity of urinary free cortisol determinations: why does it continue? J. Clin. Endocrinol. Metab. 1999;84(6):2258–9.

[45] Wartofsky L, Handelsman DJ. Standardization of hormonal assays for the 21st centu-ry. J. Clin. Endocrinol. Metab. 2010;95(12):5141–3.

[46] Soldin SJ, Soldin OP. Steroid hormone analysis by tandem mass spectrometry. Clin. Chem. 2009;55(6):1061–6.

[47] Vesper HW, Botelho JC. Standardization of testosterone measurements in humans. J. Steroid Biochem. Mol. Biol. 2010;121(3-5):513–9.

[48] Thienpont LM, Van Uytfanghe K, Blincko S, Ramsay CS, Xie H, Doss RC, et al. State-of-the-art of serum testosterone measurement by isotope dilution-liquid chromatog-raphy-tandem mass spectrometry. Clin. Chem. 2008;54(8):1290–7.

[49] Stanczyk FZ, Clarke NJ. Advantages and challenges of mass spectrometry assays for steroid hormones. J. Steroid Biochem. Mol. Biol. 2010;121(3-5):491–5.

[50] Mohler J, Bahnson RR, Boston B, Busby JE, D'Amico A, Eastham JA, et al. NCCN clinical practice guidelines in oncology: prostate cancer. J NatlComprCancNetw. 2010;8(2):162–200.

[51] Oefelein MG, Feng A, Scolieri MJ, Ricchiutti D, Resnick MI. Reassessment of the defi-nition of castrate levels of testosterone: implications for clinical decision making. Ur-ology. 2000;56(6):1021–4.

[52] Oefelein MG, Cornum R. Failure to achieve castrate levels of testosterone during lu-teinizing hormone releasing hormone agonist therapy: the case for monitoring serum testosterone and a treatment decision algorithm. J. Urol. 2000;164(3 Pt 1):726–9.

[53] Sharifi R, Browneller R. Serum testosterone suppression and potential for agonistic stimulation during chronic treatment with monthly and 3-month depot formulations of leuprolide acetate for advanced prostate cancer. J. Urol. 2002;168(3):1001–4.

[54] Soyupek F, Soyupek S, Perk H, Ozorak A. Androgen deprivation therapy for pros-tate cancer: effects on hand function. Urol. Oncol. 2008;26(2):141–6.

[55] Vickers MA Jr, Lamontagne DP, Guru KA, Satyanarayana RK, Vickers KE, Menon M. Autologous tunica vaginalis and subcapsular orchiectomy: a hormonal therapy for prostate cancer. J. Androl. 2004;25(3):375–81.

[56] Issa MM, Lendvay TS, Bouet R, Young MR, Petros JA, Marshall FF. Epididymal sparing bilateral simple orchiectomy with epididymoplasty: preservation of esthetics and body image. J. Urol. 2005;174(3):893–7.

[57] Venkateswaran S, Margel D, Yap S, Hersey K, Yip P, Fleshner NE. Comparison of serum testosterone levels in prostate cancer patients receiving LHRH agonist therapy with or without the removal of the prostate. Can UrolAssoc J. 2012;6(3):183–6.

[58] Pickles T, Hamm J, Morris WJ, Schreiber WE, Tyldesley S. Incomplete testosterone suppression with luteinizing hormone-releasing hormone agonists: does it happen and does it matter? BJU international. 2012. doi: 10.1111/j.1464-410X.2012.11190.x.

[59] Tomlinson C, Macintyre H, Dorrian CA, Ahmed SF, Wallace AM. Testosterone measurements in early infancy. Arch Dis Child Fetal Neonatal Ed. 2004;89(6):F558–F559.

[60] Eichholz A, Ferraldeschi R, Attard G, de Bono JS. Putting the brakes on continued androgen receptor signaling in castration-resistant prostate cancer. Molecular and Cellular Endocrinology. 2012;360(1-2):68-75.

[61] Oefelein MG. Words of wisdom. Re: determining dosing intervals for LHRH agonists based on serum testosterone levels: a prospective study. Eur. Urol. 2008;54(1):235–6.

[62] Mostaghel EA, Nelson PS. Intracrine androgen metabolism in prostate cancer progression: mechanisms of castration resistance and therapeutic implications. Best Pract. Res. Clin. Endocrinol. Metab. 2008;22(2):243–58.

[63] Luu-The V, Bélanger A, Labrie F. Androgen biosynthetic pathways in the human prostate. Best Pract. Res. Clin. Endocrinol. Metab. 2008;22(2):207–21.

[64] Hashimoto K, Masumori N, Hashimoto J, Takayanagi A, Fukuta F, Tsukamoto T. Serum testosterone level to predict the efficacy of sequential use of antiandrogens as second-line treatment following androgen deprivation monotherapy in patients with castration-resistant prostate cancer. Jpn. J. Clin. Oncol. 2011;41(3):405–10.

# Chapter 9

# Describing Prostate Cancer Dynamics: Second Look at PSA-Doubling Time and PSA-Specific Growth Rate

Glenn Tisman

Additional information is available at the end of the chapter

## 1. Introduction

Physicians responsible for patient care focus on readily available clinical and trending laboratory data to help direct the patient's clinical course and evaluate efficacy of therapy. Most clinicians fail to incorporate newer parameters of tumor response such as tumor growth rate when evaluating patient treatment response. Available now, is a wealth of dynamic growth parameters that shed new light on tumor biology and should be used in clinical decision-making.

What follows is in part a review of former paradigms of prostate tumor growth. Later, focus is directed to newer techniques to assist in evaluating targeted drug effects on the kinetics of prostate and other cancers. The discussion introduces the concept of tumor or marker specific growth rate (SGR) and challenges historical results obtained by use of the classic tumor or marker doubling time (PSA-DT).

As we proceed with this discussion, a mobile device App for hand-held computers including the iPhone, iPad, or iPod is presented. This conveniently facilitates a more sophisticated tumor and marker analysis at the bedside or in the clinic.

## 2. Historical perspective of tumor growth kinetics, exponential and Gompertzian kinetics

Though there is occasional homage paid to Gompertzian tumor growth, for practical purposes, when we care for patients, tumors are frequently undergoing exponential expansion.

In the absence of tumor mutation or perturbation by therapy the growth rate of exponential-ly growing tumors is constant. Rarely, there may be periods of interrupted growth.

Gompertzian growth [1, 2, 3] is best described by a sigmoid-shaped curve. At tumor initia-tion growth is occult, slow and remains subclinical for several years. A second phase is the rapid, clinically apparent exponential phase lasting for a few years followed by the slower terminal growth phase as the tumor approaches 35-40 doublings representing a volume ap-proaching 1000 cc or a tumor diameter of 10 cm Figure 1. The duration of tumor growth from inception is several years and for three quarters of that period the tumor is clinically undetectable. At the time of discovery, the oncologist is attending to the last quarter of tu-mor growth.

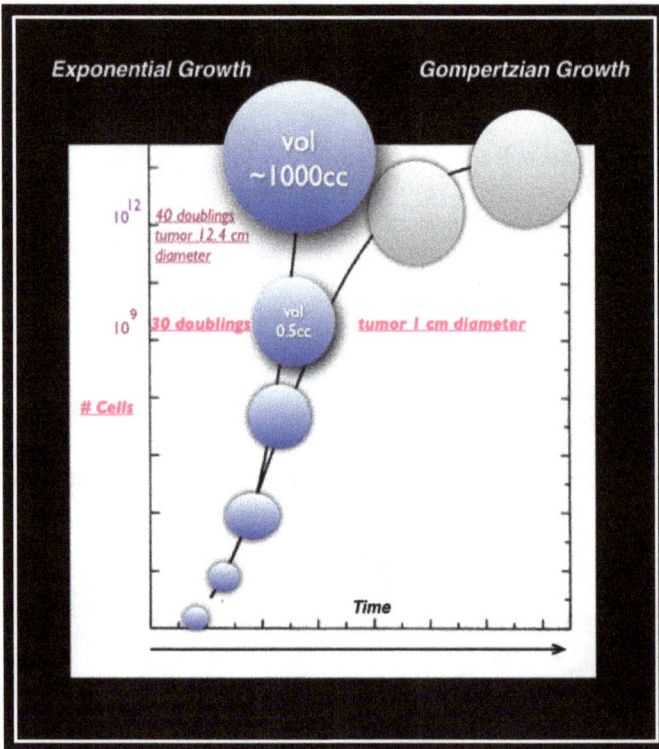

**Figure 1.** Note the differences between the exponential and Gompertzian growth curves. The lethal burden of tumor is approximately 1000 cc or ~35-40 doublings. In the clinic when tumors reach 0.5-1 cm in diameter (30 doublings or $10^9$ cells) they are measurable and follow the exponential growth curve, the steeper the slope the larger the tumor specific growth rate (SGR). Nonetheless, many feel that when looking at the entire lifespan of malignant tumors (over several years) tumor growth may better be described by Gompertzian kinetics [3].

## 3. Exponential growth

In 1934 Mottram [4, 5] reported work on the rat tar wart. Tar warts are tar-carcinogen in-duced neoplasms of the skin starting 75-100 days after the continuous painting of the rat's neck with tar. Histologically, some warts appear benign while others are clearly malignant.

Using the tar wart tumor growth model, Mottram was the first to describe tumor expansion as exponential. Exponentially growing tumors graphically produce straight lines by plotting linear time on the x-axis versus the log (at any base) of either tumor area, tumor cell number, tumor volume or tumor diameter on the y-axis see Figure 2.

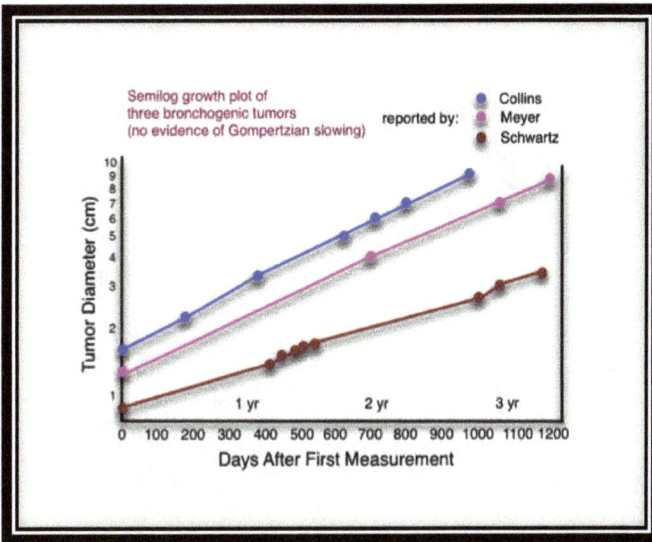

**Figure 2.** Friberg, Collins, Spratt, Steel, Schwartz affirmed that in the clinic, an exponential growth pattern adequately described tumor growth for most patients. A semi-log plot of tumor diameter vs. time illustrates the linear relationship characteristic of exponential growth.

Twenty years later Laird [6, 7] reported on the growth of transplanted tumors in the rat. Un-der her specific laboratory conditions, most tumor growth could be described in terms of the Gompertzian model. Her experiments lead her to accept that for her laboratory model; most transplantable, rapidly growing tumors could be described in Gompertzian terms.

Studies of tumor growth in clinic patients have been described in terms of both exponential and Gompertzian models. Nevertheless, several investigators reported data that was incon-sistent with the Gompertzian model for the majority of their patients. These authors engag-ed routine imaging of both metastatic and primary pulmonary lesions in an attempt to resolve whether exponential growth could be confirmed in the clinic. Friberg, Collins, Spratt, Steel, Schwartz [8, 9, 10, 11, 12,13] affirmed that in the clinic, an exponential growth pattern adequately described tumor growth for most patients Figures 2, 3.

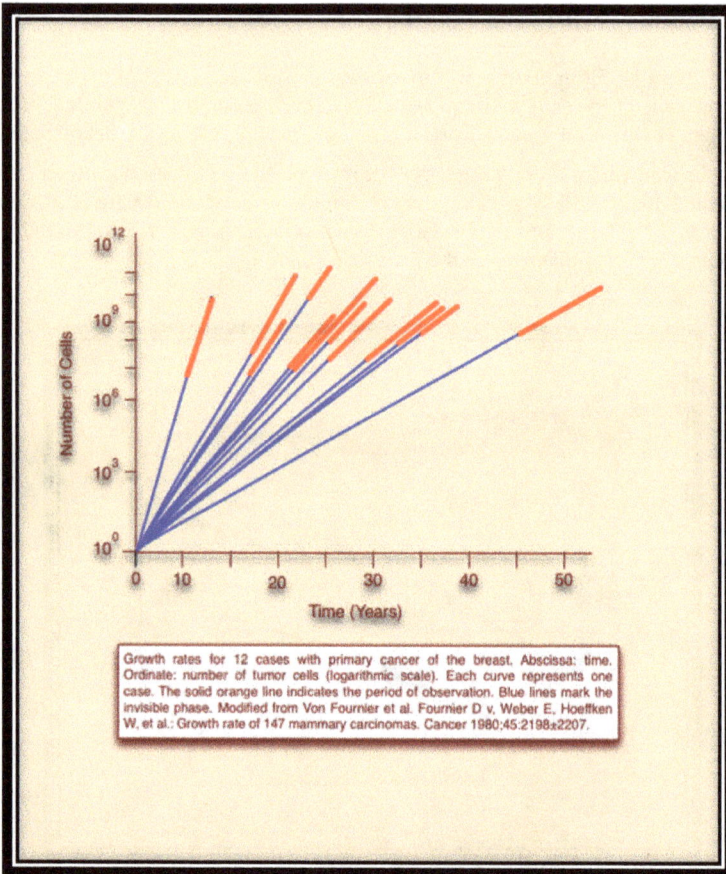

**Figure 3.** Von Fournier et al. confirm a straight-line (by semi-log plot) relationship for patients with breast tumors supporting the model of exponential growth model.

## 4. The tumor marker as a surrogate for tumor growth exemplified by PSA and prostate cancer

### 4.1. PSA Velocity (PSA-V)

PSA-V is the rate of change in serum PSA over time. PSA-V = 1/2 (($PSA_2$-$PSA_1$/$t_1$ in years) + ($PSA_3$ – $PSA_2$/$t_2$ in years)), where $PSA_1$ is the first, $PSA_2$ the second and $PSA_3$ the third PSA measurement. Time represents the interval (in years) between PSA measurements. It is recommended that three PSA measurements obtained over 24 months yields optimal accuracy. A PSA-V exceeding 0.75 ng/ml/year is highly predictive of prostate cancer. PSA-V is more useful than PSA doubling time (PSA-DT) in the pretreatment setting to help identify those men with life-threatening disease [14].

Studies confirm that the PSA tumor marker reflects prostate tumor growth and PSA dynamic changes are useful for predicting clinical outcome in several situations such as tumor recurrence and overall survival [15].

Klotz [16] reviewed the value of PSA as a tumor marker in patients with prostate cancer. He noted that use of a single serum value of PSA is inadequate for predicting patient survival. However, the PSA-V as ng/ml/yr. was a marker of disease biology. D'Amico [17] included preoperative PSA-V in determining subsequent risk of death from prostate cancer in 1095 men with clinically localized prostate cancer that underwent prostatectomy and radiation therapy [18]. A PSA-V >2 ng/ml/yr the year before prostatectomy, was associated with lymph node metastases, an advanced pathologic stage, and high-grade disease. This threshold level of PSA-V was associated with a significantly shortened time to recurrence, death from prostate cancer, and death from any cause. Strikingly, men with a PSA rise of >2.0 ng/ml had prostate cancer-specific mortality rates nine times those with a PSA-V <2 ng/ml.

## 4.2. Tumor marker Doubling Time (DT)

Miyamoto [19] studied the growth of hepatic metastases in colorectal cancer patients. He established that a tumor marker could accurately reflect tumor volume and its changes. Using the CEA tumor marker he reported an almost equal and parallel correlation between CEA doubling time and hepatic tumor volume doubling time.

PSA-DT Figure 4 is the time it takes for the serum PSA to double. Evidence indicates PSA-DT closely mirrors prostate tumor volume doubling time. Kato et al. in 2008 [20] undertook an attempt to correlate prostate tumor volume to serum PSA level. Kato's group calculated that for each ng/ml increment of serum PSA, there was a 0.302 cc increase in total tumor volume and a 0.7% increase in relative tumor volume. Total tumor volume in cc was given as V(cc) = 3.476 + 0.302 X PSA (ng/ml) while the percent tumor volume Volume(%) = 11.331 + 0.704 X PSA (ng/ml).

Babaian et. al. [21] reported that multivariate regression analysis of tumor volume as a function of PSA, grade and stage demonstrated that log PSA had the strongest association with tumor volume. Tanaka [22] reported that among significant preoperative and postoperative parameters, calculated cancer volume remained an independent predictive parameter in multivariate analysis (P <0.01). Tumor volume, as calculated by preoperative parameters, was an independent predictor of biochemical recurrence in patients who had undergone radical prostatectomy. Vollmer et al. [23] used a compartmental model and first order kinetics to develop the calculation necessary to relate serum PSA to tumor volume. They found that the resulting model was a good fit to the observed kinetic data of PSA measured after biopsy or prostatectomy. The model also predicted a linear relationship between PSA and the sum of volumes of benign and malignant tissues.

Until evidence to the contrary, it is assumed that similar to colorectal tumors and CEA, there is a reasonable relationship between serum PSA and its kinetics allowing its use as a predictor of changes of prostate tumor volume and growth kinetics.

An important point when using serum PSA in calculations is that an exact interval for testing remains controversial, some investigators stress that the interval between PSA-DT determinations should approach 3-6 months [24] to limit error due to random variation of PSA values. Using a third generation highly sensitive PSA assay, our laboratory changes in PSA are precise to the third decimal point and allow educated decision-making based on monthly determinations.

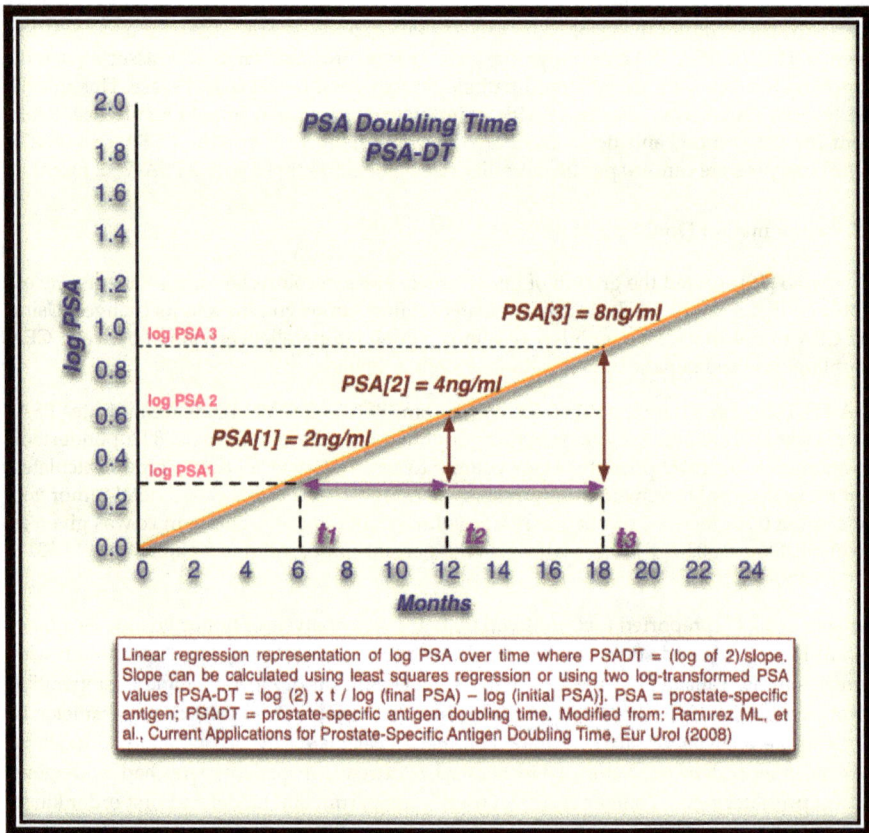

**PSA Doubling Time**
**PSA-DT**

PSA[3] = 8ng/ml
log PSA 3
PSA[2] = 4ng/ml
log PSA 2
PSA[1] = 2ng/ml
log PSA1

Linear regression representation of log PSA over time where PSADT = (log of 2)/slope. Slope can be calculated using least squares regression or using two log-transformed PSA values [PSA-DT = log (2) x t / log (final PSA) – log (initial PSA)]. PSA = prostate-specific antigen; PSADT = prostate-specific antigen doubling time. Modified from: Ramırez ML, et al., Current Applications for Prostate-Specific Antigen Doubling Time, Eur Urol (2008)

**Figure 4.** This figure is a semi-log plot of logs PSA (y-axis) vs. time (x-axis) [26]. Note the linear relationship, indicating that the rise of PSA values follows an exponential expansion of PSA.

Historically, PSA kinetics for watchful waiters included PSA-DT. A PSA-DT of >10 yr. can be considered favorable; a PSA-DT of <3-4 yr. suggests a change in biology and consideration should be given to an alternative therapy [25]. PSA kinetics should always be combined with other diagnostics such as endorectal ultrasound; endorectal MRI, digital rectal exam and repeat prostate biopsies approximately every 6-12 months.

### 4.3. PSA-DT as a surrogate for drug activity

PSA is one of the major androgen receptor-dependent target genes [27], and clinical monitoring is used to detect early stage disease as well as the emergence of recurrent tumor after therapy [28, 29, 30] and changes mirror changes in tumor bulk and indicate response to drugs. The graphic representation of PSA-DT is illustrated and its formula is given in Figure 4 [26].

Kelloff et al. [31], reviewed the use of PSA-DT as a surrogate for tumor response to drugs in patients with prostate cancer. They concluded that protocols that demonstrate significant changes in PSA-DT might be used to support accelerated approval of newer therapies. There is data to suggest PSA-DT in castrate resistant patients is predictive of outcome after chemotherapy [32]. An important caveat is expressed by Newling's review [33] of the subject which concluded that though dynamic changes in the PSA such as PSA-DT are commonly used in clinical trials of new drug therapies, PSA-DT might be affected by other factors including assay variations and false elevations of serum PSA caused by irritation of bladder catheters, prostatitis and cystitis. A substantial incidence of transient elevations of PSA (55%) was reported following combined external beam radiation and brachytherapy for prostate cancer [34]. These complicating issues should always be considered before PSA-DT is used to modify therapy.

Most recently, newer targeted and immunotherapies were found to produce paradoxical effects on PSA kinetics. Newling [33] argues that PSA should therefore be used as a secondary end point while overall survival still remains the gold standard in evaluating therapeutic efficacy for patients with hormone refractory disease.

## 5. Defining PSA response

Investigators participating in new prostate cancer drug trials commonly define PSA response according to the Bubley guidelines [35] for phase II clinical trials in androgen-independent prostate cancer. The guidelines qualify the following categories of PSA: PSA normalization, PSA <=0.2 ng/ml; PSA decrease, PSA decline ≥50%, confirmed by a second PSA value 4 or more weeks later; PSA progression, PSA ≥25% increase over the baseline (and an increase in the absolute value PSA level by at least 5 ng/mL). Though useful for evaluating clinical trials, these PSA changes lack sensitivity when evaluating subtle drug effects vs. prostate tumor growth [36,37, 38].

Therasse [39, 40], in his thesis reports on MRI and PSA as tools in a RECIST evaluation used to define tumor response in prostate cancer patients with measurable soft tissue lesions. When comparing MRI soft tissue responses to serum PSA changes, the correlation of PSA and MRI showed agreement in 14 of the 20 (70%) patients.

## 6. PSA-DT and Survival of prostate cancer patients

The importance of PSA-DT in predicting survival is illustrated by Freedland et al. [41] Figure 5. This chart presents data for a group of patients experiencing biochemical recurrence of PSA after prostatectomy. Under these circumstances, PSA-DT clearly defined prostate cancer survival into four groups: 1) PSA-DT >=15 months, 2) PSA-DT 9-14 months 3) PSADT 3-8.9 months, 4) PSA-DT <3 months. For this study, PSA-DT is clearly a surrogate for prostate cancer-specific survival.

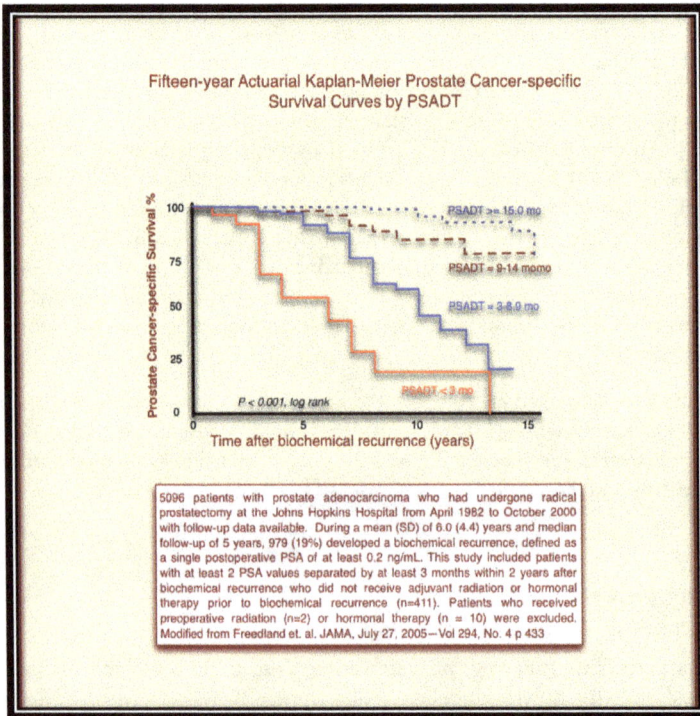

**Figure 5.**

## 7. PSA in the era of biologic and targeted therapy

A wealth of data establishes PSA as a marker of tumor aggressiveness, tumor stage, drug response and survival. Controversy and concern persists regarding PSA's role as a marker of disease stabilization and response induced by cytostatic and immunotherapies when compared to cytolytic therapies. An evaluation of the difficulties surrounding PSA interpretation has been addressed [42].

Two vaccine trials, Sipuleucel-T (Provenge) [43, 44, 45] and the TRICOM PROSTVAC [46, 47] demonstrated a significant overall survival benefit without any consistent decline in PSA, raising questions about the value of PSA response for non-hormonal, non-cytotoxic therapies. In addition, wide fluctuations have been observed in PSA values due to a transient effect of some drugs on PSA production seemingly independent of cell proliferation. The independent, non-proliferative effect of drugs on PSA expression should be considered when interpreting PSA response data. These aberrant PSA effects must be considered together with imaging results and clinical evaluation of the patient. Nevertheless, it has been consistent that post therapy a >50% PSA decline in pre-treatment PSA carries a significant overall survival advantage [48, 35].

Kelly [48] reported on 110 assessable patients treated on seven sequential protocols at Memorial Sloan-Kettering Cancer Center for hormone-refractory prostate cancer a statistically significant survival advantage in 110 patients with >50% PSA decline (>25 months survival) versus those without a 50% PSA decline (8.6 months survival). These results suggest that post therapy PSA declines can be used as a surrogate end point to evaluate new agents in hormone-refractory prostate cancer and criteria for response need prospective validation for phase III trials. Smith et al. [49] showed that a PSA decline > 50% for at least 8 weeks resulted in a longer mean survival time of 91 weeks versus 38 weeks for patients showing a smaller PSA reduction. An improved PSA response was associated with prolonged survival in the TAX 327 study (Docetaxel plus Prednisone or Mitoxantrone plus Prednisone for Advanced Prostate Cancer), with a median survival of 33 months when the PSA was normalized (<4 ng/mL) versus 15.8 months for an abnormal PSA [50, 51].

Heidenreich [52], the chair of the European Association of Urology oversaw the EAU 2012 Prostate Cancer Guidelines. He acknowledged that the PSA has been validated to be the most clinically useful tumor marker of treatment failure following local therapy and of tumor response as well as of tumor progression following hormonal treatment.

## 8. Assessment of molecularly targeted, cytostatic or anti-angiogenic agents

Bellmunt [53] and others expressed concern that PSA response criteria are not established to properly evaluate molecularly targeted cytostatic or anti-angiogenic agents [54]; therefore, certain drug-specific limitations may exist when using PSA or PSA-DT as an indicator of progression or response. One clear example was noted in a study of sorafenib (Nexavar) in castrate resistant prostate cancer, in which two patients with PSA progression were found to have dramatic resolution of bony disease [55]. Therapy-associated PSA "surge" has been described after effective chemotherapy. PSA surge occurs with Samarium[153] radiotherapy, androgen deprivation and chemotherapy and is generally transient. The surge may be due to rapid lysis of prostate cancer cells thus spilling intracellular contents into the intravascular space [56]. Similarly, 10 of 16 patients who discontinued sorafenib and did not receive other therapy demonstrated post-discontinuation PSA declines of 7–52% [57]. The review by Bellmunt [58, 59] notes that several targeted therapies caused prolongation of the PSA-DT as well as significant suppression of PSA levels. The era of targeted therapy for prostate cancer is just beginning and will require changes in how we interpret PSA kinetics.

## 9. Considerations in evaluating tumor growth effects of targeted therapies

Newer targeted therapies are often cytostatic or cytolentic (slowing proliferation) [60], resulting in disease stabilization, improved quality of life and extended survival. Examples of such drugs include sorefinib (Nexavar) [61], axitinib (Inlyta) for renal cell carcinoma [62], and mTOR inhibitors (everolimus (Afinitor) [63] and temsirolimus (Torisel)). Dasitinib (Sprycel) and sorefinib (Nexavar) are active in prostate cancer. Dasatinib is active in chronic granulocytic leukemia and GIST, inhibits BCR/ABL tyrosine kinase, KIT, PDGFR and Src tyrosine kinase amongst other targets. The Src tyrosine kinase is instrumental in driving hormone-independent prostate cancers [64]. Dasatinib is active in castrate resistant prostate cancer and may be administered safely with docetaxel [65, 66].

These newer therapies target not only the tumor cell but also modify the supporting stroma and microvasculature. The cytostatic/cytolentic effects may leave the tumor dimensionally intact, stable on imaging studies but with slower or absent growth for extended periods of time. Some imaging techniques such as PET and MRI [67], able to quantify such metabolic effects, may enhance clinical evaluation while CT images appear unchanged.

There is mounting evidence that stabilization of tumor growth significantly prolongs overall survival to a degree similar to patients experiencing an objective response judged by RECIST or RECIST 1.1 criteria (Response Evaluation Criteria in Solid Tumors). This raises concern and new calls for modification of current RECIST categories to include new definitions for targeted responses [68].

Simple reductions in PSA levels as defined by Bubley [35] have not yet been validated as a surrogate end point for use in clinical trials of agents with novel mechanisms of action. As indicated, cytotoxic chemotherapy alone, in combination with molecular-targeted agents, or the sole use of targeted therapies, produces different and at times transient and paradoxical changes in serum PSA and further studies are needed to further define this issue.

As questions have emerged concerning the utility of PSA levels as a surrogate end point, the Prostate Cancer Clinical Trials Working Group reviewed the criteria for outcome measures in clinical trials that evaluate systemic treatment for patients with progressive prostate cancer. Recommendations conclude that PSA responses may be delayed in trials of non-cytotoxic agents, and rising PSA levels in the absence of other signs of progression should not lead to discontinuation of trials. This recommendation might lead to much consternation between the patient and doctor where discussion of the latest PSA value is often the primary subject during follow-up visits.

# 10. Projected tumor size and projected PSA uncover hidden drug activity

Now that surrogacy of static values of PSA and PSA-DT is being questioned for targeted therapies, new techniques of response evaluation are under study. One attempt to quantitate treatment efficacy redirects attention from PSA-DT to PSA-specific growth rate (PSA-SGR) [69, 70, 71]. Generally ignored, **projected tumor and marker value** play a particularly important role in uncovering and quantifying hidden, cytostatic or cytolentic drug effects. Projected tumor volume or marker value is calculated prior to the initiation of therapy and based on the specific growth rate constant (SGR) before the start of therapy. The projected value is illustrated in Figure 7. This growth projection captures the inherent tumor SGR before therapy and predicts what the outcome (projected tumor or marker volume/value) would be at any future date in the absence of treatment or tumor mutation. Older cytotoxic drugs, when effective, inhibit innate growth by programmed cell death and apoptosis resulting in autophagy and tumor cell lysis [60, 72]. This results in a measurable reduction of tumor size. Interestingly, these drugs are often in part cytostatic or cytolentic and depending on dose may result in stable disease. Keep in mind that prolongation of cytostatic or cytolentic suppression by any drug may eventually induce cytotoxicity and cell lysis [60] Figure 6.

Different combinations of static/lytic drug activity may result in reduced tumor/marker size or complete tumor growth inhibition without clinically detectable change in tumor size. Under these circumstances, use of **projected** growth uncovers hidden suppression of proliferation. A common clinical scenario occurs when during treatment, a tumor increases in size but much less than **projected**. Unless the clinician calculates what the **projected** tumor size should be, the true degree of tumor suppression is not appreciated Figure 7.

## 10.1. Mathematical relationships of exponentially growing tumors and projected tumor marker or tumor size/volume

The mathematical expression for exponential expansion of growth is: $V_t = V_0 e^{\alpha t}$ where the tumor volume at time $V_t$ is predictable and is the product of the starting tumor volume [$V_0$] and [e = 2.71828, the base of the natural logarithm raised to the product of the specific growth rate constant $\alpha$ or (SGR) and the duration of growth $\Delta t$ or $(t_1 - t_0)$].

This is given as $V_t = V_0 e^{SGR \cdot \Delta t}$ and mathematical rearrangement yields $SGR = \dfrac{\ln(\frac{V2}{V1})}{t2 - t1}$

Inhibitory drug effects slow SGR and are precisely quantifiable by calculating changes of SGR and the tumor size before and after therapy. Tumor size after therapy should be compared to the **projected** tumor size the same time after therapy. The current standard for clinical oncologists is comparison of tumor size before and after therapy while neglecting comparison with the **projected** tumor size. Differences between post therapy tumor size and the post therapy projected tumor size are the clue to hidden responses that are almost never evaluated by the clinical oncologist. These often-subtle differences between projected and post therapy tumor sizes may reveal hidden growth stimulation (mutation or idiosyncratic drug effect) as well as subtle growth inhibition, which may lead to prolonged clinical stability.

The following relationships, extracted from Mehrara's analysis [69,70,71] define projected tumor volume: $\int_{ti}^{t} \triangle SGR\,(t) * dt = \ln(\frac{Vn}{Vi}) - \ln(\frac{Vt}{Vi})$ where $V_n$ = **projected** tumor volume, $V_t$ = volume of tumor at the time of response evaluation and $V_i$ is the volume at the initiation of therapy. The tumor response or TR = - $\ln(V_t/V_n)$ where $V_t$ is the volume of treated tumor and $V_n$ is the hypothetical or projected tumor volume, both evaluated at the time of efficacy assessment. These relationships are the model for the growth kinetics of exponentially growing tumors and generally require the use of at least a handheld computer to facilitate evaluation in the clinic. This is further discussed in the appendix.

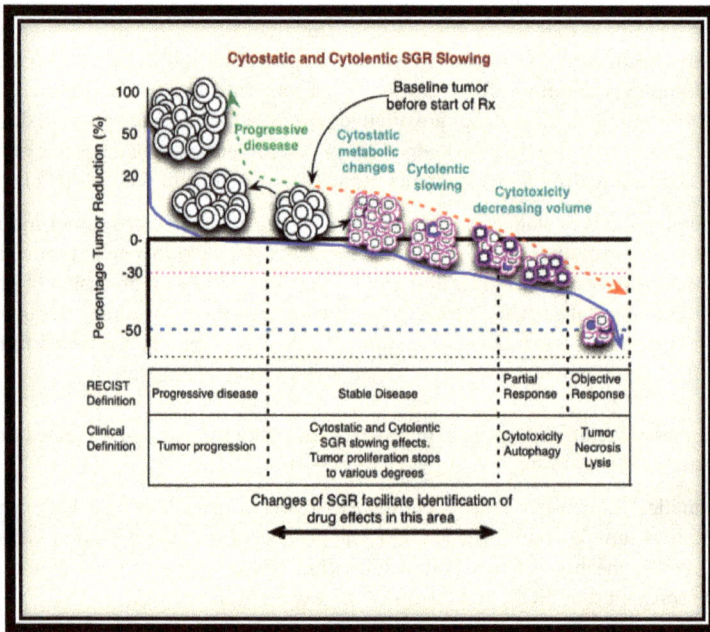

**Figure 6.** *In vitro and in vivo*, a clear distinction between cytostatic and cytolytic drugs does not exist. Low-dose cytolytic chemotherapy may exert cytostasis or so-called cytolentic slowing of cell proliferation leading to cell lysis, while targeted therapy's prolonged cytostatic metabolic effects (or large doses of targeted therapy) may induce cytolysis and autophagy (autophagocytosis). Regardless of mechanism of cell inhibition, the SGR and the TR (treatment response) calculations clearly and objectively define and quantitate drug efficacy (TR value).

Picture a 4.0 cm diameter (14.1 cc) pulmonary metastasis. At the time of discovery two months before the start of therapy the tumor was 3 cm (33.5 cc). The pre-therapy SGR for this tumor = 1.46%/d (tumor volume was expanding by 1.46%/d). Sixty-one days of therapy was administered and the tumor grew to 4.5 cm (47.7 cc). SGR decreased from 1.46%/d to 1%/d. Clinicians unaware of SGR and the projected tumor volume at this point might declare drug resistance however; **the projected tumor volume was actually 80.6 cc and the tu-**

mor reached only 47.7 cc. Even though the tumor grew, therapy was significantly effective in slowing growth (59% of intrinsic tumor growth was inhibited)! The parameter for treatment efficacy, TR was +0.5. A positive value for TR means that therapy had some inhibitory activity against the tumor, the larger the value the better. A negative value means therapy was associated with growth stimulation. The value of TR is useful as an objective standard comparator to help evaluate efficacy between different treatments.

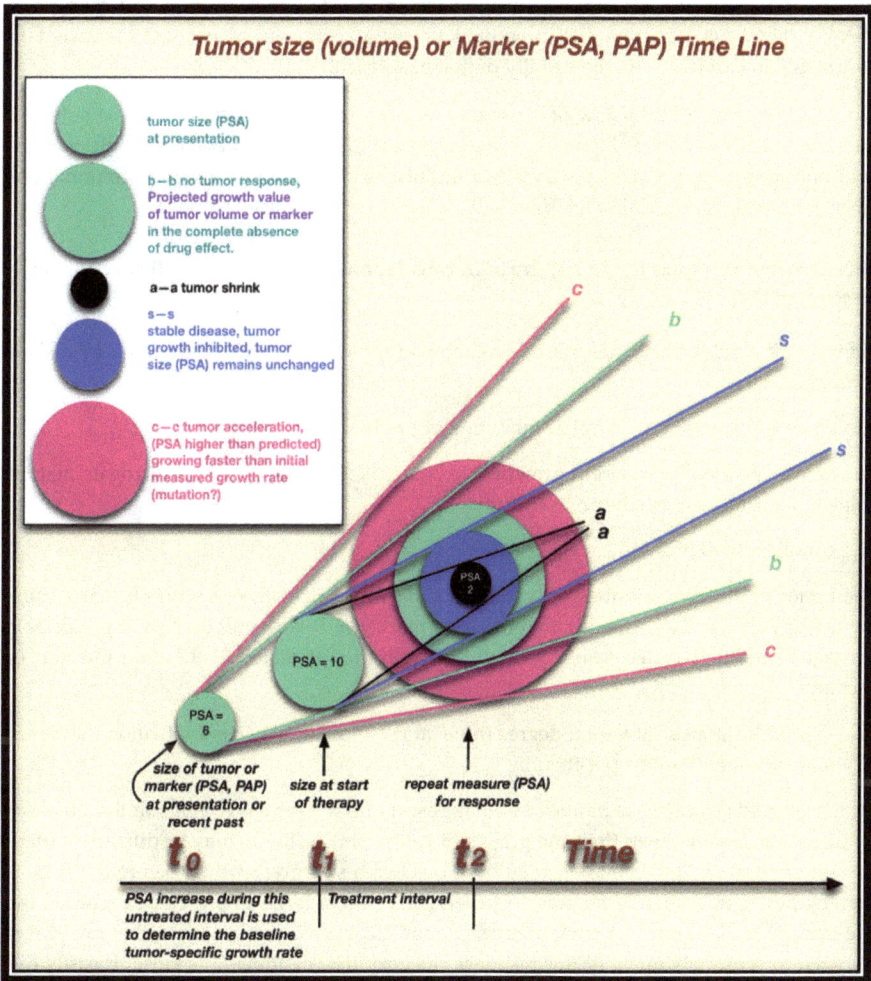

**Figure 7.** Tumor size (volume) or Marker (PSA, PAP) Time Line

Figure 7 illustrates potential tumor responses to drug treatment. Some of the responses such as positive and negative deviation from the **projected PSA** value or **projected tumor volume** are routinely overlooked in the clinic because **projected sizes** for these parameters must be calculated in advance (projected volume is illustrated by the largest b-b green circle at $t_2$). SGR is calculated based on tumor or PSA growth between $t_0$ and $t_1$. Deviations from **projected values** reveal subtle drug-tumor interactions. In the appendix we discuss straightforward evaluation of all five-treatment outcome scenarios illustrated above by a hand-held computer.

Until now, most attempts to capture drug effects vs. prostate tumors employed changes of PSA-DT. However, Mehrara [70] presented newer assessments of PSA-DT compared to PSA-SGR that cast doubt on the validity of that historic collection of work.

What follows is a general listing of consequences of drug-tumor interaction. These potential tumor or marker responses Figures 6, 7 are important to understand because subtle changes in tumor proliferation may be the only drug-induced tumor response and may go unnoticed when evaluating targeted therapy by RECIST/RECIST 1.1 response criteria.

### 10.2. Targeted therapies might require SGR calculations to evaluate the full spectrum of tumor response

Figures 6, 7 display tumor responses evaluable in the clinic. RESIST 1.1 criteria follow for comparison.

**1.** Disease stabilization (complete inhibition of pre-therapy SGR)

The marker or tumor's **inherent growth rate** is inhibited causing it or its surrogate marker value to remain unchanged during therapy.

**2.** Uninterrupted growth

The tumor or marker continues its calculated pre-therapy growth rate without change during therapy. The growth noted in the surrogate marker or tumor after therapy is predictable and equal to the projected tumor growth based on the calculated SGR before the start of therapy.

**3.** Tumor "response" of varied degree (note: at the time of response evaluation the tumor may be larger than the pre-therapy value)

Tumor or marker growth is inhibited and at post-therapy response evaluation the tumor or its surrogate marker is **less than the projected value**. This response may be difficult to identify since the tumor or its marker may have reached a size greater than before the start of therapy however, tumor or marker post therapy is **not as large as projected** based on the pre-therapy SGR Figure 7. A computer calculation comparing pre- and post-therapy SGR is required to accurately quantify this response category. TR (treatment response) is easily calculable and offers an objective and continuous value for the degree of response. TR is used as either a "tumor response" or "tumor marker response", to quantitate the effect of therapy. This continuous variable is useful to directly compare treatment efficacy between differing therapies.

Mehrara [71] defined some limitations for the current use of treatment response including: 1) PR and CR as defined in RECIST and other methods are no longer of value for quantifying responses to cytostatic/cytolentic drugs. Combinations of cytolytic and cytostatic/cytolentic therapies add further difficulty to response interpretation. A further problem arises when drugs are used at the extremes of dosing where tumor-killing activity may change from cytostatic/cytolentic to cytolytic and vise versa. 2) Classically, no consideration is given to the persistence of tumor SGR and or its inhibition during the course of therapy. Clinically, this is a trap for the oncologist if response is based solely in terms of whether the tumor marker or size is decreased at the end of therapy 3) The advantage of TR as a continuous variable (as opposed to a discrete variable used to compartmentalize responses such as CR, PR, SD) is that TR is a measurement of inhibitory (+TR) as well as accelerating (-TR) drug effects and is directly comparable between therapies and independent of mechanism of drug action.

A simple statement that the marker or tumor is larger post therapy is no longer adequate to evaluate tumor responses.

**4.**     The size of the tumor or its surrogate marker decreases after therapy.

This may be a partial or complete return to normal, manifest by partial or complete disappearance of tumor/marker abnormality.

**5.**     Tumor acceleration and deceleration

Tumor **acceleration** occurs when the tumor or marker growth rate (SGR) after therapy is greater than the pre-therapy or baseline SGR and SGR = (SGR after Rx − SGR before Rx) / (t2−t1) is a negative value. Tumor growth rate acceleration is positive and may indicate the presence of a tumor-accelerating mutation or an unexpected untoward drug effect.

Tumor **deceleration** occurs when SGR before therapy is greater than SGR after therapy and is expressed as: $SGR$ deceleration = $(SGR$ after Rx − $SGR$ before Rx$) / (t2−t1)$  this is a negative value.

The rate of change calculations are based on the pre-therapy calculated SGR and its rate of change is calculated at the end of therapy and is expressed as: Acceleration or deceleration of the SGR: $\Delta SGR / \Delta t$. Or EDITOR use $(SGR_2 - SGR_1)/(T_2 - T_1)$.

Note: In the presence of multiple tumor targets the sum of tumor diameters or volumes is used as an approximation. Clonal heterogeneity (a mosaic of tumors growing at different growth rates and or demonstrating a mixed response) may make some tumors inadequate for analysis.

In 1999 an attempt to write a specific dogma evaluating tumor response resulted in the RECIST 1.0 criteria, later updated 2009 as RECIST 1.1 [73]. Note the absence of drug-response based on the concept of projected tumor growth.

RECIST 1.1 criteria

**Complete Response (CR):** Disappearance of all target lesions. Any pathological lymph nodes (whether target or non-target) must have reduction in short axis to <10 mm.

**Partial Response (PR):** At least a 30% decrease in the sum of diameters of target lesions, taking as reference the baseline sum of diameters.

**Progressive Disease (PD):** At least a 20% increase in the sum of diameters of target lesions, taking as reference the smallest sum on study (this includes the baseline sum if that is the smallest on study). In addition to the relative increase of 20%, the sum must also demonstrate an absolute increase of at least 5 mm. (Note: the appearance of one or more new lesions is also considered progression).

**Stable Disease (SD):** Neither sufficient shrinkage to qualify for PR nor sufficient increase to qualify for PD, taking as reference the smallest sum diameters while on study.

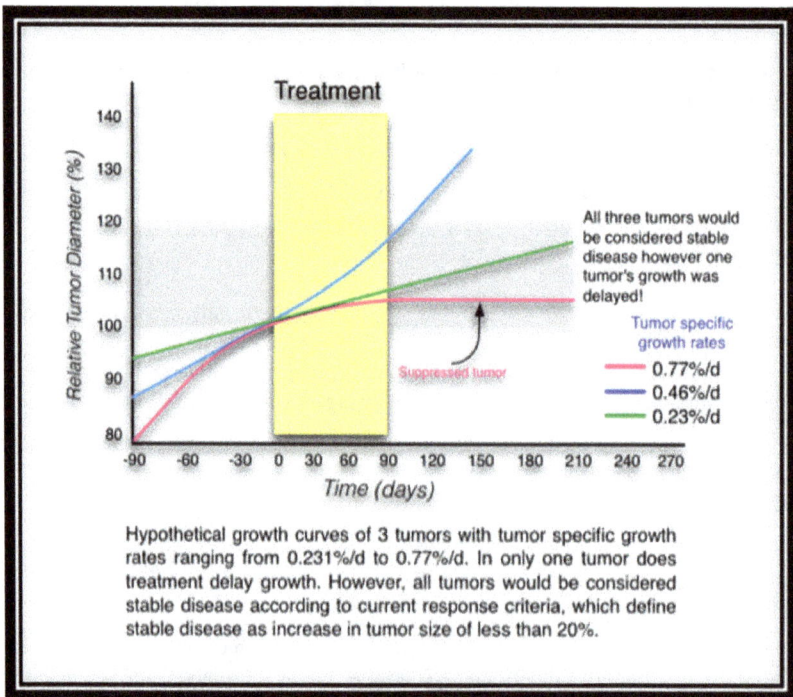

Hypothetical growth curves of 3 tumors with tumor specific growth rates ranging from 0.231%/d to 0.77%/d. In only one tumor does treatment delay growth. However, all tumors would be considered stable disease according to current response criteria, which define stable disease as increase in tumor size of less than 20%.

**Figure 8.** Weber [74] reveals the difficulty of classifying real growth inhibition within the RECIST1.1 criteria of stable disease. Real or suppressed tumor growth is illustrated by the pink growth curve only.

Weber noted that the RECIST 1.1 disease stabilization category does not differentiate between a drug that slows tumor growth and the complete lack of drug effect Figure 8. The RECIST 1.1 definition for disease progression is >5 mm absolute increase in size in addition to >20% increase compared with the nadir. In this figure, though all three tumors do not meet the progressive disease criteria and thus would be termed stable, the growth of the third was slowed by therapy. Though all three are termed stable, note the subtle difference between the two tumors showing a continued and uninterrupted pre-therapy growth rate (SGR), compared to the slowed growth rate of the tumor depicted by the red line. Surely there is a drug effect vs. the red tumor. This active drug could be overlooked in spite of its potential to increase survival if maintained for a sufficient period of time.

In a review of a group of patients treated with targeted therapies, Tourneau [75] revealed clinical evidence where investigators overlooked subtle cytostatic/cytolentic (slowing of SGR) drug activity Figure 6, 8. The group analyzed 50 patient participants in 18 targeted therapy drug trials. Among the 44 patients who withdrew from study because of disease progression according to the investigators' assessment, 18 patients (41%) demonstrated a favorable slowing trend in tumor specific growth rate. Among the 18, 5 had disease progression according to RECIST 1.1 according to retrospective reassessment of on-study imaging and occurrence of no new lesion during study treatment. Their preliminary evaluation concluded that a substantial proportion of patients treated with targeted agents were removed from protocol in spite of possibly benefitting from therapy.

Ferte et al. [76] studied metastatic renal cell carcinoma patients treated with sorafenib (Nexavar) and everolimus (Afinitor). Analysis of tumor SGR clearly revealed drug effects that would have been missed had RECIST response criteria been applied. Tumor response was assessed before, during, at the time of tumor progression and after drug discontinuation. Tumor growth rate was computed by dividing tumor shrinkage by the time between two related evaluations (% RECIST x 100 /day).

In two different patient populations (IGR and TARGET) tumor growth rate significantly decreased following sorafenib (-23.6 vs. 20 (IGR) and -19 vs. 22 (TARGET)) and everolimus (-5.2 vs. 30 (IGR)). The great majority of patients (IGR) had a decrease in the tumor growth rate during vs. before therapy, regardless of the RECIST evaluation, both with sorafenib (28/29) or everolimus (36/37). Growth rate after sorafenib or everolimus interruption was significantly higher than at the time of progression in both settings (IGR) (14.6 vs. 31 and 17.9 vs. 32.1 respectively). No significant difference was observed between growth rate before or after therapy for either sorafenib or everolimus (IGR). They concluded that SGR evaluation revealed: 1) better evaluation of tumor response, regardless of RECIST criteria, 2) had independent prognostic value, 3) the possibility that continuation of sorafenib or everolimus after disease progression might be beneficial to patients by sustaining a continued suppression of tumor growth.

The following section presents a model of tumor growth rate expressed as an executable algorithm in the form of an Apple App that quantitates subtle changes of tumor specific growth rate (SGR).

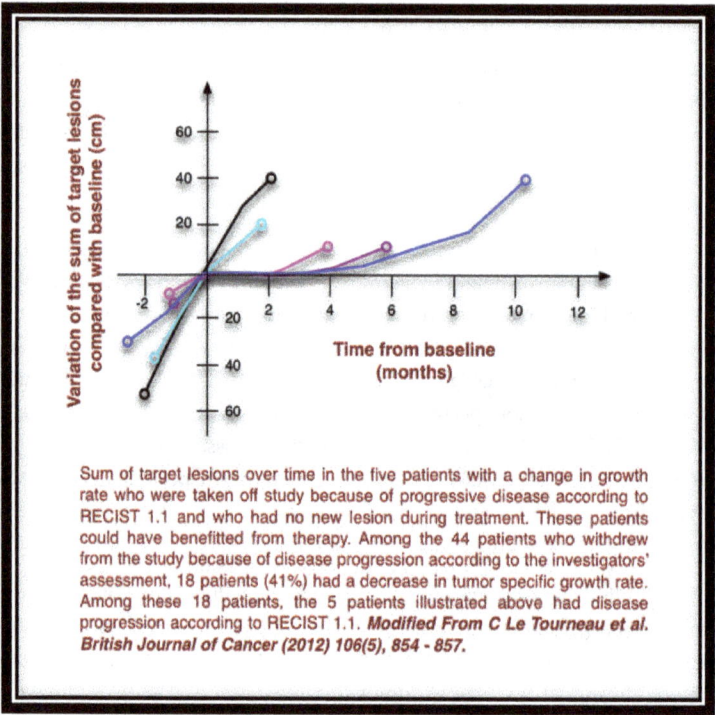

Sum of target lesions over time in the five patients with a change in growth rate who were taken off study because of progressive disease according to RECIST 1.1 and who had no new lesion during treatment. These patients could have benefitted from therapy. Among the 44 patients who withdrew from the study because of disease progression according to the investigators' assessment, 18 patients (41%) had a decrease in tumor specific growth rate. Among these 18 patients, the 5 patients illustrated above had disease progression according to RECIST 1.1. *Modified From C Le Tourneau et al. British Journal of Cancer (2012) 106(5), 854 - 857.*

**Figure 9.** Following a patient's tumor size often reveals subtle changes in the slope of the tumor measurement or marker growth curve as revealed above. These subtle changes in growth rate are not associated with a significant decrease of tumor size or marker value. As Le Tourneau et al. and Ferte et al. demonstrate, subtle changes in tumor growth rate are not evaluated as a response when applying RECIST 1.1 criteria nevertheless, they do represent a true cytostatic effect of targeted therapies that may translate into a meaningful prolonged survival.

## 11. SGR is a useful tool to identify subtle drug-associated tumor or marker kinetic changes of tumors

Mehrara, as part of his PhD thesis at the Department of Radiation Physics, University of Gothenburg, Goteborg, Sweden presented an analysis of tumor growth kinetics based on the tumor specific growth rate constant (SGR). The analysis assumes that for most practical purposes clinically observable tumor growth follows exponential growth. Additionally, this is true for the surrogate PSA tumor marker. SGR is rapidly calculable by hand-held mobile devices and facilitates the rapid identification of tumor responses easily overlooked in the clinic, many of which are not readily apparent without computer analysis. Occasionally, changes of SGR uncover subtle tumor stimulation.

Construction of the exponential growth curve, similar in shape to the mid portion of the Gompertzian curve Figure 1, requires just two different measurements of tumor volume (or diameter, area, cell number) or a surrogate marker at two different times to satisfy the exponential growth equation: $Vt = V0e^{at}$. Here "$a$" is the exponential growth constant, and $V_t$ and $V_0$ are the tumor volume at times t and $t_0$, respectively. This model implies that tumor volume can increase indefinitely and the growth rate of a tumor is proportional to its volume and $dV/dt = aV$.

SGR is the relative change in tumor volume per unit time calculable as percent increase or decrease of tumor volume per unit time. Excluding mutations, for exponentially growing tumors, SGR is constant, *i.e.*, SGR or $a$ is independent of tumor volume or age. Faster growing tumors have higher SGR values, SGR=0 represents non-growing tumors; a negative SGR represents tumor regression. In 1956 Collins et al. [9] graphically introduced the concept of tumor doubling time. The DT formulation was proposed in 1961 [10]: DT = $(t_2-t_1)$ * ln(2) / [ln($V_2/V_1$)]. Other relationships of importance include the specific growth rate, SGR = ln($V_2/V_1$)/($t_2-t_1$) and DT = ln(2)/SGR. These equations are descendants of the primary exponential growth equation, $V_t = V_0e^{at}$

Mehrara expresses concerns based on his mathematical treatment of SGR and DT suggesting that for clinical studies, SGR is the best indicator of tumor growth. Tumor growth rate, especially but not limited to urology circles, is usually quantified as DT i.e. PSA-DT. Because of the subtle mathematical relationship between SGR and DT, use of DT alone to evaluate therapeutic effects may give erroneous results.

Mehrara's studies revealed that DT has several drawbacks when used to describe tumor or tumor marker growth rates. The shortfalls include 1) for brief measurement time intervals, or high volume and very small measurement uncertainties the mean DT can either overestimate or underestimate the average growth rate; 2) DT approaches infinity for very slow growing tumors and is mathematically limited while SGR is a continuous variable no mater the speed and 3) the non normal frequency distribution of DT values restricts use of parametric statistics thus reducing use of more discriminatory statistics especially when studying small samples [77]. Unlike DT, SGR is definable for all tumor volume changes no matter how small, and it is Gaussian (normally) distributed allowing use of parametric statistics. SGR is more accurate to use when considering growth fraction, cell loss rate, and tumor growth rate heterogeneity. For these reasons, Mehrara opines that SGR be used instead of DT, to quantify tumor growth rate.

Accuracy and clinical outcome analysis comparing SGR and DT would be a valuable area of research in light of the cytostatic changes leading to subtle changes of growth rate characteristic of targeted therapies. Later, an in depth illustration of the differences between DT and SGR will help illuminate this issue.

Collins and Schwartz [9, 10] both analyzed several tumors in patients as they defined the use of tumor volume doubling time. Note that for bronchogenic lung cancers a semi-logarithmic plot of tumor diameter (y-axis) versus a linear time period (x-axis) produces a near straight line Figure 2.

## 12. Measuring tumor growth

It is imperative to depend on sensitive and precise marker assays. Guess [38] tried to address this problem by use of splines or line segments to average all PSA-DT values in an attempt to better detect therapy-induced changes of PSA-DT. Unfortunately, this computerized technique is cumbrous for most to apply.

The accurate and reproducible measurement of tumor diameters from imaging studies is critical. Keep in mind that occasionally plain radiographs of larger lesions are preferred because CT imaging may slice through a lesion at variable levels producing aberrant results for elliptical lesions.

A closer look at differences between DT and SGR.

The mathematical relationship between DT and SGR as revealed by the exponential growth model is important because as displayed in Figure 10, sole use of tumor volume doubling time (TV-DT) or tumor marker doubling time (PSA-DT) rather than tumor or marker specific growth rate as a measure of treatment outcome may be destined for failure depending on the magnitude of differences in the clinical study. Applying the exponential model of tumor growth to published studies reporting only DT as displayed here Table 1,2 and Figures 11,12 reveals discordant conclusions from those using SGR. Note that the DT is mathematically logarithmically related to the inverse of the exponential growth constant (SGR): SGR = ln(2)/DT.

The opposite results using SGR compared to those obtained with DT are critical since prostate cancer research is steeped in the use of the PSA-DT to predict survival, tumor dissemination, relapse, and tumor response to drugs and hormones and to radiation efficacy. In the prostate cancer literature use of DT as a parameter of response is established canon.

Mehrara reveals that DT is not normally symmetrically distributed (non-Gaussian distribution) and its use as an indicator of treatment response could yield inaccurate conclusions. Changes in DT over-predict drug effects in slow growing tumors while they under-predict in rapidly growing tumors and DT is essentially of no value for tumor volumes (or markers) that show no change in value (stable disease) where DT approaches infinity see Figure 10.

Work by others confirms the importance of the tumor or marker-specific growth rate. Stein et al. [46] studied a combination of equations that simultaneously modeled both tumor/ PSA regression and tumor/PSA exponential growth. They found that only the exponential growth equation with its specific growth rate constant (PSA-SGR) predicted a statistically significant high mortality hazard ratio of 5.14 (95% confidence interval, 3.10 - 8.52) in his study group of patients with prostate cancer. The disease regression formula was unable to predict patient mortality.

## 13. Why PSA-SGR is more useful than PSA-DT

As noted in Figure 10, when SGR is fast and increases 1% from 4 to 5%/day, the doubling time changes 1.3-fold from 4 to 3 days (a slight change). However, when the SGR is slower and increases 1% from 1 • 2%/d, doubling time changes four-fold from 69 to 17 days (a large change). A DT of 1-day does not represent the same growth rate when the tumor is slowing as when the tumor is rapidly growing. As the absolute value of SGR approaches zero, DT approaches infinity and is of no practical use other than to say the tumor or marker is stable. Because of the DT-SGR relationship at the extremes of tumor or marker growth, therapy-induced changes in doubling times at the extremes of SGR do not accurately represent the magnitude of the impact of therapy.

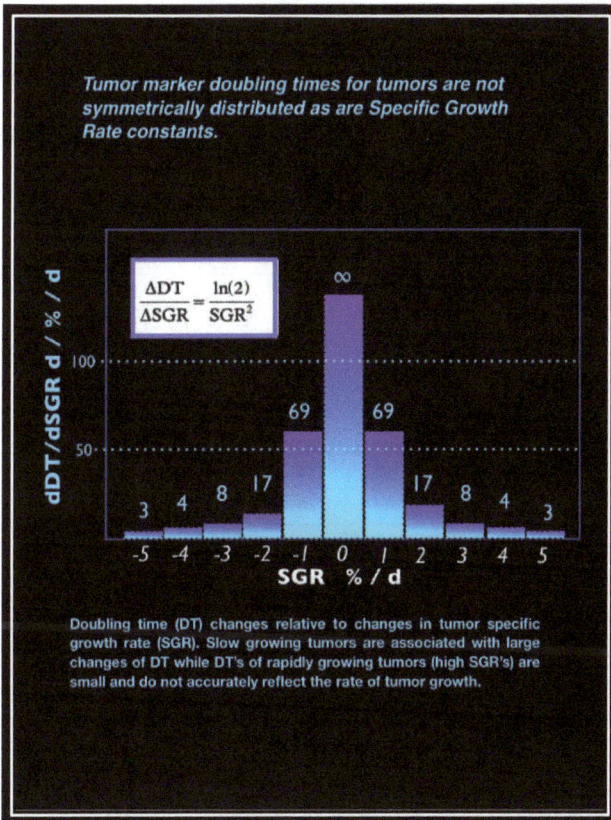

**Figure 10.** This figure, modified from Mehrara [70], displays the variation of tumor volume doubling time or tumor marker doubling time (DT) per unit change of tumor specific growth rate (SGR) based on:.

## 14. Clinical application of DT and SGR: Discordant results

Mehrara retrieved data from two previously published clinical studies [70]. The first by Guess et al. [38] Table 1 who studied the effect of modified citrus pectin (MCP) on PSA-DT of 12 prostate cancer patients. Mehrara extracted data and analyzed for both PSA-DT and PSA-SGR before and after therapy. The difference between PSA-DT before and after treatment was not found to be statistically significant by the paired t-test (p = 0.27). Nevertheless, when transforming PSA-DT to PSA-SGR the difference before and after MCP treatment is statistically significant by the paired t-test (p = 0.003) and nonparametric Wilcoxon matched pairs signed rank test: p = 0.002. Thus, a therapy initially deemed ineffective by PSA-DT analysis, when analyzed for a group of patients based on PSA-SGR proved to be highly significant Table 1.

| | Effect of modified citrus pectin (MCP) on PSA-DT and PSA-SGR | | | |
|---|---|---|---|---|
| Patient | Before Rx PSA-DT (mo) | After Rx PSA-DT (mo) | Before Rx PSA-SGR (%/mo) | After Rx PSA-SGR (%/mo) |
| A | 3.97 | 13.34 | 17.46 | 5.16 |
| B | 5.67 | 10.11 | 12.22 | 6.86 |
| C | 1.14 | 2.91 | 60.80 | 23.82 |
| D | 3.37 | 7.71 | 20.57 | 8.99 |
| E | 1.58 | 16.49 | 43.87 | 4.20 |
| F | 10.5 | 7.97 | 6.60 | 8.70 |
| G | 2.66 | 11.95 | 26.06 | 5.80 |
| H | 3.64 | 3.27 | 19.04 | 21.20 |
| I | 2.04 | 4.96 | 33.98 | 13.97 |
| J | 2.33 | 3.24 | 29.75 | 21.39 |
| K | 6.29 | -155.49 | 11.02 | -0.45 |
| L | 5.12 | -645.51 | 13.54 | -0.11 |

Nonparametric Wilcoxon matched pairs signed rank: p = 0.42
Parametric Paired t-test p = 0.2704

Nonparametric Wilcoxon matched pairs signed rank: p = 0.002
Parametric Paired t-test p = 0.0027

**Table 1.** Guess et al. [38] studied the effect of modified citrus pectin (MCP) on PSA-DT of 12 prostate cancer patients. Mehrara extracted that data and analyzed both PSA-DT and PSA-SGR before and after therapy. The difference between PSA-DT before and after treatment was not statistically significant by the paired t-test (p = 0.27). Nevertheless, when transforming PSA-DT to PSA-SGR the difference before and after MCP treatment is statistically significant by the paired t-test (p = 0.003) and nonparametric Wilcoxon matched pairs signed rank test: p = 0.002.

A second analysis of original data by Nishida et al. (1999) [78] was based on a study of the correlation of tumor volume and the CA19-9 tumor marker of pancreatic cancer patients Table 2. The correlation between CA19-9-DT and tumor volume-DT was statistically significant (p<0.0001). However, after converting tumor-volume-DT to TV-SGR and CA19-9-DT to CA19-9-SGR, correlation between CA19-9-SGR and TV-SGR was no longer statistically significant (p>0.3). Since SGR is the preferred parameter, the initial analysis of Nishida may benefit from a second look.

| Relationship between CA19-9-DT and TV-DT vs. CA19-9-SGR and TV-SGR | | | | |
|---|---|---|---|---|
| Patient | CA19-9 DT (Days) | Tumor-DT (Days) | CA19-9-SGR %/day | Tumor-SGR %/day |
| A | 8.3 | 34.8 | 8.4 | 2 |
| B | 39.7 | 44.6 | 1.7 | 1.6 |
| C | 46.3 | 34.5 | 1.5 | 2 |
| D | 36.5 | 21.2 | 1.9 | 3.3 |
| E | 30.4 | 47.7 | 2.3 | 1.5 |
| F | 67.1 | 112.8 | 1 | 0.6 |
| G | 44.7 | 70.6 | 1.6 | 1 |
| H | 24.7 | 18.4 | 2.8 | 3.8 |
| I | 42.7 | 50.6 | 1.6 | 1.4 |
| J | 137.5 | 231.6 | 0.5 | 0.3 |
| K | 42.3 | 39.3 | 1.6 | 1.8 |
|  | Linear regression: $r^2 = 0.89$ p < 0.0001 | | Linear regression: $r^2 = 0.09$ p = 0.37 | |

**Table 2.** This table displays the extracted data from Nishida's study [78] of the correlation of tumor volume and the CA19-9 tumor marker of pancreatic cancer patients. The correlation between CA19-9-DT and tumor volume-DT was statistically significant (p<0.0001). However, after converting tumor-volume-DT to TV-SGR and CA19-9-DT to CA19-9-SGR, correlation between CA19-9-SGR and TV-SGR was no longer statistically significant (p>0.3).

Most prostate cancer studies employ changes in the PSA-DT. PSA-DT values are not normally distributed and thus not readily subject to more sensitive parametric statistical analysis. However, PSA-specific growth rate is normally distributed and parametric statistics can be applied. Nonparametric statistical methods lose discriminatory power especially for clinical studies of smaller groups of patients [77].

During a cursory review of the literature we found two additional studies, one dealing with the effects of celecoxib on PSA-DT Figure 11 and the other investigating the effects of a combination of calcitriol and naproxin on PSA-DT of prostate cancer patients Figure 12.

Smith et al. [79] Figure 11 studied the biologic activity of celecoxib, a selective cyclooxygenase-2 inhibitor, in men with recurrent prostate cancer using change in PSA-DT as the primary outcome variable. We carefully extracted the data from his graphic report. We applied the Wilcoxon matched-pairs signed rank test [two tailed] (for nonparametric distribution of

PSA-DT) to the data. PSA-DT before versus after celecoxib was highly significant: p = 0.0006. After transformation of PSA-DT to PSA-SGR, the Paired t-test [two tailed] for parametric distribution of PSA-SGR suggests that the celecoxib effect lacked statistical significance p = 0.213!

A second study by Srinivas [80] Figure 12 evaluated naproxen in combination with calcitriol in patients with early recurrent prostate cancer. All patients received 45 µg of calcitriol (DN101, Novacea, South San Francisco, CA, USA) orally once a week with naproxen 375 mg twice a day and were evaluated for a biochemical PSA response and a change in PSA doubling time (PSA-DT). Testing the efficacy of the combination therapy using changes of PSA-DT by the non-parametric Wilcoxon matched-pairs signed rank test [two tailed] p = 0.037 a significant difference. However, after transforming PSA-DT to PSA-SGR ($SGR_{PSA}$ = ln(2)/$DT_{PSA}$), analysis with the parametric Paired t-test [2-tailed] indicate naproxen plus calcitriol was not effective in slowing tumor growth, p = 0.213.

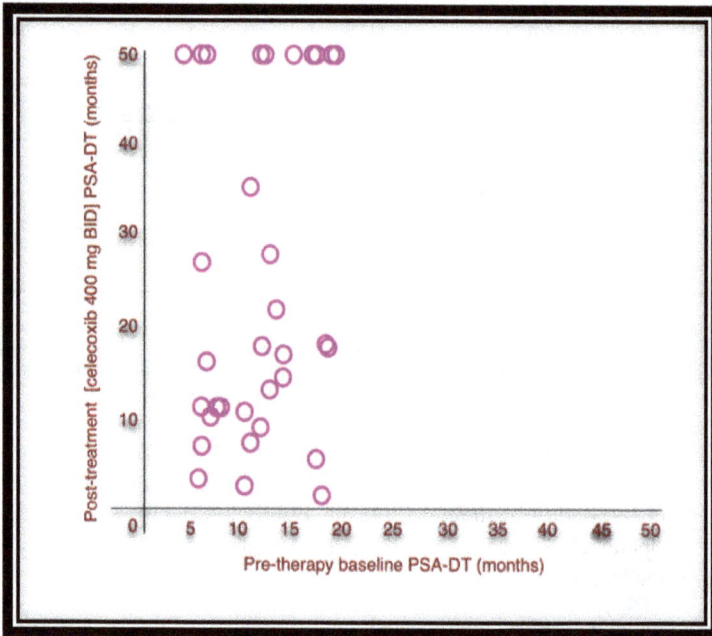

Figure 11. Smith et al. [79] studied the biologic activity of celecoxib, a selective cyclooxygenase-2 inhibitor, in men with recurrent prostate cancer using change in PSA-DT as the primary outcome variable. We retrieved their graphic data for our own analysis. A histogram of the PSA-DT paired differences for before and after celecoxib appears normally distributed. Applying the parametric Paired t-test statistic for significance of the difference yields p = 0.0002. Next, we transformed the same (before-after celecoxib PSA-DT data with to PSA-SGR before and after pairs and applied the paired t-test. Contrary to the statistical analysis for celecoxib induced change of PSA-DT, changes of PSA-SGR revealed that the celecoxib difference was no longer significant, p = 0.213!

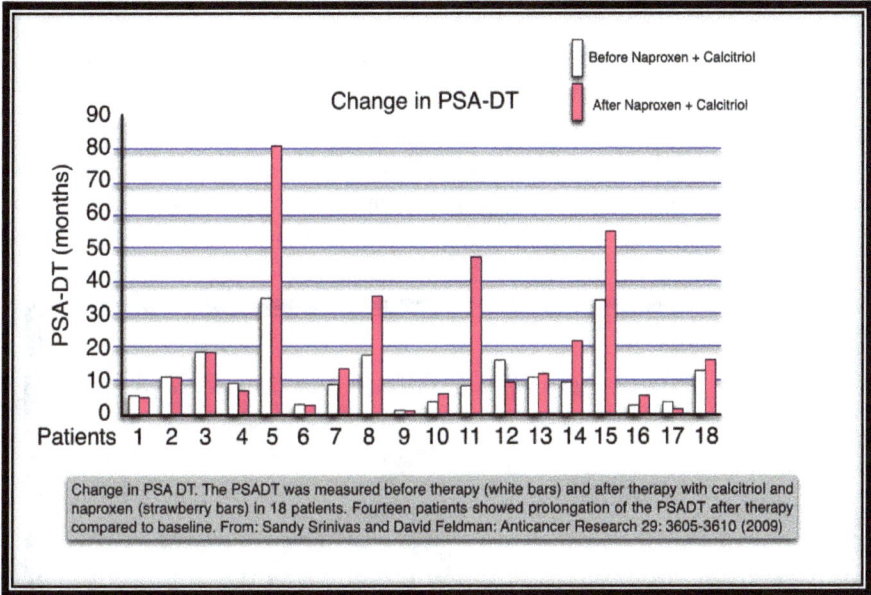

Change in PSA DT. The PSADT was measured before therapy (white bars) and after therapy with calcitriol and naproxen (strawberry bars) in 18 patients. Fourteen patients showed prolongation of the PSADT after therapy compared to baseline. From: Sandy Srinivas and David Feldman: Anticancer Research 29: 3605-3610 (2009)

**Figure 12.** Sinivras and Feldman [80] evaluated naproxen in combination with calcitriol in patients with early recurrent prostate cancer. All patients received 45 μg of calcitriol (DN101, Novacea, South San Francisco, CA, USA) orally once a week with naproxen 375 mg twice a day and were evaluated for a biochemical PSA response and a change in PSA doubling time (PSA-DT). Applying the paired t-test for statistical significance (before PSA-DT and after PSA-DT) resulted in p = 0.034. Nevertheless, after transforming PSA-DT to PSA-SGR (PSA-SGR = ln(2)/PSA-DT), analysis with the paired t-test [2-tailed] suggested naproxen plus calcitriol was not effective in slowing tumor growth, p = 0.213.

The non-linear relationship between the SGR and DT may be responsible for erroneous interpretations of treatment effects reported in prior prostate cancer trials that published results solely in terms of changes in PSA-DT Figure 10.

## 15. Evaluation of tumor and surrogate marker drug responses, rate of change of response:
*SGR* acceleration = (*SGR* after Rx − *SGR* before Rx) / (*t*2−*t*1) ; A positive number

The dynamic of PSA change was used as an early predictor of overall survival after a short exposure to docetaxel therapy (4 doses). Knowledge that a drug may extend survival after just a short exposure would minimize toxicity from ineffective drugs. Hannenin's work [81] found that a rapid rate of PSA decline expressed as PSA half-life <70 days was associated with a longer overall-survival Figure 13. This result was independent of other known markers of survival and allowed for a greater survival differentiation than PSA suppression alone. Response-time evaluations may play a new role in determining drug efficacy earlier than usual. I would propose study of an alternate expression for tumor acceleration or deceleration in terms of SGR as: SGR (accel...decal) = $\text{SGR2-SGR1}/(t_2\text{-}t_1)$. The value of this expression may be positive for acceleration or negative for deceleration.

De Crevoisier [82] found that a PSA decline 6 weeks after the start of EBRT when used as monotherapy and 3 months after the start of androgen deprivation therapy (ADT) in patients treated with combined ADT and external beam radiation is predictive of progression and specific survival.

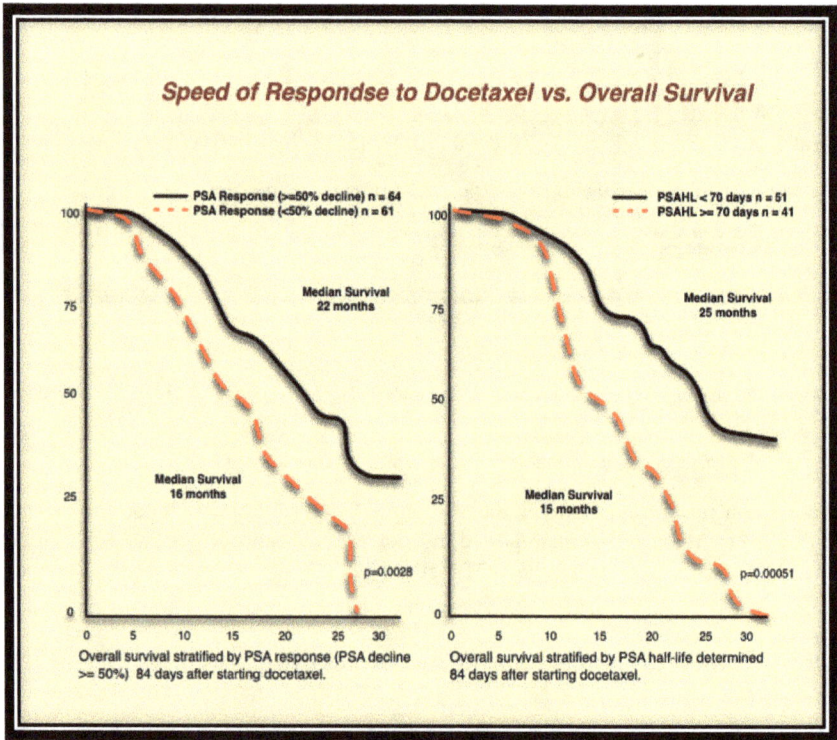

**Figure 13.** Treatment-associated tumor/marker deceleration in response to docetaxel. The magnitude of rate of change (acceleration-deceleration) of SGR resulting from therapy is an early predictor of prostate-specific survival.

Figure 14 illustrates a computer analysis of a prostate cancer patient treated with docetaxel. A pelvic node is noted to grow over 4.5 months from 1.3 to 1.6 cm in greatest dimension. This establishes the pre-therapy SGR of 0.46%/d and the tumor volume (assuming a sphere) before starting therapy is 2.1 cc. Fifty-one days of therapy induces a decrease of tumor diameter to 0.9 cc and a decrease of tumor volume to 0.38 cc. Had the tumor grown uninterrupted the projected tumor volume would have been 2.7 cc. In this case, the value for deceleration of SGR for the tumor: is given as $(SGR2$ after Rx $- SGR1$ before Rx$) / (t2 - t1) = -0.021\% / d / d$.

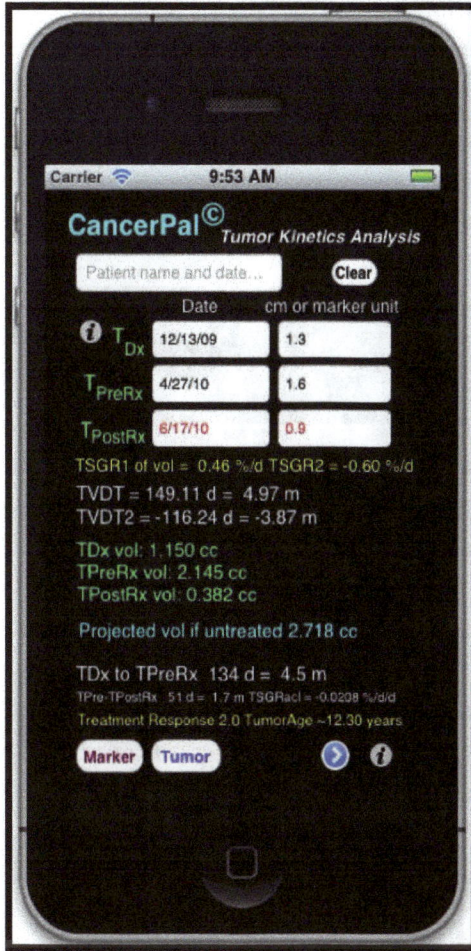

**Figure 14.** This calculation displays results for a patient treated with docetaxel (see text).

This is an objective measure of the rate of change of SGR. The treatment response is displayed as $= + 2.0$. This assigns a calculated continuous variable as a measure of the degree of response and is used to objectively compare docetaxel efficacy to any other administered drug. Positive TR values represent tumor reduction compared to the **projected** tumor size while a negative TR represents tumor growth relative to the **projected** size. Estimated age of tumor, here approximated ~ 12.3 years, is a calculated value based on the initial SGR of 0.46%/d in the absence of therapy. This assumes constant, continuous exponential growth over many years. Tumor age calculations are gross approximations and notoriously subject to large error.

Figure 15 illustrates the evaluation for a 68 year-old man undergoing watchful waiting for a Gleason score 3+3 = 6, T1c prostate cancer. Three PSA values are displayed for three sequential dates. When the patient was asked if he had changed medication between 3/2/11 and 5/1/11 he noted he was ingesting a new Chinese herbal mixture sold to enhance energy and libido.

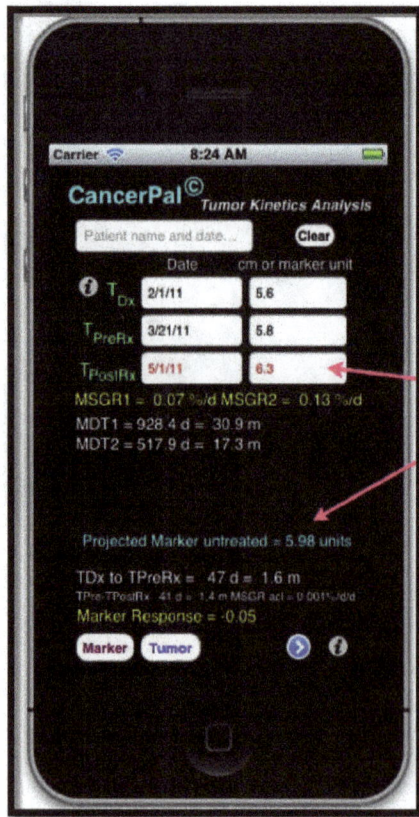

**Figure 15.** Evaluation of a 68 year-old man undergoing watchful waiting for a Gleason score 3+3 = 6, T1c prostate cancer. The patient was ingesting a stimulatory Chinese herb.

Subtle acceleration of the tumor marker value was uncovered by inspection of the projected PSA value for 5/1/11 as compared to the actual measured value for that date. Notice the confirmative quantitative measures given by the calculation Figure 14 of the marker specific growth rate $MSGR_2 = 0.13\%/d$ compared to $MSGR_1 = 0.07\%/d$; marker doubling time MDT2 = 17.3 months compared to the initial $MDT_1 = 30.9$ months; by both the positive value for MSGR acceleration = +0.001%/d/d and by the negative value for marker response MR = -0.05. Based on the marker-specific growth rate (MSGR) for the first interval TDx thru TPRx (the date at initiation of therapy) of 0.07%/d, the App calculated the expected PSA on 5/1/11 to be 5.98 ng/ml. However, the measured value was higher = 6.3 ng/ml. The negative value for MR of -0.05 indicates a negative marker response thus PSA expansion (marker acceleration confirmed this = +0.001%/d/d). We suspected that the Chinese herb might have caused subtle acceleration of PSA production and or tumor growth. Other explanations for acceleration of the PSA value include decreased clearance of PSA or the subtle appearance of a mutated, faster growing clone of PSA-producing tumor cells. Note that in the absence of knowledge of the inherent initial PSA-SGR between 2/1/11 and 3/2/11 and calculation of the expected **projected** value of PSA for 5/1/11, the subtle PSA acceleration would have been missed.

## 16. Predicting approximate tumor size or marker value for any arbitrary date in the future

Assuming untreated clinical cancers and their markers expand at a relatively constant exponential rate, it is possible to predict values for tumor diameter, volume and marker for any arbitrary future date. Figure 16 displays a PSA projection made for a patient with newly diagnosed prostate cancer who asked if a preplanned three-month holiday before initiation of therapy could jeopardize his chance for a curative procedure. The prediction, assuming constant exponential expansion of serum PSA, is that the PSA value upon returning from sabbatical would increase from 9.4 to 16.28 ng/ml. This alarmed the patient and he cancelled the trip to initiate therapy.

## 17. Unique treatment paradigms may be suggested by analysis of tumor growth rate

Figure 17 illustrates results for a patient with pancreatic cancer post Whipple procedure who was found on 6/4/10 to have an enlarged peri-aortic mass = 1.8 cm (3.1 cc). Repeat CT on 8/27/10 noted increased size to 2.9 cm (12.8 cc). Therapy with gemcitabine was initiated on 8/27/10. Post therapy reevaluation of the mass on 12/24/10 revealed growth to 3.1 cm (15.6 cc). The patient was discouraged and frightened and thought he had wasted precious

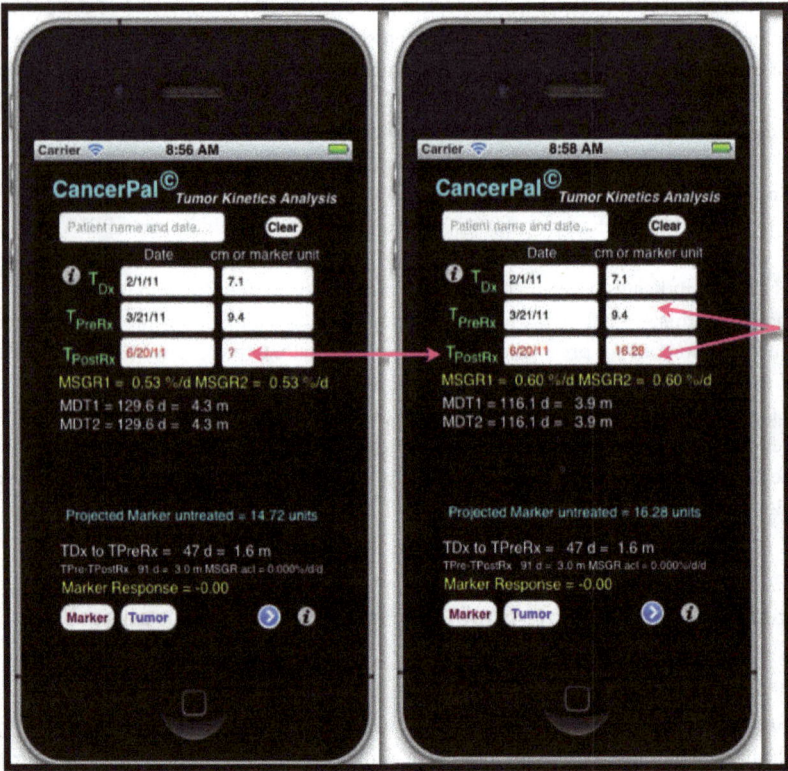

**Figure 16.** PSA projection made for a patient with newly diagnosed prostate cancer

time and subjected himself to undo toxicity for no gain. However, evaluation revealed that had the tumor never been treated with gemcitabine it would have reached the **projected volume** of 96.9 cc by 12/24/10. Thus, based on the initial exponential growth rate from 6/4/10 thru 8/27/10, the tumor volume was actually 84% **less than what it would have been** had no drug been given (15.6 cc vs. 96.9 cc).

This patient experienced substantial tumor suppression by gemcitabine in spite of its growth. Under these circumstances, when there are poor second choices for effective therapy, instead of discarding gemcitabine, perhaps addition of another compound with differing toxicity might be a reasonable option.

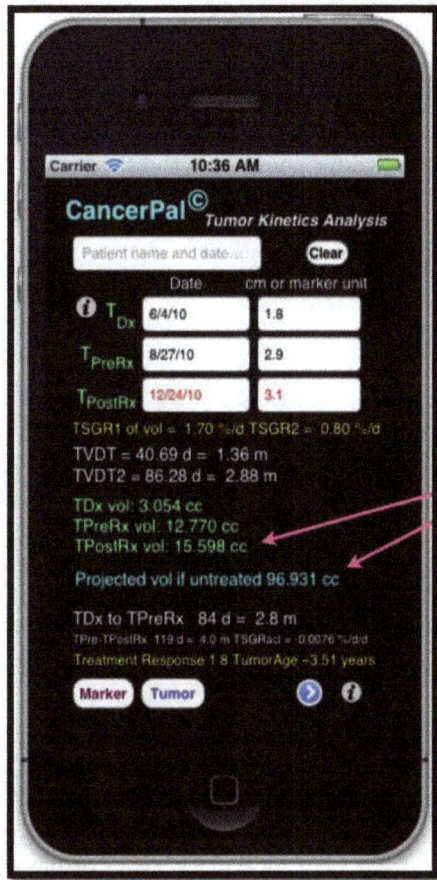

**Figure 17.** The tool we developed to facilitate calculation of tumor kinetics is named CancerPal©. The software App is available from Apple Corporation's App store. The App analyzes kinetic changes of tumor markers and or tumor diameter/volume/area and is run on the iPhone, iPad, or iPod. Clinical use is facilitated by the small size and portability of the new hand-held devices. The App is routinely used in our clinic for objectively measuring subtle drug effects on tumor and the dynamics of surrogate tumor markers. A video tutorial of the App is available at www.healthsciencereports.com.

## 18. Conclusion

Several principles of prostate cancer management rely on the absolute and dynamic values of various formulations of PSA i.e. PSA-V, PSA-DT and PSA-SGR. This review introduces SGR, a parameter that is underused and closely reflects the true growth rate of tumors undergoing exponential expansion. Several instances are presented where results of studies employing PSA-DT yield statistically divergent results after converting PSA-DT to PSA-SGR. It is recommended that for some studies results be reevaluated in terms of PSA specific growth rate, PSA-SGR.

Newly introduced targeted therapies require innovative techniques to evaluate drug efficacy. Tumor or tumor marker specific growth rate and the concept of **projected** tumor or marker value are tools capable of quantitatively evaluating subtle effects of targeted drugs. Calculation of the **projected** tumor size and tumor marker values is critical to properly evaluate subtle drug-tumor proliferative outcomes.

# Appendix

CancerPal©

It is important to realize that CancerPal© remains an experimental tool used strictly for analysis of clinical and laboratory data by cancer researchers, pharmacists or clinical research radiation and medical oncologists. The methods used in designing this tool have been discussed primarily in the references listed below with special attention given to the work of Mehrara et al. PNA, A Limited Liability Corporation, cannot be held responsible for any treatment modifications or recommendations made based on this research tool.

What CancerPal© does

CancerPal© evaluates whether a chemotherapy or targeted therapy should be continued alone, possibly dropped or added to by revealing concealed drug activity causing suppression of the tumor specific growth rate. The app uncovers occult efficacy of drugs by comparing the measured drug-induced tumor size vs. the projected tumor size or projected tumor-marker value that would occur in the absence of any therapy. Sudden changes in tumor growth rate suggesting drug related tumor stimulation or a detrimental, growth-promoting mutation is rapidly identified. CancerPal© may uncover hidden tumor acceleration unexpectedly caused by drugs, immunosuppression or alternative therapies thought to be harmless

CancerPal© uses a tumor's specific growth rate (TSGR) defined as percentage increase in volume per day or percentage increase in the specific tumor marker per day thus avoiding errors inherent in the doubling time calculation which consistently overestimates the growth rate of slowly growing tumors and underestimates the growth rate of rapidly growing tumors.

This app predicts the tumor diameter or tumor marker value at any time in the future assuming constant exponential tumor or tumor marker growth over the period of observation. This, when compared to the actual measured tumor diameter or marker value, identifies tumor response, stability or acceleration. The app predicts a tumor marker or diameter at any time point in the future based on patient-specific tumor kinetics. CancerPal© may quickly alert the clinician of emergence of a mutant, more aggressive, rapidly dividing clone of tumor cells suggesting a review of therapy. Analysis based on continual exponential growth for the relatively short time (several months) in the multi-year history of tumor growth has been found to be more useful for kinetic calculations in spite of some tumors demonstrating Gompertzian growth over the long haul (several years)

Continuous variables for Tumor Response (TR) and Marker Response (MR) allow for quantitation of drug/biological response modulator effects. Negative values of TR and MR indicate tumor acceleration, values close to or equal to zero indicate lack of response while positive values confirm beneficial tumor response. Responses are numerically quantitated and elusive disease stability may now numerically be defined by a continuous variable. Drugs previously thought to be of no value may be found to induce useful and profound disease stability

The software is helpful for those patients followed by watchful waiting/active surveillance for prostate or any other cancer. Prostate tumors changing biological behavior are immediately identified in a quantitative and objective manner by rapidly uncovering changes in PSA kinetics without the errors inherent in the PSA doubling time (PSA-DT) parameter. The software can help determine whether metastectomy is a reasonable treatment modality for some patients with pulmonary metastasis [83].

CancerPal© uses the exponential growth constant as described by John Spratt to extrapolate backwards to approximate the time of tumor initiation in years based on the rate of growth

Patient data required for analysis

Three dates and three associated measurements of a tumor marker or tumor diameter

- TDx (date at diagnosis + marker value or tumor diameter in cm)
- TPreRx (date of initiation of Rx + marker value or tumor diameter in cm)
- TPostRx (date of measurement of drug effect + tumor marker value or diameter in cm).

CancerPal© information output:

- Tumor Specific Volume Growth Rates for two intervals ($TSGR_1$ and $TSGR_2$)
- Tumor Marker Specific Growth Rates for two intervals ($MSGR_1$ and $MSGR_2$)
- Tumor Specific Growth Rate acceleration and deceleration
- Tumor Volume Doubling Times for two intervals (TVDT)
- Tumor Marker Doubling Time for two intervals (MDT)
- Projected TSGR and MSGR at any user designated time in the future
- Treatment Response as both Tumor Response and Tumor Marker Response, both as continuous numerical values used to quantitate the effect of therapy. Negative numbers reveal growth acceleration; values of zero reveal no effect and positive values indicate varying degrees of therapeutic efficacy.

- Tumor volumes in cc are calculated for TDx, TPreRx and TPostRx.

- Extrapolates back to the time of tumor initiation thus calculating how long it took for the tumor to reach the initial tumor diameter.

- Calculates approximate time to death in the absence of therapy, assuming constant tumor growth rate.

## Acknowledgements

Peter Jahn, Whittier, CA for manuscript review and discussion, mathematical suggestions and statistical considerations.

## Author details

Glenn Tisman

Whittier Cancer Research Building, Whittier, CA, USA

## References

[1] Bassukas ID. Comparative gompertzian analysis of alterations of tumor growth patterns. Cancer Res 1994, Aug 15; 54(16): 4385-92.

[2] Demicheli R, Foroni R, Ingrosso A, Pratesi G, Soranzo C, Tortoreto M. An exponential-gompertzian description of lovo cell tumor growth from in vivo and in *vitro data*. Cancer Res 1989, Dec 1; 49(23): 6543-6.

[3] Norton L. A gompertzian model of human breast cancer growth. Cancer Res 1988, Dec 15;48(24 Pt 1):7067-71.

[4] Mottram JC. On the correlation between malignancy and the rate of growth of tar warts in mice. Cancer Res 1934, Dec; 22(4): 801-30.

[5] Mottram JC. A further consideration of the growth rates of tar warts in mice and of their autografts. The American Journal of Cancer 1936; 28(1): 115-20.

[6] Laird AK. Dynamics of normal growth. Annual Report 1964; 6971:52.

[7] Laird AK. Dynamics of tumour growth: Comparison of growth rates and extrapolation of growth curve to one cell. Br J Cancer 1965; 19(2): 278.

[8] Friberg S, Mattson S. On the growth rates of human malignant tumors: Implications for medical decision-making. J Surg Oncol 1997, Aug; 65(4): 284-97.

[9]  Collins VP, Loeffler RK, Tivey H. Observations on growth rates of human tumors. Am J Roentgenol Radium Ther Nucl Med 1956, Nov; 76(5): 988-1000.

[10] Schwartz M. A biomathematical approach to clinical tumor growth. Cancer 1961; 14:1272-94.

[11] Spratt JS, Spjut HJ, Roper CL. The frequency distribution of the rates of growth and the estimated duration of primary pulmonary carcinomas. Cancer 1963, Jun; 16:687-93.

[12] Spratt Jr JS, Spratt TL. Rates of growth of pulmonary metastases and host survival. Ann Surg 1964; 159(2): 161.

[13] Steel GG, Lamerton LF. The growth rate of human tumours. Br J Cancer 1966, Mar; 20(1): 74-86.

[14] Loeb S, Kettermann A, Ferrucci L, Landis P, Metter EJ, Carter HB. PSA doubling time versus PSA velocity to predict high-risk prostate cancer: Data from the Baltimore longitudinal study of aging. Eur Urol 2008, Nov; 54(5): 1073-80.

[15] Tosoian J, Loeb S. PSA and beyond: The past, present, and future of investigative biomarkers for prostate cancer. ScientificWorldJournal 2010; 10:1919-31.

[16] Klotz L, Teahan S. Current role of PSA kinetics in the management of patients with prostate cancer. European Urology Supplements 2006, Apr; 5(6): 472-8.

[17] D'Amico AV, Chen MH, Roehl KA, Catalona WJ. Preoperative PSA velocity and the risk of death from prostate cancer after radical prostatectomy. N Engl J Med 2004, Jul 8; 351(2): 125-35.

[18] D'Amico AV, Chen MH, de Castro M, Loffredo M, Lamb DS, Steigler A, et al. Surrogate endpoints for prostate cancer-specific mortality after radiotherapy and androgen suppression therapy in men with localised or locally advanced prostate cancer: An analysis of two randomised trials. Lancet Oncol 2012, Feb; 13(2): 189-95.

[19] Miyamoto S. A chronological study of hepatic metastasis from colorectal cancer. Jpn J Gastroenterol Sur 1991;24:1990-6.

[20] Kato RB, Srougi V, Salvadori FA, Ayres PP, Leite KM, Srougi M. Pretreatment tumor volume estimation based on total serum psa in patients with localized prostate cancer. Clinics (Sao Paulo) 2008, Dec; 63(6): 759-62.

[21] Babaian RJ, Troncoso P, Steelhammer LC, Lloreta-Trull J, Ramirez EI. Tumor volume and prostate specific antigen: Implications for early detection and defining a window of curability. J Urol 1995, Nov; 154(5): 1808-12.

[22] Tanaka N, Fujimoto K, Hirayama A, Nakai Y, Chihara Y, Anai S, et al. Calculated tumor volume is an independent predictor of biochemical recurrence in patients who underwent retropubic radical prostatectomy. Adv Urol 2012; 2012:204215.

[23] Vollmer RT, Humphrey PA. Tumor volume in prostate cancer and serum prostate-specific antigen. Analysis from a kinetic viewpoint. Am J Clin Pathol 2003, Jan; 119(1): 80-9.

[24] Carter HB, Pearson JD, Waclawiw Z, Metter EJ, Chan DW, Guess HA, Walsh PC. Prostate-specific antigen variability in men without prostate cancer: Effect of sampling interval on prostate-specific antigen velocity. Urology 1995, Apr; 45(4): 591-6.

[25] Van den Bergh RC, Roemeling S, Roobol MJ, Wolters T, Schröder FH, Bangma CH. Prostate-specific antigen kinetics in clinical decision-making during active surveillance for early prostate cancer--a review. Eur Urol 2008, Sep; 54(3): 505-16.

[26] Ramírez ML, Nelson EC, Devere White RW, Lara PN, Evans CP. Current applications for prostate-specific antigen doubling time. Eur Urol 2008, Aug; 54(2): 291-300.

[27] Lonergan PE, Tindall DJ. Androgen receptor signaling in prostate cancer development and progression. J Carcinog 2011; 10:20.

[28] Bidart JM, Thuillier F, Augereau C, Chalas J, Daver A, Jacob N, et al. Kinetics of serum tumor marker concentrations and usefulness in clinical monitoring. Clin Chem 1999, Oct; 45(10): 1695-707.

[29] Nash AF, Melezinek I. The role of prostate specific antigen measurement in the detection and management of prostate cancer. Endocr Relat Cancer 2000, Mar; 7(1): 37-51.

[30] Ryan CJ, Smith A, Lal P, Satagopan J, Reuter V, Scardino P, et al. Persistent prostate-specific antigen expression after neoadjuvant androgen depletion: An early predictor of relapse or incomplete androgen suppression. Urology 2006;68(4):834-9.

[31] Kelloff GJ, Coffey DS, Chabner BA, Dicker AP, Guyton KZ, Nisen PD, et al. Prostate-specific antigen doubling time as a surrogate marker for evaluation of oncologic drugs to treat prostate cancer. Clin Cancer Res 2004, Jun 1; 10(11): 3927-33.

[32] Oudard S, Banu E, Scotte F, Banu A, Medioni J, Beuzeboc P, et al. Prostate-specific antigen doubling time before onset of chemotherapy as a predictor of survival for hormone-refractory prostate cancer patients. Ann Oncol 2007, Nov; 18(11): 1828-33.

[33] Newling DW. Issues with the use of prostate-specific antigen as a surrogate end point in hormone-resistant prostate cancer. European Urology Supplements 2009, Jan;8(1): 13-9.

[34] Singh AK, Guion P, Susil RC, Citrin DE, Ning H, Miller RW, et al. Early observed transient prostate-specific antigen elevations on a pilot study of external beam radiation therapy and fractionated MRI guided high dose rate brachytherapy boost. Radiat Oncol 2006; 1:28.

[35] Bubley GJ, Carducci M, Dahut W, Dawson N, Daliani D, Eisenberger M, et al. Eligibility and response guidelines for phase II clinical trials in androgen-independent

prostate cancer: Recommendations from the prostate-specific antigen working group. J Clin Oncol 1999, Nov; 17(11): 3461-7.

[36] WOO TCS, Richard Choo MD, Mary Jamieson RN, Chander BSNDS. Vitamin D3 (cholecalciferol) in the treatment of biochemically-relapsed prostate cancer. .

[37] Guess BW, Scholz MC, Strum SB, Lam RY, Johnson HJ, Jennrich RI. Modified citrus pectin (MCP) increases the prostate-specific antigen doubling time in men with prostate cancer: A phase II pilot study. Prostate Cancer Prostatic Dis 2003;6(4):301-4.

[38] Guess B, Jennrich R, Johnson H, Redheffer R, Scholz M. Using splines to detect changes in PSA doubling times. Prostate 2003, Feb 1; 54(2): 88-94.

[39] Therasse P, Arbuck SG, Eisenhauer EA, Wanders J, Kaplan RS, Rubinstein L, et al. New guidelines to evaluate the response to treatment in solid tumors. European organization for research and treatment of cancer, national cancer institute of the United States, national cancer institute of canada. J Natl Cancer Inst 2000, Feb 2; 92(3): 205-16.

[40] Therasse, P. Response assessment in cancer clinical trials. Doctorate thesis; Erasmus University, Rotterdam, 2006.

[41] Freedland SJ, Humphreys EB, Mangold LA, Eisenberger M, Dorey FJ, Walsh PC, Partin AW. Risk of prostate cancer-specific mortality following biochemical recurrence after radical prostatectomy. JAMA 2005, Jul 27; 294(4): 433-9.

[42] Armstrong AJ, Eisenberger MA, Halabi S, Oudard S, Nanus DM, Petrylak DP, et al. Biomarkers in the management and treatment of men with metastatic castration-resistant prostate cancer. Eur Urol 2012, Mar; 61(3): 549-59.

[43] Gupta S, Carballido E, Fishman M. Sipuleucel-T for therapy of asymptomatic or minimally symptomatic, castrate-refractory prostate cancer: An update and perspective among other treatments. Onco Targets Ther 2011; 4:79-96.

[44] Garcia JA. Sipuleucel-T in patients with metastatic castration-resistant prostate cancer: An insight for oncologists. Ther Adv Med Oncol 2011, Mar; 3(2): 101-8.

[45] Bitting RL, Armstrong AJ, George DJ. Management options in advanced prostate cancer: What is the role for sipuleucel-t? Clinical Medicine Insights: Oncology; 5:325-32.

[46] Stein WD, Gulley JL, Schlom J, Madan RA, Dahut W, Figg WD, et al. Tumor regression and growth rates determined in five intramural NCI prostate cancer trials: The growth rate constant as an indicator of therapeutic efficacy. Clin Cancer Res 2011, Feb 15; 17(4): 907-17.

[47] Madan RA, Bilusic M, Heery C, Schlom J, Gulley JL. Clinical evaluation of TRICOM vector therapeutic cancer vaccines. Semin Oncol 2012, Jun; 39(3): 296-304.

[48]  Kelly WK, Scher HI, Mazumdar M, Vlamis V, Schwartz M, Fossa SD. Prostate-specific antigen as a measure of disease outcome in metastatic hormone-refractory prostate cancer. J Clin Oncol 1993, Apr; 11(4): 607-15.

[49]  Smith DC, Dunn RL, Strawderman MS, Pienta KJ. Change in serum prostate-specific antigen as a marker of response to cytotoxic therapy for hormone-refractory prostate cancer. Journal of Clinical Oncology 1998; 16(5): 1835-43.

[50]  Berthold DR, Pond GR, Soban F, de Wit R, Eisenberger M, Tannock IF. Docetaxel plus prednisone or mitoxantrone plus prednisone for advanced prostate cancer: Updated survival in the TAX 327 study. J Clin Oncol 2008, Jan 10; 26(2): 242-5.

[51]  Berthold DR, Pond GR, de Wit R, Eisenberger M, Tannock IF, TAX 327 Investigators. Survival and PSA response of patients in the TAX 327 study who crossed over to receive docetaxel after mitoxantrone or vice versa. Ann Oncol 2008, Oct; 19(10): 1749-53.

[52]  Heidenreich A, Bolla M, Joniau S, Van Der Kwast TH, Matveev V, Mason MD, et al. Guidelines on prostate cancer. Eur Urol 2008; 53(1): 68-80.

[53]  Bellmunt J, Rosenberg JE, Choueiri TK. Recent progress and pitfalls in testing novel agents in castration-resistant prostate cancer. Eur Urol 2009; 56(4): 606.

[54]  Loriot Y, Massard C, Fizazi K. Recent developments in treatments targeting castration-resistant prostate cancer bone metastases. Ann Oncol 2012, May; 23(5): 1085-94.

[55]  Dahut WL, Scripture C, Posadas E, Jain L, Gulley JL, Arlen PM, et al. A phase II clinical trial of sorafenib in androgen-independent prostate cancer. Clin Cancer Res 2008, Jan 1; 14(1): 209-14.

[56]  Thuret R, Massard C, Gross-Goupil M, Escudier B, Di Palma M, Bossi A, et al. The postchemotherapy PSA surge syndrome. Ann Oncol 2008, Jul; 19(7): 1308-11.

[57]  Chi KN, Ellard SL, Hotte SJ, Czaykowski P, Moore M, Ruether JD, et al. A phase II study of sorafenib in patients with chemo-naive castration-resistant prostate cancer. Ann Oncol 2008, Apr; 19(4): 746-51.

[58]  Bellmunt J, Rosenberg JE, Choueiri TK. Recent progress and pitfalls in testing novel agents in castration-resistant prostate cancer. Eur Urol 2009; 56(4): 606.

[59]  Bellmunt J, Oh WK. Castration-resistant prostate cancer: New science and therapeutic prospects. Ther Adv Med Oncol 2010, May; 2(3): 189-207.

[60]  Rixe O, Fojo T. Is cell death a critical end point for anticancer therapies or is cytostasis sufficient? Clin Cancer Res 2007, Dec 15; 13(24): 7280-7.

[61]  Nabhan C, Tolzien K, Lestingi T, Kelby SK, Galvez AG, Bitran JD. Activity of sorafenib (SOR) in chemotherapy-failure castration-resistant prostate cancer (CRPC). ASCO/GU Proceedings 2010; 122.

[62]  Carmichael C, Lau C, Josephson DY, Pal SK. Comprehensive overview of axitinib development in solid malignancies: Focus on metastatic renal cell carcinoma. Clin Adv Hematol Oncol 2012 May; 10(5): 307-14.

[63]  Baselga J, Campone M, Piccart M, Burris HA, Rugo HS, Sahmoud T, et al. Everolimus in postmenopausal hormone-receptor-positive advanced breast cancer. N Engl J Med 2012, Feb 9; 366(6): 520-9.

[64]  Kung HJ. Targeting tyrosine kinases and autophagy in prostate cancer. Horm Cancer 2011, Feb; 2(1): 38-46.

[65]  Adamo V, Noto L, Franchina T, Chiofalo G, Picciotto M, Toscano G, Caristi N. Emerging targeted therapies for castration-resistant prostate cancer. Front Endocrinol (Lausanne) 2012; 3:73.

[66]  Agarwal N, Sonpavde G, Sternberg CN. Novel molecular targets for the therapy of castration-resistant prostate cancer. Eur Urol 2012, May; 61(5): 950-60.

[67]  Brindle K. Watching tumours gasp and die with MRI: The promise of hyperpolarised 13C MR spectroscopic imaging. Br J Radiol 2012, Jun; 85(1014): 697-708.

[68]  Rosen MA. Use of modified RECIST criteria to improve response assessment in targeted therapies: Challenges and opportunities. Cancer Biol Ther 2010, Jan; 9(1): 20-2.

[69]  Mehrara E, Forssell-Aronsson E, Ahlman H, Bernhardt P. Specific growth rate versus doubling time for quantitative characterization of tumor growth rate. Cancer Res 2007, Apr 15; 67(8): 3970-5.

[70]  Mehrara E, Forssell-Aronsson E, Ahlman H, Bernhardt P. Quantitative analysis of tumor growth rate and changes in tumor marker level: Specific growth rate versus doubling time. Acta Oncol 2009; 48(4): 591-7.

[71]  Mehrara E, Forssell-Aronsson E, Bernhardt P. Objective assessment of tumour response to therapy based on tumour growth kinetics. Br J Cancer 2011, Aug 23; 105(5): 682-6.

[72]  Elmore S. Apoptosis: A review of programmed cell death. Toxicol Pathol 2007, Jun; 35(4): 495-516.

[73]  Eisenhauer EA, Therasse P, Bogaerts J, Schwartz LH, Sargent D, Ford R, et al. New response evaluation criteria in solid tumours: Revised RECIST guideline (version 1.1). Eur J Cancer 2009, Jan; 45(2): 228-47.

[74]  Weber WA. Assessing tumor response to therapy. J Nucl Med 2009, May; 50 Suppl 1:1S-10S.

[75]  Le Tourneau C, Servois V, Diéras V, Ollivier L, Tresca P, Paoletti X. Tumour growth kinetics assessment: Added value to RECIST in cancer patients treated with molecularly targeted agents. Br J Cancer 2012, Feb 28; 106(5): 854-7.

[76]  Ferte C, Albiges L, Soria JC, Loriot Y, Fizazi K, Escudier BJ. The use of tumor growth rate (TGR) in evaluating sorafenib and everolimus treatment in mrcc patients: An in-

tegrated analysis of the TARGET and RECORD phase III trials data. J Clin Oncol 30, 2012 (suppl; Abstr 4540).

[77]  Motulsky H. Intuitive statistics a nonmathematical guide to statistical thinking. Second Ed. New York: Oxford University Press; 2010k.

[78]  Nishida K, Kaneko T, Yoneda M, Nakagawa S, Ishikawa T, Yamane E, et al. Doubling time of serum CA 19-9 in the clinical course of patients with pancreatic cancer and its significant association with prognosis. J Surg Oncol 1999, Jul; 71(3): 140-6.

[79]  Smith MR, Manola J, Kaufman DS, Oh WK, Bubley GJ, Kantoff PW. Celecoxib versus placebo for men with prostate cancer and a rising serum prostate-specific antigen after radical prostatectomy and/or radiation therapy. J Clin Oncol 2006, Jun 20; 24(18): 2723-8.

[80]  Srinivas S, Feldman D. A phase II trial of calcitriol and naproxen in recurrent prostate cancer. Anticancer Res 2009, Sep; 29(9) : 3605-10.

[81]  Hanninen M, Venner P, North S. A rapid PSA half-life following docetaxel chemotherapy is associated with improved survival in hormone refractory prostate cancer. Can Urol Assoc J 2009, Oct; 3(5): 369-74.

[82]  De Crevoisier R, Slimane K, Messai T, Wibault P, Eschwege F, Bossi A, et al. Early PSA decrease is an independent predictive factor of clinical failure and specific survival in patients with localized prostate cancer treated by radiotherapy with or without androgen deprivation therapy. Ann Oncol 2010, Apr; 21(4): 808-14.

[83]  Lee JH, Gulec SA, Kyshtoobayeva A, Sim MS, Morton DL. Biological factors, tumor growth kinetics, and survival after metastasectomy for pulmonary melanoma. Ann Surg Oncol 2009, Oct; 16(10): 2834-9.

# Medical Treatment

# Chapter 10

# Rational Categorization of the Pipeline of New Treatments for Advanced Cancer – Prostate Cancer as an Example

Sarah M. Rudman, Peter G. Harper and
Christopher J. Sweeney

Additional information is available at the end of the chapter

## 1. Introduction

### 1.1. The problem

Whilst improvements in patient survival have been realized for a number of haematological and solid malignancies in the last 30 years, new efficacious systemic anti-cancer treatments are still needed. The current, widely used drug development paradigm is often associated with a poor conversion rate from experimental to licensed drug. This process involves a significant investment of resources from sponsors, investigators and patients and to date has only lead to a limited chance of success. At present there are in excess of 800 anti-cancer agents in development and less than 10 new FDA approvals each year [1]. In order to address this problem there has been considerable debate concerning the best trial methodology to rationalize this process, with discussion of the timing, sequence and design of appropriate trials [2]. At present in many tumour types including breast, lung, renal cell and prostate cancer, the pipeline of new agents is crowded. In order therefore to use the available financial and patient resource wisely, it is crucial to identify the key important pathways in oncogenesis that in turn may help and prioritize the drugs with the most promise.

### 1.2. A promising future

In recent years advances in molecular biology have aided our understanding of the pathogenesis of cancer. This has occurred concurrently with technological advances allowing rational drug design and development (such as tyrosine kinase inhibitors, monoclonal antibodies and anti-sense oligonucleotides). Combining these two advances has been very beneficial in the drug development process such that we now have a wealth of opportunities. The challenge now is how to rationally categorize and prioritize the many strategies that can be deployed. In the discussion below, we propose a rational process to evaluate the merits of different strategies and use prostate cancer as an example. The different strategies include focusing on cytotoxic agents, synthetic lethality strategies, angiogenesis, oncogene addiction pathways and activated survival pathways such as those driven by systems of inflammation and/or metabolism.

## 2. Building on past successes – Cytotoxics and agents targeting key biological pathways

### 2.1. Cytotoxic agents

Cytotoxic chemotherapy has had an established role for many cancer types for many decades with the ability to eradicate some cancers, prevent relapse from micrometastatic disease in others and offer life prolonging or palliative benefit in other cancers. With respect to prostate cancer, a role for cytotoxic chemotherapy in the treatment of metastatic castrate refractory prostate cancer (CRPC) was first established using mitoxantrone in 1996, when it was shown to provide effective palliation of pain symptoms compared to prednisolone alone without prolongation of overall survival [3]. This was not associated with a survival benefit and to date the only class of cytotoxic agents to improve survival in metastatic prostate cancer are the taxanes [4]. Docetaxel was licensed in metastatic CRPC patients in 2004 following a phase III study of docetaxel plus prednisone versus mitoxantrone plus prednisone. The taxanes block cells in the G2/M phase of the cell cycle by stabilizing microtubules in the mitotic spindle thereby rendering them unable to separate during mitosis. Cancer cells sensitivity to taxanes is often short lived and resistance develops. The mechanism of this is poorly understood, although over expression of P-glycoprotein and mutations in the tubulin gene have been described [5]. Whilst the non-specific targeting of cycling cells by cytotoxic agents is not classed as targeted therapy, ongoing efforts do exist to introduce new cytotoxic agents to the prostate cancer arena. The aim of improving efficacy and delivery whilst minimizing toxicity underlies this development. In this era of personalized medicine, cytotoxic agents may continue to have a role especially where tumours do not harbour an obvious upregulated or mutated pathway to target. This approach has already led to the development and approval of the synthetic taxane - cabazitaxel for use in the second line metastatic CRPC setting. In the international multicentre phase III TROPIC trial, patients who had progressed on docetaxel were randomized to receive cabazitaxel plus prednisone or mitoxantrone plus prednisone. An improvement in overall survival of 2.4 months was seen (15.1 months versus 12.7 months HR=0.7 p<0.001) [6].

In addition to new members of existing cytotoxic drug classes, new mechanisms of drug delivery continue to be developed. Nanoparticle albumin bound (nab) paclitaxel and docetaxel use albumin as a vehicle to improve drug delivery to the tumour. This approach has proven to be successful using nab-paclitaxel (Abraxane®) in metastatic breast cancer where it delivered a 49% higher dose of drug to patients than a conventional solvent based approach. In addition, higher response rates were seen with an overall response rate of 33% (versus 19% for standard paclitaxel) and increased time to progression from 16.9 to 22 weeks [7]. Both agents are also in development in prostate cancer, where phase II trials are currently evaluating nab-paclitaxel and nab-docetaxel in the CRPC population. Other novel drug delivery strategies include water soluble biodegradable polyglutamate polymer with linked chemotherapeutic molecules (e.g. paclitaxel poligumex, Opaxio®) [8,9] and a nanoparticle bound docetaxel agent (BIND014) has also recently entered phase I clinical trials [10] (Table 1)

| Drug | Class | Study Design | Results | Current phase of clinical development | Reference |
|------|-------|--------------|---------|----------------------------------------|-----------|
| **Androgen receptor blockers** | | | | | |
| Abiraterone | CYP 17 lyase inhibitor | Randomised placebo controlled phase III trial in post-docetaxel and chemo naïve CRPC pts. | Overall survival adv 3.9 months in post chemo population Chemo naïve study stopped early. Median OS not yet reached for Abiraterone | Licensed in post-docetaxel pts Awaiting license in chemo naïve pts | [26, 28, 29] |
| Enzalutamide /MDV3100 | Androgen receptor antagonist | Phase III randomized placebo controlled AFFIRM study | Overall survival adv 4.8 months. Favourable toxicity profile. 0.6% seizure rate | Phase III trials in chemo-naïve setting completed accrual | [33, 34] |
| Orteronel/ TAK700 | 17,20 lyase inhibitor | Phase I-II dose escalation study in metastatic CRPC pts accrued. | RPIID is 400mg BID, no DLTs | Phase II trial accruing in asymp CRPC pts, pts without mets but rising PSA & in combination with docetaxel in met CRPC pts. | [30, 31] |
| TOK-001 | AR antagonist, CYP 17 lyase inhibitor, ↓AR levels | | | Phase I-II in CRPC pts (ARMOR1) currently accruing | [113] |
| **Histone deacetylase (HDAC) inhibitors** | | | | | |
| Panobinostat | HDAC inhibitor | Phase I completed in combination with docetaxel/pred and phase II completed as single agent in CRPC pts | Safe as single agent and in combination. IV formulation going forward | Phase I-II with Bicalutamide in CRPC pts accruing | [37] |

| Vorinostat | HDAC 6 inhibitor | Phase I with safety study with docetaxel q21 days and vorinostat q1-14 days Phase II in post chemo CRPC pts receiving 400mg vorinostat orally | 12 pts enrolled but 5 DLTs reported. Trials suspended due to excess toxicity 27 pts but terminated due to excess toxicity. Significant toxicity seen. 44% G3 AE's | Phase I in combination with temsirolimus planned | [38, 39] |
| SB939 | HDAC inhibitor (multiple classes) | Phase I dose escalation trial in solid malignancies | MTD 80mg, RPIID 60mg, DLTs were fatigue, troponin elevation & QTc prolongation | Phase II single agent study in recurrent/met prostate cancer accruing | [114] |
| Romidepsin | Depsipeptide HDAC inhibitor | Phase II in chemo naïve met CRPC pts. 13 mg/m2 q1,8,15 every 28 days | 35 pts enrolled. 2 pts had PR "/>6months. 11 pts stopped due to toxicity. N&V, fatigue & anorexia | Combination studies with cytotoxic agents planned | [115] |
| **HSP90 inhibitors** | | | | | |
| IPI-504 (Retaspmycin) | 17-AAG analogue HSP90 inhibitor | Phase II study in CRPC patients stratified by prior chemotherapy at 400mg/m$^2$ | No PSA or RECIST responses seen. G5 ketoacidosis and hepatic failure observed | Clinical development ongoing in NSCLC | [43] |
| STA9090 | 2$^{nd}$ gen HSP90 inhibitor | Phase I dose escalation studies with IV wkly and twice wkly admin | Wkly admin - MTD 216mg/m$^2$ DLTs due to amylase elevation, diarrhoea & fatigue Twice weekly – MTD as yet not reached | Phase II prostate trials planned | [44] |
| 17AAG (Tanespimycin) | 1$^{st}$ gen HSP90 inh | Phase II in metastatic CRPC pts. 300mg/m$^2$ weekly for ¾ weeks | Trial stopped after 1$^{st}$ phase due to lack of PSA response. G3 fatigue | No further prostate trials | [41, 42] |
| siRNA against AR | Nanoparticle technology | In pre-clinical development | | | [10] |

**Table 1.** The Androgen Receptor pathway

New classes of cytotoxic agents are also in development in prostate cancer. These are members of the epothilone family and the halichondrin B analogue - eribulin. The epothilones are macrolide antibiotics that also act by stabilizing microtubules. They are water soluble and as such do not have to be administered in a lipophilic solution, therefore reducing the allergic reaction rate compared to taxanes. To date the epothilone - ixabepilone is licensed for use in metastatic chemo-refractory breast cancer, although it has also shown activity and acceptable toxicity in a phase II study in a mixed chemo naïve and post chemotherapy CRPC population [11]. Clinical development of several members of this family in prostate cancer continues. Patupilone or naturally occurring Epothilone B and sagopilone (a fully synthetic compound) have also shown activity in post docetaxel and chemo naïve CRPC patients respectively [12, 13].

Eribulin mesylate (or Halaven, Eisai Co.) is a synthetic analogue of the marine sponge natural product Halichondrin B that is a potent naturally occurring mitotic inhibitor. Eribulin binds predominantly with high affinity to the ends of microtubules leading to mitotic arrest and ultimately apoptosis. Eribulin is also licensed for use in metastatic chemotherapy refractory breast cancer patients although a phase II study in both chemotherapy naive and pretreated prostate cancer patients has been performed. Most activity was demonstrated in the chemotherapy naïve cohort with a 22.4% PSA response rate and 8.8% overall response rate [14].

Another successful cytotoxic strategy for targeting prostate cancer metastases with radiation has been the studies using the alpha-emitter Radium 223. This radiopharmaceutical that acts as a calcium mimic can selectively target bone lesions from prostate cancer whilst its low penetrance alpha-emissions are cytotoxic to cancer cells. Its half life of 11.4 days also favours its use as a cancer treatment. Having proven its safety in phase I and II trials [15], the phase III ALSYMPCA trial was stopped early after a pre-planned efficacy interim analysis following recommendations from the independent data monitoring committee on the basis of a significant improvement in overall survival and favourable toxicity profile. In this large study of 922 patients, Radium-223 significantly improved overall survival in patients by 2.8 months (HR 0.695 95% CI 0.552-0.875) in addition to delaying the time to first skeletal-related event by 5.2 months (HR 0.610 95% CI 0.461-0.807) [16].

## 2.2. Targeting key biological pathways

A leading premise for the treatment for advanced prostate cancer is to target the androgen receptor (AR) axis or to identify cases where a single pathway mutation is thought to drive carcinogenesis. It is proposed that triaging the current pipeline of agents can be directed by building on prior successes. In light of recent advances in our knowledge of AR pathway signaling, further exploration of this pathway is warranted. Moreover, since molecular interrogation of distinct clones driving individual prostate cancers is now possible, treatment of these tumours with agents targeting these mutations would also be desirable. In the past the prostate cancer treatment paradigm has been to expose the patient to an established sequence of agents in a 'one size fits all' approach – which may have missed identifying a drug with major activity in a few patients. A strategy that is being increasingly more recognized is the need to characterize a patient's cancer and select the most appropriate treatment for that cancer phenotype. It is also important to ensure that critical appraisal of pre-clinical and clinical research continues to help guide these endeavors to identify oncogene addiction pathways.

## 3. Extinguishing the AR axis

The androgen dependence of prostate cancer on testosterone was first observed as early as 1941 when the effect of castration on androgen levels in prostate cancer was studied [17]. This lead to the introduction of androgen deprivation therapy and the generation of the cas-trate state where serum levels of testosterone are reduced to <50ng/dl or 1.7nmol/l. This treatment is initially effective in 80-90% of patients and results in PSA or radiological re-sponses and clinical improvement in the patient's symptoms. Eventually, the patient's can-cer progresses despite serum testosterone levels continuing to be low. The current term used to describe this state is 'castrate resistant prostate cancer' which has replaced the misleading term 'hormone-refractory prostate cancer'. CRPC more accurately describes the ongoing de-pendence of the cancer on AR signaling despite low measureable testosterone levels.

Ligand independent AR signaling is thought to occur in the majority of CRPC tumours via activation of oncogenes such as ERBB2 or H-*ras* and through MAP kinase signaling [18, 19]. A small proportion of CRPC tumours will also harbour amplifications or point mutations in the ligand-binding domain of the androgen receptor gene leading to altered responsiveness to ligands [20]. A third mechanism of action bypasses androgen receptor in favour of an alternative signaling pathway [21].

The evidence for ongoing androgen sensitivity is also strengthened by the observation of up regulation of AR protein levels in hormone resistant versus hormone sensitive paired xenografts [21] as well as in patient tumour samples [22, 23]. Maintained intra-tumoural levels of testosterone and dihydrotestosterone are also observed despite castrate serum an-drogen levels [24].

In addition to testicular androgen production, extragonadal sites of androgen synthesis also contribute to testosterone levels. These *de novo* adrenal and intra-tumoural pathways utilize the 17α-hydroxylase and C17, 20-lyase activity of the CYP17A1 enzyme involved in the ste-roid biosynthesis pathway. The importance of this pathway was initially clinically exploited with the use of ketoconazole, a weak reversible inhibitor of CYP17. Anti-tumour activity was demonstrated with a PSA response rate of 20-62% in phase II trials and a median dura-tion of response of 3-7 months [25]. However its use was associated with significant toxicity and up to 20% of patients discontinued treatment. This toxicity profile has not been ob-served with the more potent CYP17 inhibitor abiraterone acetate. This agent has successfully reawakened interest in further manipulation of the AR axis in CRPC patients. After success-ful phase I and II clinical trial development [26, 27] randomized double blind placebo con-trolled phase III trials of abiraterone plus prednisolone versus placebo plus prednisolone in chemotherapy naïve and post docetaxel patients were conducted. Results in post docetaxel patients revealed a statistically significant increase in median overall survival of 3.9 months in favour of abiraterone as well as improvements in time to PSA progression, radiological PFS and PSA response rate [28]. More recent results from the interim analysis of chemother-apy naïve patients have also shown significant activity in favour of abiraterone with the in-terim data monitoring committee recommending unblinding and crossover for patients receiving prednisone alone [29]. Abiraterone was also well tolerated with the predominant toxicities being hypertension, hypokalaemia and fluid retention. These are the expected consequences of the mineralocorticoid excess resulting from the accumulation of precursors upstream of CYP17. These have subsequently been managed with the concomitant use of steroids or the mineralocorticoid antagonist eplerenone.

Orteronel (or TAK 700, Takeda Pharmaceuticals) is another 17,20 lyase inhibitor which has also advanced to phase III CRPC trials after successful phase I and II development [30, 31]. This inhibitor is now in phase III trials as a single agent in asymptomatic CRPC patients and in patients with a rising PSA but no detectable metastatic disease as well as in phase I/II trials in a number of prostate cancer settings including in combination with docetaxel in metastatic CRPC patients.

In addition to steroid biosynthesis inhibitors, further manipulation of the AR axis in castrate patients has been demonstrated using MDV3100 or enzalutamide. First generation anti-androgens such as bicalutamide, flutamide and nilutamide competitively inhibit the AR ligand binding domain. This response is often transient as castration resistance develops which may in part be a consequence of the partial agonist activity of this class [21]. These observations led to the rational design of enzalutamide, an orally available anti-androgen with superior AR binding compared to bicalutamide, and no AR agonist activity in bicalutamide-resistant and AR-over expressing cell lines [32]. A phase I/II study of enzalutamide in 140 post-chemotherapy metastatic CRPC patients demonstrated a PSA response rate of 56% (78/140 patients), soft tissue responses in 22% (13/59 patients), and a median time to progression of 47 weeks. enzalutamide was well tolerated with the most common grade 3 or 4 adverse events being fatigue that resolved with a dose reduction [33]. This activity was confirmed in the multicentre double blind placebo controlled phase III AFFIRM trial comparing enzalutamide against placebo. This trial of 1199 docetaxel pre-treated patients was also stopped early due to a 4.8 months overall survival benefit for enzalutamide compared to placebo with all subgroups benefiting [34].

Other agents in development that manipulate the androgen receptor axis are shown in table 1. In addition to agents intrinsic to the androgen receptor pathway, inhibitors of chaperone proteins may also be important targets. Histone deacetylases (HDAC) are enzymes which remove acetyl groups from proteins and in so doing modulate the protein-protein interactions of co-activators associated with AR binding. HDAC enzymes are over expressed in certain solid tumours including prostate cancer, where high expression levels are associated with poor outcome [35]. HDAC over expression in prostate cancers is also often co-existent with genetic rearrangements in the ETS (E-twenty six) gene family. These genetic alterations have been found in up to 70% of prostate cancers and may interact with HDAC's already known to be upstream regulators and downstream transducers of the ETS transcription factors family [36]. The preclinical rationale for HDAC inhibition in prostate cancer has led to early phase clinical development of several HDAC inhibitors. Phase I/II studies of panobinostat both as a single agent and in combination with docetaxel confirmed the safety of this approach [37]. In the single arm study, all patients developed progressive disease despite evidence of acetylated histones in peripheral blood mononuclear cells, however 5 out of 8 (63%) patients in the combination study had a ≥ 50% reduction in PSA value. At present a study in combination with bicaluta-mide in CRPC patients is recruiting. However trials involving single agent vorinostat (an HDAC6 inhibitor known to acetylate tubulin and stabilize microtubules) have been ter-minated early due to excess toxicity with no significant activity [38, 39].

The other major group of agents that are involved in post-translational modification of the AR axis are heat shock proteins. These are proteins that ensure the maintenance of oncogenic protein homeostasis in the presence of stress factors such as hypoxia or acidot-ic conditions. Heat shock protein 90 (HSP 90) is an ATP-dependent multi-chaperone complex implicated in the function of the AR. The AR is stabilized by the interaction with HSP 90 that allows it to interact with androgens [40]. Pre-clinical models have shown HSP 90 inhibition leads to decreased AR expression and function and a phase I trial of 17-AAG both as a single agent and in combination with cytotoxic chemotherapy demonstrated drug safety [41]. The subsequent phase II study however failed to reach its primary endpoint and was terminated [42]. Significant toxicity was observed with the 17-AAG analogue retaspmycin (or IPI-504) [43] although clinical development of the second generation HSP90 inhibitor STA9090 has confirmed safety in phase I trials and is pro-ceeding [44]. Studies are planned to determine whether the newer HSP90 agents can hit target and decrease activity with a suitable toxicity profile or whether the therapeutic window is too narrow for safe use of these agents.

In addition, small interfering RNA's (siRNA's) are a class of double stranded RNA mole-cules that are now known to exist as important gene regulatory factors in both plant and an-imal systems. Selective targeting of the androgen receptor by siRNA molecules may further silence the AR signaling pathway in prostate cancer. This may be made viable by nanoparti-cle technology being able to facilitate use of otherwise undeliverable agents. The develop-ment of these agents is currently hampered by the need for safe systemic delivery of these agents without the off target and immune stimulation problems encountered with other nu-cleic acid medicines such as plasmid DNA and anti-sense oligonucleotide [45].

# 4. An advanced understanding of cancer biology comes of age

### 4.1. Specific targeting of DNA repair mechanisms

In recent years one successful targeted approach has been to exploit the vulnerability of tu-mors with an impaired DNA damage repair mechanism by inhibiting a second DNA repair pathway and as such commit the cancer cell to die. This concept of synthetic lethality has been most successfully demonstrated in patients bearing tumors with BRCA-1/-2 mutations where homologous recombination (HR) mechanisms are already known to be inadequate. This hypothesis has reactivated the development of poly (ADP-ribose) polymerase (PARP) inhibitors. PARP is an enzyme that is crucial in the base excision repair pathway. When this repair mechanism is inhibited in the presence of pre-existing impaired HR then efficient

DNA repair is prevented and apoptosis occurs. Following pre-clinical and more recently proof of concept clinical trials in patients with BRCA mutated breast and ovarian carcinoma, the PARP inhibitor olaparib has demonstrated significant activity [46]. Whilst it is hoped that the application of these agents may broaden to include sporadic tumours in which mutations in DNA pathways may also be found, there has also been considerable interest in other tumours types where these mutations may be found. The inherited BRCA-2 mutation is associated with a 20% lifetime risk of developing prostate cancer that often occurs before 65 years of age. The subsequent tumors are often of high Gleason score, more advanced stage at diagnosis and patients have a shorter survival than patients with sporadic prostate cancers [47]. One of three prostate cancer patients with germ-line BRCA variant had a prolonged response to olaparib in a phase 1 trial [48]. In addition to BRCA mutated cancers, pre-clinical evidence has also demonstrated a sensitivity of tumours with phosphatase and tensin homolog (PTEN) deficiency to PARP inhibition [49]. This is one of the most commonly mutated genes in human cancers where it has a role in genome stability. PTEN deficiency is associated with an HR defect that sensitizes tumours cells to PARP inhibition using the same mechanism as BRCA mutated cancers.

At present, the clinical development of olaparib has been focused on breast and ovarian cancer. Studies in prostate cancer are underway with the PARP inhibitor veliparib (or ABT888) in combination with temozolamide in a phase I study recruiting patients with metastatic prostate cancer. In addition a phase I study using the Merck PARP inhibitor - MK4827 is currently recruiting to a prostate cancer enriched second stage following encouraging phase I study data in advanced solid malignancies [50].

### 4.2. Oncogene addiction pathways

The development of drugs targeting tumours driven by so-called 'oncogene addictions' has lead to some success. Examples include imatinib targeting the bcr-abl translocation in CML and mutated c-kit in GIST, trastuzumab and laptinib in HER-2 positive breast cancers BRAF inhibitors in melanomas with BRAF mutations. Molecular studies in prostate cancer have to date identified mutations of this type in less than 20% of all sporadically occurring prostate cancers. Analysis of a cohort of 206 prostate cancer cases found the common BRAF mutation V600E in 10.2% (or 21/206 cases) [51], whilst PI3 kinase mutations were found in only 3% of a separate cohort [52]. Drugs inhibiting BRAF as well as PI3 kinase mutations may lead to meaningful responses in patients with tumors been driven by these mutations. It is hoped that further "oncogene addiction" pathways will be uncovered and be able to be drugged.

### 4.3. Ligand and transcription factor driven survival pathways

Whilst it is often hoped that mutations in a single molecular pathway will be uncovered as the crucial oncogenic event in tumour development and its abrogation lead to meaningful anticancer activity, to date this has been rarely found to be the case for sporadic tumours. Another approach is to consider the factors that cause and/or are associated with the development as well as the survival of cancer. The role of androgens and androgen receptor is clear for prostate cancer. Other biological approaches associated with cancer development and survival include the metabolism and inflammatory systems. In both cases, there is epidemiological, preclinical and pathological data implicating these systems in the development of prostate cancer. In comparison to the "oncogene addiction" phenomenon, these cancers are driven by altered expression of ligands and control mechanisms (such as transcription factors). Knowledge of these pathways has provided valuable clues for the treatment of cancer.

## 5. Targeting the metabolism system

Incidence and disease specific mortality in prostate cancer exhibit marked global variation with the highest levels seen in Western Europe, North America and the lowest in Asia [53]. It is assumed that whilst this is accounted for by a significant genetic component, that diet and lifestyle factors may also contribute. Epidemiological studies also support an association between dietary fat intake, poor prognosis and risk of relapse [54]. In order to identify new pathways that are important in prostate cancer pathogenesis, evaluating a role for the metabolism system and its key components is crucial.

Cancer cells are already known to differ from normal cells in some of the fundamental metabolic pathways they employ. Most cancer cells generate energy by primarily metabolizing glucose by glycolysis followed by lactate production. This occurs in contrast to normal cells in which glucose is catabolised by oxidative phosphorylation, a primarily aerobic process. Proliferating cancer cells also exhibit increased glucose uptake compared to normal cells. This results in tumour cells with glycolytic rates over 200 times higher than those of normal tissues and allows efficient generation of macromolecules needed for new cancer cell production. This so-called Warburg hypothesis was initially thought to be the fundamental cause of cancer, however it is now thought to explain how tumours may flourish in low oxygen environments [55]. These observations suggest that differences in metabolism between normal tissues and cancer cells may be important in oncogenesis.

Insulin and insulin-like growth factors (IGF-1) are extracellular hormones and growth factors that regulate important metabolic pathways such as fatty acid and sterol synthesis as well as growth factor signaling via the PI3 kinase and MAP kinase pathways. Their activation may stimulate tumourigenesis by activating one or both of these mitogenic pathways and disrupting fat metabolism.

IGF-I and IGF-II bind to the IGF-1 receptor, a tyrosine kinase receptor that is known to be upregulated following castration in animal models [56]. It has been implicated in the development of the castrate resistant state with evidence that inhibition of the IGF-1 receptor may enhance the effect of castration in xenograft models [57]. Targeting the IGF-1 receptor is therefore an attractive therapeutic target in CRPC. Several IGF-1 receptor inhibitors are currently being evaluated in clinical trials and candidates include both monoclonal antibodies and small molecule tyrosine kinase inhibitors. Cixutumumab (or IMC-A12) is a fully human IgG1 subclass monoclonal antibody that has reached phase II of clinical development. A single agent study of chemotherapy naïve asymptomatic patients noted that the drug was well tolerated with grade 3 fatigue and hyperglycaemia the worst toxicity seen and 29% of patients had stable disease [58]. Future trials with this agent are planned or ongoing including in the first line metastatic setting with androgen deprivation therapy (SWOG S0925) based on supporting preclinical data [57].

| Drug | Class | Study Design | Results | Current phase of clinical development | Reference |
|---|---|---|---|---|---|
| **Insulin-like growth factor receptor inhibitors** | | | | | |
| Cixitumumab /IMC-A12 | IGF-1 R inh | Phase II study in chemo naïve CRPC Asx pts 10mg/kg q2 wkly or 20mg/kg q3 wkly | 29% disease stab >6 mths. Worst toxicity G3 fatigue & ↑glycaemia | Phase II Neoadj +ADT in high risk pts + Temsiro in met CRPC + 1st line met+ADT | [58] |
| Figitumumab /CP-751871 | IGF-1 R inh | Phase Ib in adv solid tumours in comb with docetaxel 75mg/m2 | 46 pts - MTD not reached. 4PR and 12 pts with disease stab >6months. G3/4 febrile neutropenia, fatigue 10/18 CRPC pts had >5 CTC with 60% response | Phase III studies recruiting in NSCLC (ADVIGO 1016). Phase II in breast, prostate, colorectal & Ewings sarcoma | [59, 60] |
| Ganitumab/ AMG 479 | IGF-1 R inh | Phase I dose escalation study in adv solid malign of IV q2 wkly | 53 pts - 1DLT – G3 ↓plts & transminitis. MTD not reached – maxdose 20mg/kg. ↑ in serum IGF-1 | Phase II studies recruiting in Ex Stage small cell with platinum, +Everolimus in colorectal, in carcinoid & pNETs | [61] |
| Lisitinib/ OSI-906 | Dual kinase inhibitor of Insulin & IGF-1 R | Phase I continuous dose escalation study in adv solid tumours using BID & QD dosing Phase I intermittent dosing in adv solid tumours | 57 pts – MTD reached 400mg QD, 150mg BID. DLTs were ↑ QTc & G3 hyperglycaemia SD >12 weeks seen in 18/43 pts MTD 600 mg | Phase III recruiting in Adrenocortical Ca Phase II + Erlotinib in Breast | [62, 116] |
| **AMP Kinase activators** | | | | | |
| AICAR (Aminoimidazole-4 -caboxamide-1-b- riboside | AMP mimetic | Preclinical studies show inhibition of prostate cancer cell proliferation | Inhibition of tumour growth in prostate cancer xenograft models | | [78, 117] |

| A-769662 | AMP K subunit act. | Delay tumour development & decrease tumour incidence in PTEN def mice | | | [79] |
|---|---|---|---|---|---|
| Metformin | Indirect | 44% reduction in prostate cancer cases compared to Caucasian controls | | Phase II recruiting in loc adv or met CRPC and in loc disease as prevention against MS with ADT | [80] |
| Resveratrol | Indirect | Phase I single dose safety study in colon ca pts with hepatic metastases | Results are awaited | Phase I/II currently recruiting as neoadj in colon carcinoma pts | [82] |
| **mTOR inhibitors** | | | | | |
| Temsirolimus | mTOR inhibitor | Phase II study in CRPC patients post first line docetaxol chemotherapy. Pts receive maintenance temsirolimus 25mg/m2 weekly | Currently recruiting | Phase II recruiting in chemo naïve CRPC pts, in comb with cixutumumab in met CRPC, in CRPC after no response to chemo with bevacizumab & PI/II with docetaxel | [118] |
| Everolimus | mTOR inhibitor via mTORC1 | Phase II study in castrate resistant prostate cancer of bicalutamide and everolimus compared to bicalutamide alone | *In vivo* evidence of synergy between mTOR and AR pathways. Study ongoing but 8 pts enrolled. 6/8 responses in PSA. Well tolerated with no unexpected toxicity | Phase I/II in met CRPC with docetaxel & bevacizumab, in post chemo pts with carbo/pred, in neoadj setting in int/high risk localized disease & in first line met/ locally adv setting | [72, 73, 74] |
| **PI3 kinase inhibitors** | | | | | |
| XL-147 | Class I PI3K isoform inhibitor | Phase I dose escalation study in adv solid malig of continuous daily dosing or d1-21 of 28 day cycle | 68pts – DLT G3 rash. Inhibition of PI3K & ERK demonstrated. Prolonged stable disease observed | Recruiting to Phase I study in solid tumours and Phase I/II in breast & endometrial carcinoma | [65] |

| GDC-0941 | Pan PI3K inhibitor | Phase I dose escalation study. GDC-0941 given QD for 21 out of 28 day cycle. BID cohorts also recruited | 36 pts enrolled, dose escalation ongoing. QD dosing safe up to 254mg, BID dosing safe up to 180mg. 3 DLTs – headache, pl eff and red TLCO | Phase I study recruiting in NSCLC & Met breast cancer in comb. With paclitaxel or carbo +/- bevacizumab | [66] |
| --- | --- | --- | --- | --- | --- |
| BKM120 BEZ235 | Pan class I PI3K inhibitor | Phase I dose escalation study. BKM120 PO QD | 30 pts enrolled from 12.5-150mg. MTD 100mg. PD data suggests active drug at 100mg. 8/10 PR on FDG-PET | Phase I/II currently accruing in HER2+ Met breast ca. Also recruiting in combination with GSK 1120212 | [67] |
| **Akt inhibitors** | | | | | |
| GSK 2141795 GSK 2110183 | Akt inhibitor | | | First-in-human phase I study of GSK 2141795 in advanced solid malig, also recruiting in combination with GSK 1120212 | |
| Perifosine | Oral Akt inhibitor | CRPC pts with rising PSA but no detectable mets. 900mg loading dose then 100mg daily | 20% pts had a PSA reduction but did not meet PSA response criteria. DLTs included hypoNa, arthritis, photophobia, hyperuricaemia | Recruiting phase III in multiple myeloma with bortezomib +/- dex , phase I in recurrent paediatric solid tumours | [70] |
| MK2206 | Highly selective non ADP comp Akt inhibitor | Phase I dose escalation study 30-90mg QOD in 28 day cycles in tx-refractory solid tumours | MTD established at 60mg QOD. PD efficacy confirmed with dec pAKT levels. SD seen in 6/19 pts | Phase II bicalutamide +/- MK2206 in pts after local therapy + rising PSA, Phase I in com with docetaxel is recruiting | [71] |

**Table 2.** The Metabolic Syndrome

A second IGF-1 receptor antibody is the human IgG2 subclass antibody figitumumab. This was evaluated in a phase I dose escalation trial during which the maximum feasible dose was estab-lished as 20mg/kg intravenously every 21 days [59]. A phase Ib dose escalation study in combination with docetaxel then enrolled 46 predominantly metastatic CRPC patients. This combination was well tolerated with no MTD reached and the toxicity profile included nausea, febrile neutropenia, anorexia, fatigue and hyperglycaemia. A 22% response rate was observed with a disease stabilization rate of 44% for ≥ 6 months [60]. A phase II study of this combination has completed accrual and results are awaited. A third monoclonal antibody ganitumumab (or AMG478, Amgen) is also in clinical development and whilst safe in phase I dose escalation studies, its focus for ongoing development is in lung and colorectal carcinoma [61]. OSI-906 or linsitinib is a first in class inhibitor of both the insulin and IGF-1 receptors. It has been evaluated in phase I dose escalation safety studies where MTDs of 400mg QD and 150 mg BID were reached. The dose limiting toxicities were the known class effects hyperglycaemia and prolongation of the QTc interval. Whilst further development of this compound continues in adrenocortical and breast carcinomas [62], a phase II study of linsitinib in asymptomatic or mildly symptomatic CRPC patients has completed accrual and results are awaited.

An important downstream intracellular signaling pathway that has been implicated in prostate cancer pathogenesis, progression and the development of castration resistance is the PI3K/Akt/mTOR pathway. Phosphatidylinositol-3 kinase (PI3K) activation results in the phosphorylation of phosphatidylinositol 4,5-bisphosphate (PIP2) to generate the second messenger phosphatidylinositol 3-5triphosphate (PIP3) that activates the Akt signal transduction cascade. Reports suggest that PI3K signaling may play a critical role in castration resistance allowing prostate cancers to maintain continued proliferation in low androgen environments [63]. In addition, the PI3K isoforms p85 and p110b appear to have a role in regulating AR-DNA interactions and the assembly of the AR based transcriptional complex [64]. There are numerous PI3K inhibitors in clinical development, XL147 (Exelixis) is a class I isoform inhibitor whilst SF1126 (Semafore), GDC0941 (Genentech) and BEZ234 (Novartis) are pan PI3K inhibitors. All agents have successfully completed phase I dose escalation studies and preliminary results suggest that these agents are well tolerated and have favourable pharmacokinetic-pharmacodynamic profiles [65 - 67]. Further tumour specific phase I/II studies are ongoing, although at present no prostate specific studies are in progress.

The Akt's are a family of three serine/threonine kinases – AKT-1, AKT-2, & AKT-3. Phosphorylation of AKT modulates multiple downstream cellular functions including apoptosis, metabolism and proliferation. Enhanced pAKT correlates with more aggressive histological and pathological prostate cancer stage, and a worse prognosis underlining its importance as a druggable target and possible role as a prognostic biomarker [68, 69]. There are several classes of Akt inhibitors currently in clinical development including those inhibiting the catalytic and the pleckstrin homology (PH) domains. Perifosine, an alkylphospholipid inhibiting the PH domain has reached phase II in CRPC patients. Unfortunately although well tolerated this agent did not exhibit significant activity [70]. The pan-AKT inhibitors GSK2141795 and MK2206 with simultaneous targeting of both AKT-1 and AKT-2 are considered potentially superior to single isoform inhibitors. MK2206 was well tolerated in a phase II dose escalation study with an observed MTD of 60mg. Pharmacodynamic endpoints were met with a measurable reduction in pAKT levels. In addition, 6 of 19 patients achieved stable disease [71]. Further development continues in a number of tumour types both as single agent and in combination with chemotherapy. Of note a phase I study in combination with docetaxel is currently recruiting, as is a randomized phase II study of bicalutamide +/- MK2206 in prostate cancer patients with a rising PSA after definitive local therapy. GSK2141795 and GSK 2110183 also entered phase I development with results of first in human safety studies pending.

Mammalian target of rapamycin (mTOR) is also a serine/threonine kinase downstream of PI3K which interacts with the mTOR complexes mTORC1 and mTORC2 to regulate cell proliferation and inhibit apoptosis. Proof of principle that the PI3K pathway can be successfully targeted for clinical use in cancer has been demonstrated by the development of the rapamycin analogs - temsirolimus and everolimus that inhibit the mTORC1 kinase. Temsirolimus is an intravenous formulation which was the first compound in this class to be approved by the FDA for first line treatment in poor risk patients with advanced renal cell cancer. Everolimus an oral formulation is also approved for use in advanced renal cell cancer but in the second line setting. Single agent studies of these agents in the prostate cancer setting have been performed but were considered disappointing with a short time to progression (2.5 months) and no radiographic or PSA responses [72]. Everolimus has also been evaluated in combination with docetaxel in CRPC patients. The recommended phase II dose was 10mg everolimus and 70mg/m2 docetaxel, 3 patients had a PSA response and the combination was well tolerated with fatigue and haematological toxicities the most common [73]. Further studies with both agents in prostate cancer continue with a similar study involving temsirolimus in combination with docetaxel, as well as studies with cixitumumab and bevacizumab. A randomized study in hormone responsive patients of bicalutamide +/- everolimus is currently recruiting with early results suggesting the combination was well tolerated with PSA responses observed in six of eight patients [74]. Studies in the neoadjuvant and localized disease setting are also ongoing.

Finally, AMP kinase is a serine/threonine kinase that is activated by metabolic stressors that deplete ATP and increase AMP levels. Its activity is also under the control of hormones such as adiponectin and leptin as well as cytokines [75]. The activation of AMP kinase reduces insulin levels, as well as increasing ATP producing activities (glucose uptake, fatty acid oxidation) and suppressing ATP-consumption (synthesis of fatty acids, sterols, glycogen and proteins). AMP kinase therefore acts as a metabolic switch controlling glucose and lipid metabolism. Decreased AMP kinase activity is thought to contribute to the metabolic abnormalities involved in the metabolic syndrome [76]. In addition polymorphisms in a gene locus encoding one of the AMPK subunits correlates with prostate cancer risk [77].

Activators of AMP kinase activity may be direct or indirect. Several direct AMP kinase activators act either by allosteric binding to AMP kinase subunits or as an AMP mimetic. These agents aminoimidazole-4-caboxamide-1-b-riboside (AICAR), A-769662 and PT1 are at an early stage of clinical development. AICAR has been shown to inhibit prostate cancer cell proliferation and tumour growth in xenograft models [78]. However its further development may be limited by its poor specificity for AMPK and low oral bioavailability. To date no interventional oncology studies have been undertaken. The recent publication of the crystal structure of AMP kinase subunits has allowed rational drug design of A-769662 and

PT1. A769662 has been shown to delay tumour development and decrease tumour incidence in PTEN deficient mice [79].

The indirect activator metformin is a well established treatment for type II diabetes mellitus. Its use is associated with a 44% risk reduction in prostate cancer cases compared with controls in Caucasian men [80]. The mechanism of metformin's antitumour effect is not completely understood, although it is hypothesized that metformin may decrease circulating glucose, insulin and IGF-1 levels by inhibiting hepatic gluconeogenesis resulting in increased signaling through the insulin/IGF-1 pathway [81]. Its action in prostate cancer is currently under evaluation in a number of clinical trials, these include as a preventative treatment for metabolic syndrome in men on androgen deprivation therapy and as first line therapy in locally advanced or metastatic prostate cancer patients. Finally, resveratrol is a phytoalexin produced by plants when under attack by pathogens. It is found in the skin of grapes, grape products, red wine and mulberries and is thought to have anticancer properties. These were first identified when it was shown to inhibit tumourigenesis in a mouse skin cancer model [82]. Its indirect action on AMP kinase remains to be elucidated although its anticancer action has been explored in a number of tumour types. Clinical trials using resveratrol have explored potential roles in preventing and treating diabetes, Alzheimers disease and weight loss. In addition safety studies of its use in colorectal carcinoma patients with liver metastases have been conducted and the results are awaited. As yet no studies in prostate cancer are planned.

# 6. Inflammation

Numerous studies have implicated inflammation in the development of prostate cancer and its metastases. Pathologists have recognized focal areas of epithelial atrophy in the periphery of the prostate (proliferative inflammatory atrophy - PIA), where prostate cancers typically arise and these areas are associated with acute or chronic inflammation and can show morphological transitions in continuity with high grade PIN [83]. This could indicate a role of PIA as a cancer precursor [84]. Putative causes of these lesions are infection or dietary oxidants. To date, the identification of an infectious agent directly involved in prostate carcinogenesis has been elusive. However, it is possible that one or more infectious agents may be indirectly involved in prostate carcinogenesis by being initiators of the inflammatory lesion (PIA). Interesting data includes serologic evidence of *T. vaginalis* infection being associated with a higher prostate cancer risk overall, and an almost two-fold risk for poorly differentiated disease [85] as well as greater prostate cancer specific mortality (HR: 1.5; 95% CI: 1.0, 2.2) [86]. It is also of note that hereditary susceptibility genes which encode proteins with infectious response function: RNASEL and MSR1 (macrophage scavenger receptor 1) have been associated with prostate cancer [83]. Single nucleotide polymorphism's of anti-oxidant genes have also been associated with prostate cancer and include OGG1 (repair from oxidized DNA), MnSOD [88]. Also the incidence of prostate cancer has been decreased with anti-oxidants such as lycopene and NSAIDs [87].

One possible mediator of the inflammation that leads to cancer and is instigated by oxidative stress from a diverse arrays of causes is NFκB activation. Specifically, it has been shown that a vicious cycle of oxidative stress causing DNA damage and consequent influx of inflammatory cytokines into the microenvironment results in further production of proteases, angiogenic factors, growth factors and immunosuppressive cytokines. Examples of NFκB controlled proteins found in prostate cancer include COX-2, XIAP, CXCR4, macrophage inhibitory cytokine-1 (MIC-1), IL-6, IL-8, IL-1, CXCL12, and the CXCR4 [89].

NFκB is a protein complex that controls DNA transcription and is activated by numerous factors including cytokines, free radicals, receptor activator of nuclear factor kappa-B (RANK), and microbial pathogens [90]. Upon activation, the NFκB dimers translocate to the nucleus with activation of numerous genes controlling cell growth, differentiation, inflammatory responses and apoptosis. Aberrant regulation of NFκB has previously been linked to inflammatory states and cancer. Moreover, NFκB controls many of the hallmarks of cancer including: invasion (IL-6); angiogenesis (IL-8, VEGF); propagation through the cell cycle (cyclin D1); and evasion of apoptosis (cIAP-1, TRAF-2, Bcl-$X_L$) [91 - 95]. As such, NFκB activation has clear-cut biological plausibility as a driver of cancer progression and CRPC. In tumor cells, NFκB is constitutively active either due to mutations in genes encoding the NFκB transcription factors themselves or in genes that control NFκB activity (such as IκB genes) or due to tumor cells secreting activation factors (e.g. IL-1). Constitutive NFκB activation in prostate cancer is found in both tumor and its associated stroma and occurs early in the disease process [96 - 100]. It is of note that preclinical work has mechanistically connected NFκB activation to development of prostate cancer with a metastatic phenotype [97]. Specifically, loss of the Ras GTPase-activating protein (RasGAP) gene DAB2IP lead to increased EZH2 and in turn induced NFκB activation which in turn resulted in metastatic prostate cancer in an orthotopic mouse tumor model.

Drugs targeting the inflammatory system are in preclinical and clinical development. The agents can be classified as upstream or direct inhibitors of nuclear factor kappa B or inhibitors of products of NFκB activation Table 3. This is a very new area but one which may lead to significant improvements.

| Drug | Class | Study Design | Results | Current phase of clinical development | Reference |
|---|---|---|---|---|---|
| **Upstream agents** | | | | | |
| EZH2inhibitor (Enhancer of Zeste protein) | Polycomb grp protein | Pre-clinical studies only Ectopic expression of miRNAs impt in EZH2 action inhibit cell growth & tumourigenesis | | | [119] |

| Custirsen OGX-011 | Clusterin Inhibitor (antisense oligo) | Randomised phase II in mCRPC with PD on or within 6m docetaxel (D) D/Pred/C or Mito/Pred/C | 42 pts – 3/23pts with PR in D/P/C OS 15.8 mths M/P/C OS 11.5 mths Toxicity similar in both arms | Phase III Docetaxel +/- Custirsen in mCRPC as 1st & 2nd line recruiting | [120] |
|---|---|---|---|---|---|
| Bortezomib | Proteosome inhibitor | Phase II study of bortezomib with addition of MAB on progression. Bortezomib given d1,4,8,11 for 3 cycles | No activity in addition to docetaxel or paclitaxel (phase I) and high rates of PN observed. When given as single agent or MAB – 11/15 CR with TTP 5.5 months | Results awaited for phase I study with mitoxanthrone | [121, 122, 123] |
| Carfilzomib | Selective proteosome inhibitor | Phase I trial in relapsed or refractory haem malig, d1-5 IV 1.2-20mg/m2 | MTD 15mg/m2 – DLT of feb neutropenia & G4 thrombocytopenia. 2/29 responses | No prostate specific trials recruiting | [124] |
| Denosumab (bone) | Anti-RANKL antibody | Randomised phase III trial denosumab vs zoledronic acid in mCRPC with bone mets | Median time to first SRE 20.7m denosumab vs 17.1m zoledronic acid HR 0.82 p=0.00002 | Phase III study investigating lens opacification in men on demosumab and ADT | [125] |
| **Direct agents** | | | | | |
| Silibinin (derived from Milk Thistle) | Via down regulation of epithelial-mesenchymal transition regulators | Phase II single arm study in PC pts with localized disease prior to prostatectomy. Pts given 13g/day | Transient high blood concentration observed but low tissue concentration. Response results awaited | | [126] |
| Flavopiridol (Alvocidib) | Cyclin dependent kinase inhibitor | Phase II single agent study in met CRPC pts. 72 hour IV infusion at 40-60 mg/m2/day | 36 pts enrolled. No objective responses. 14% pts met 6 month PFS endpoint. | Further development in germ cell tumours & gastric/GOJ ca | [127] |
| Thalidomide | IkB kinase inhibitor | Phase II studies docetaxel (75mg/m2) and docetaxel/bevacizumab (15mg/m2) +/- thalidomide (200mg/m2) | 60 pts enrolled. 90% PSA decline of >50%. Median TTP 18.3 months, median OS 28.2 months. Manageable toxicity but all pts had G3/4 neutropenia | Phase III placebo controlled trial in recurrent hormone sensitive non metastatic PC | [128, 129] |

| Lenolidamide | | Phase II trial after biochemical relapse with LHRH agonists & phase I/II trial as single agent 5mg or 25 mg | 159 pts enrolled. Med TTP PSA 15 vs 9.6 mths. Thalidomide well tolerated, 47% DR. 60 pts enrolled, 25mg ass with greater change in PSA slope but higher toxicity | Phase III in met CRPC pts, docetaxel/ prednisone +/- lenolidamide | [130, 131] |
|---|---|---|---|---|---|
| Parthenolide analogue (derived from *Tanacetum parthenium*) | NFκB inhibitor | Dimethylamino-partehnolide (DAMPT) with superior solubility & bioavailability | DAMPT inhibited NFkB DNA binding & expression of NFkB regulated anti-apoptotic proteins | Phase I dose escalation trial currently recruiting in pts with haem malig | [132] |
| **Downstream agents** | | | | | |
| Siltuximab | αIL-6 Ab | Phase II study in met CRPC pts post docetaxel. 6mg/kg IV q14d for 12 cycles | 53 pts enrolled. PSA response rate 3.8%, RECIST SD rate 23%. High baseline IL-6 levels ass with poor prognosis | Phase I study in combination with docetaxel in met CRPC pts | [133] |
| Celecoxib | NSAID | | | | |
| CNTO888 | α-chemokine ligand 2 Ab | Preclinical studies of CNTO888 2mg/kg twice weekly ip in vivo prostate cancer model | Reduced tumour burden by 96% at 5 weeks also synergistic with docetaxel | Phase II in met CRPC pts post docetaxel results awaited | [134] |
| Plerixafor BKT140 | αCXCR4 | | | Focus of clinical dvpt in AML, phase I/II studies recruiting | |

**Table 3.** The Inflammatory System

# 7. Other key pathways

With time, it is anticipated that more pathways and targets key to prostate cancer growth will be identified. Angiogenesis inhibition has been successful in other cancers but minimal activity was seen in trials with Sunitinib [101] and Bevacizumab [102]. Similarly, targeting the HGF-MET axis is supported by preclinical work [103] and some activity has been seen with MET inhibition. However, Cabozantinib – a tyrosine kinase inhibitor that inhibits multiple receptor tyrosine kinases (RTKs) with growth-promoting and angiogenic properties (MET ($IC_{50}$ in enzymatic assays= 1.8nM), VEGFR2 (0.035nM), RET (3.8nM), and KIT (4.6nM) has significant and intriguing clinical activity in bony disease and some activity in soft tissue disease. This suggests the effect may be due to concurrent inhibition of two relevant pathways.

Cabozantinib has been studied in multiple solid tumors and has shown a broad spectrum of activity with tumour regression in patients with a variety of diseases. It's activity in medullary thyroid cancer is based on RET inhibition [104]. Of particular relevance to prostate cancer, a phase II discontinuation study of 168 men with progressive metastatic CRPC received Cabozantinib initially for 12 weeks [105]. Patients with PR continued open-label cabozantinib, patients with stable disease were randomized to cabozantinib or placebo, whilst patients with progression were discontinued. Trial accrual was halted after enrollment of 168 patients due to the significant activity observed. 78% patients had bone metastasis and significantly 86% of these had a complete or partial response on bone scan as early as week 6. 64% patients had improved pain and 46% patients reported lower narcotic analgesia use. To date the median PFS has not been reached. Most common related Grade 3/4 AEs were fatigue (11%), HTN (7%), and hand-foot syndrome (5%). Osteoclast and osteoblast effects were observed: 55% had declines of $\geq$50% in plasma C-Telopeptide; 56% of patients with elevated tALP had declines of $\geq$50%.

Interestingly numerous lines of preclinical and clinical evidence implicate MET and VEGFR activation in bone metastases as well as prostate cancer, especially castration resistant disease. Specifically, androgen deprivation increases MET expression in prostate cancer cells [106, 107] and c-met has been shown to be upregulated in CRPC and may be a factor that supports CRPC cells in the castrate state [106, 108]. Androgen deprivation also increases expression of c-met's ligand, Hepatocyte Growth Factor (HGF) in the stroma. Increased expression of MET and HGF may contribute to disease progression following androgen deprivation therapy. This may be a compensatory mechanism as HGF/cMET activity enhances Leydig cell steroidogenetic activity [109]. It is also of note that increased expression of MET and/or HGF correlate with prostate cancer metastasis and disease recurrence [110, 111]. In addition, VEGF has been shown to activate MET signaling via neuropilin-1. Osteoblasts and osteoclasts also express MET and VEGFRs and osteoclasts secrete HGF. This supports the notion that MET signaling not only supports the tumor, but also bone turnover which provides a fertile microenvironment for prostate cancer growth [112]. These observations provide a strong rationale for dual inhibition of VEGFR2 and MET as a therapeutic strategy in men with CRPC and bone metastases. As such, cabozantinib may not only have single agent activity but also enhance abiraterone activity by simultaneously blocking a putative resistance/survival mechanism to hormonal therapy and abrogating bone turnover and making the microenvironment less hospitable for cancer growth. Given these many reasons, it is logical to hypothesize that combining these two active agents against CRPC will result in even more substantial clinical benefit.

## 8. Conclusion & future directions

It is clear from the foregoing discussion that increased biological knowledge and drug development technologies has resulted in a vast number of agents for clinical trial testing. However, it is paramount that judicious trial designs are employed and match the drug to the tumor by ensuring that the target is present. It is also quite certain that no single drug will work given the inherent multiple redundant survival pathways. This is probably more apparent for castration resistant disease. Therefore, one can argue that waiting for metastatic disease or castrate resistant disease to assess a new drug is a defeatist approach, and that an assessment earlier in the disease spectrum to prevent the emergence of resistance is a more proactive and promising approach to improve outcomes in prostate cancer. The conduct of a study in patients with a biochemical relapse after definitive localized therapy provides a major opportunity for drug development. This approach allows the analysis of a drug in isolation and as well as an assessment and effective triage of the numerous new agents that are now available for testing. Also the primary pathology can be interrogated to look for activation of the pathway and provides an opportunity to biologically direct the evaluation of drugs relevant to a given a pathway in an individual's cancer. Ultimately, key combinations simultaneously targeting the essential and multiply redundant pathways driving cancer survival and resistance mechanisms can be developed. This has been a successful strategy for treatment of HIV and AIDS where the early use of Highly Active Anti-retroviral Therapy (HAART) has made major advances. With time and judicious clinical development, it is possible to develop a similar strategy such as Highly Effective Early Prostate Cancer Therapy (HEEPT) for patients with rapidly progressive PSA rises after definitive local therapy and have a long life expectancy. Early use of a highly effective combination therapy will hopefully eradicate the disease and prevent patients from dying from recurrent disease that may otherwise have been lethal and more difficult to treat if waited until later in the disease

## Author details

Sarah M. Rudman[1], Peter G. Harper[1] and Christopher J. Sweeney[2]

1 Dept of Oncology, Guys & St Thomas' NHS Foundation Trust, Great Maze Pond, London, SE1 9RT, UK

2 Lank Center for Genitourinary Oncology, Dana Farber Cancer Institute, 450 Brookline Ave, Boston, MA, USA

## References

[1] Sridhara R, Johnson J R, Justice R et al: Review of oncology and haematology drug product approvals at the US Food and drug administration between July 2005 and December 2007. J Natl Cancer Inst 2010 102(8) 578-9

[2] Lo Russo P M, Anderson A B, Boerner S A et al. Making the investigational oncology pipeline more efficient and effective: are we headed in the right direction? Clin Cancer Res 2010 16(24) 5956-62

[3] Tannock IF, Osoba D, Stockler MR et al: Chemotherapy with mitoxantrone plus prednisone or prednisone alone for symptomatic hormone resistant prostate cancer: a

Canadian randomized trial with palliative end-points. J Clin Oncol 1996 14(6) 1756-64

[4]  Tannock I F, de Wit R, Berry WR et al: Docetaxel plus prednisone or mitoxantrone plus prednisone for advanced prostate cancer. N Engl J Med 2004 351 1502-12 2004

[5]  Morris PG & Fornier MN: Microtubule active agents: beyond the taxane frontier. Clin Cancer Res 2008 14 7167-7172

[6]  De Bono J S, Oudard S, Ozguroglu M et al: Prednisone plus cabazitaxel or mitoxantrone for metastatic castrate resistant prostate cancer progressing after docetaxel treatment: a randomized open label trial. Lancet 2010 376 (9747) 1147-54

[7]  Gradishar WJ, Tjulandin S, Davidson N et al: Phase III trial of nanoparticle bound paclitaxel with polyethylated castor oil based paclitaxel in women with breast cancer. J Clin Oncol 2005 23(31) 7794-803

[8]  Mita M, Mita A, Sarantopoulos J et al: Phase I study of paclitaxel poliglumex administered weekly for patients with advanced solid malignancies. Cancer Chemother Pharmacol 2009 64(2) 287-295

[9]  Beer TM, Ryan C, Alumkal J et al: A phase II study of paclitaxel poliglumex in combination with transdermal oestradiol for the treatment of metastatic castrate resistant prostate cancer after docetaxel chemotherapy. Anticancer drugs 2010 21(4) 433-438

[10] Farokhzad OC, Cheng J, Teply BA et al: Targeted nanoparticle aptamer bioconjugates for cancer chemotherapy in vivo. Proc Natl Acad Sci USA 2006 103(16) 6315-6320

[11] Liu G, Chen YH, Dipaola R et al: Phase II trial of weekly ixabepilone in men with metastatic castrate-resistant prostate cancer (E3803): a trial of the eastern co-operative oncology group. Clin Genitourin Cancer 2012 10(2) 99-105

[12] Chi KN, Beardsley E, Eigl BJ et al: A phase II study of patupilone in patients with metastatic castrate-resistant prostate cancer previously treated with docetaxel: Canadian Urologic Oncology group study P07a. Ann Oncol 2012 23(1) 53-58

[13] Beer TM, Smith DC, Hussain A et al: Phase II study of sagopilone plus prednisone in patients with castrate-resistant prostate cancer: a phase II study of the Department of Defense Prostate Cancer Clinical Trials Consortium. Br J Cancer 2012 doi 10.1038/bjc. 2012.339

[14] De Bono J S, Molife R, Sonpavde G et al: Phase II study of eribulin mesylate (E7389) in patients with metastatic castration-resistant prostate cancer stratified by prior taxane therapy. Ann Oncol 2012 23(5) 1241-1249

[15] Nilsson S, Parker C, Haugen I et al: Alpharadin, a novel, highly targeted alpha pharmaceutical with a good safety profile for patients with CRPC and bone metastases: Combined analyses of phase I and II clinical trials. 2010 Genitourinary cancer symposium abstract 106

[16] Sartor AO, Heinrich D, O'Sullivan JM et al: Radium-223 chloride (Ra-223) impact on skeletal-related events (SREs) and ECOG performance status (PS) in patients with castration-resistant prostate cancer (CRPC) with bone metastases: Interim results of a phase III trial (ALSYMPCA). J Clin Oncol 2012 30 suppl abstrc 4551

[17] Huggins C & Hodges CV. Studies on prostate cancer, I: the effect of castration of estrogen and of androgen injection on serum phosphatases in metastatic carcinoma of the prostate. Cancer Res 1941 1 293-297

[18] Craft, N, Shostak Y, Carey M et al: A mechanism for hormone-independent prostate cancer through modulation of androgen receptor signaling by the HER-2/neu tyrosine kinase. Nat. Med. 1999 5 280–285

[19] Gioeli, D, Ficarro SB, Kwiek JJ et al: Androgen receptor phosphorylation. Regulation and identification of the phosphorylation sites. J Biol Chem. 2003 277 29304–29314

[20] Veldscholte, J Ris-Stalpers C, Kuiper GG et al: A mutation in the ligand binding domain of the androgen receptor of human LNCaP cells affects steroid binding characteristics and response to anti-androgens. Biochem. Biophys. Res. Commun. 1990 173 534–540

[21] Chen CD, Welsbie DS, Tran C et al: Molecular determinants of resistance to anti-androgen therapy. Nature Medicine 2004 10 (1) 33-39

[22] Mitsiades N, Schultz B, Taylor S et al: Increased expression of androgen receptor and enzymes involved in androgen synthesis in metastatic prostate cancer: targets for novel personalized therapies. J Clin Oncol 2009 27: (15 suppl) abstr 5002

[23] Koivisto PA & Hellin H J: Androgen receptor gene amplification increases tissue PSA protein expression in hormone-refractory prostate carcinoma. Am J Pathol 1999 189(2) 219-223

[24] Mohler JL, Gregory CW, Ford OH. The androgen axis in recurrent prostate cancer. Clin Cancer Res 2004 10 440-448

[25] Figg WD, Liu Y, Arlen P et al. A randomized phase II trial of ketoconazole plus alendronate versus ketoconazole alone in patients with androgen independent prostate cancer and bone metastases. J Urol 2005 173 790-796

[26] Attard G, Reid A H M, A'Hern R et al: Selective inhibition with Cyp 17 with abiraterone acetate is highly active in the treatment of castrate-resistant prostate cancer. J Clin Oncol 2010 27 (23) 3742-3748

[27] Reid AH, Attard G, Danila DC et al. Significant and sustained anti-tumour activity in post docetaxel castration resistant prostate cancer with the CYP17 inhibitor abiraterone acetate. J Clin Oncol 2010 28 1489-1495

[28] De Bono JS, Logothetis CJ, Molina A et al: Abiraterone and increased survival in metastatic prostate cancer. N Engl J Med 2011 364(21) 1995-2005

[29]  Ryan CJ, Smith MR, De Bono JS et al: Interim analysis (IA) results of COU-AA-302, a randomized, phase III study of abiraterone acetate (AA) in chemotherapy-naive patients (pts) with metastatic castration-resistant prostate cancer (mCRPC). J Clin Oncol 2012 suppl. Abstrc LBA 4518

[30]  Petrylak DP, Gandhi JG, Clark WR et al: Phase I results from a phase I/II study of orteronel, an oral, investigational, nonsteroidal 17,20-lyase inhibitor, with docetaxel and prednisone (DP) in metastatic castration-resistant prostate cancer (mCRPC). J Clin Oncol 2012 30 suppl abstrc 4656

[31]  Dreicer R, Agus DB, Bellmunt J et al: A phase III, randomized, double-blind, multicenter trial comparing the investigational agent orteronel (TAK-700) plus prednisone (P) with placebo plus P in patients with metastatic castration-resistant prostate cancer (mCRPC) that has progressed during or following docetaxel-based therapy. J Clin Oncol 2012 20 suppl abstrc TPS4963

[32]  Chen Y, Clegg NJ, Scher HI. Anti-androgens and androgen-depleting therapies in prostate cancer: new agents for an established target. Lancet Oncol 2009 10 981-991

[33]  Scher HI, Beer TM, Higano CS et al: Antitumour activity of MDV3100 in castration-resistant prostate cancer: a phase 1-2 study. Lancet 2010 375 (9724) 1437-1446

[34]  De Bono JS, Fizazi K, Saad F et al: Primary, secondary, and quality-of-life endpoint results from the phase III AFFIRM study of MDV3100, an androgen receptor signaling inhibitor. J Clin Oncol 2012 30 suppl abstrc 4519

[35]  Bolden JE, Peaert MJ, Johnstone RW. Anticancer activities of histone deacetylase inhibitors. Nat Rev Drug Discov 2006 5 769-784

[36]  Welsbie DS, Xu J, Chen H et al: Histone deacetylases are required for androgen receptor function in hormone-sensitive and castrate – resistant prostate cancer. Cancer Res 2009 69 958-966

[37]  Rathkopf D, Wong BY, Ross RW et al: A phase I study or oral panobinostat alone and in combination with docetaxel in patients with castration-resistant prostate cancer. Cancer Chemother Pharmacol 2010 66 (1) 181-9

[38]  Bradley D, Rathkopf D, Dunn R et al: Vorinostat in advanced prostate cancer patients progressing on prior chemotherapy (National Cancer Institute Trial 6862): trial results and interleukin-6 analysis: a study by the Department of Defense Prostate Cancer Clinical Trial Consortium and University of Chicago Phase 2 Consortium. Cancer 2009 115 (23) 5541-9

[39]  Schneider BJ, Kalemkerian GP, Bradley D et al. Phase I study of vorinostat in combination with docetaxel in patients with advanced and relapsed solid malignancies. Invest New Drugs 2012 30(1) 249-257

[40]  Powers MV, Workman P: Targeting of multiple signaling pathways by heat shock protein 90 molecular chaperone inhibitors. Endocr Relat Cancer 2006 13 (Suppl 1): S125-S135

[41] Solit DB, Egorin M, Valentin G et al: Phase I pharmacokinetic and pharmacodynamic trial of docetaxel and 17-AAG (17-allylamino-17-demethoxygeldanamycin). J Clin Oncol 2004 22 (14 Suppl) Abstr 3032

[42] Heath EI, Hillman DW, Vaishampayam U et al: A phase II trial of 17-allylamino-17-demethoxygeldanamycin in patients with hormone-refractory metastatic prostate cancer. Clin Cancer Res 2008 14 (23) 7940-7946

[43] Oh W, Stadler WM. Srinivas S et al: A single arm phase II trial of IPI-504 in patients with castration resistant prostate cancer (CRPC). Presented at ASCO Genitourinary symposium 2009 Abstract 219

[44] Goldman JW, Raju RN, Gordon GA et al: A Phase 1 dose-escalation study of the Hsp90 inhibitor STA-9090 administered once weekly in patients with solid tumors. J Clin Oncol 2010 28:15s (suppl; abstr 2529)

[45] Oh Y K & Park T G. siRNA delivery systems for cancer treatment. Adv Drug Deliv Rev 2009 61(10) 850-862

[46] Tutt A, Robson M, Garber J E et al. Oral poly(ADP-ribose) polymerase inhibitor olaparib in patients with BRCA1 or BRCA2 mutations and advanced breast cancer: a proof of concept trial. Lancet 2010 376 235-244

[47] Gallagher DJ, Gaudet MM, Pal P et al: Germline BRCA mutations denote a clinicopathologic subset of prostate cancer. Clin Cancer Res 2010 16 (7) 2115-21

[48] Fong PC, Boss DS, Yap TA et al: Inhibition of poly(ADP-ribose) polymerase in tumours from BRCA mutations carriers. N Engl J Med 2009 361 123-134

[49] Mendes-Pereira AM, Martin SA, Brough R et al: Synthetic lethal targeting of PTEN mutant cells with PARP inhibitors. EMBO Mol Med 2009 1 (6-7) 315-22

[50] Sandhu SK, Wenham RM, Wilding G et al: First-in-human trial of a poly(ADP-ribose) polymerase (PARP) inhibitor MK-4827 in advanced cancer patients (pts) with antitumor activity in BRCA-deficient and sporadic ovarian cancers. J Clin Oncol 28:15s 2010 (suppl abstr 3001)

[51] Cho N Y, Choi M, Kim B H et al: Braf and Kras mutations in prostatic adenocarcinoma. Int J Cancer 2006 119(8) 1858-62

[52] Sun X, Huang J, Homma T et al: Genetic alterations in the PI3K pathway in prostate cancer. Anticancer Res 2009 29(5) 1739-43

[53] Hsing A W & Devesa S S: Trends and patterns of prostate cancer: what do they suggest? Epidemiol Rev 2001 23 3-13

[54] Strom S S, Yamamura Y, Forman MR et al: Saturated fat intake predicts biochemical failure after prostatectomy. Int J Cancer 2008 122 2581-5

[55] Warburg O. On the origin of cancer cells. Science 1956 123 309-314

[56]  Nickerson T, Pollak M Huynh H: Castration-induced apoptosis in the rat ventral prostate is associated with increased expression of genes encoding insulin-like growth factor binding proteins 2,3,4 and 5. Endocrinology 1998 139(2) 807-810

[57]  Plymate S R, Haugk K, Coleman I et al: An antibody targeting the type I insulin-like growth factors receptor enhances the castration induced response in androgen-dependent prostate cancer. Clin Can Res 2007 13(21) 6429-39

[58]  Higano CS, Alumkal JJ, Ryan CJ et al: A phase II study of cixutumumab (IMC-A12), a monoclonal antibody (MAb) against the insulin-like growth factor 1 receptor (IGF-IR), monotherapy in metastatic castration-resistant prostate cancer (mCRPC): Feasibility of every 3-week dosing and updated results. Presented at the ASCO Genitourinary Symposium 2010 Abstract 189

[59]  Haluska P, Shaw H M, Batzel G N et al: Phase I dose escalation study of the anti insulin-like growth factor-I receptor monoclonal antibody CP-751,871 in patients with refractory solid tumours. Clin Cancer Res 2007 13 5834-55840

[60]  Molife LR, Fong PC, Pacagnella L et al: The insulin-like growth factor-I receptor inhibitor figitumumab (CP-751, 871) in combination with docetaxel in patients with advanced solid tumours: results of a phase Ib dose-escalation, open-label study. Br J Cancer 2010 103 (3) 332-9

[61]  Tolcher AW, Sarantopoulos J, Patnaik A et al: Phase I, pharmacokinetic, and pharmacodynamic study of AMG 479, a fully human monoclonal antibody to insulin-like growth factor receptor 1. J Clin Oncol 2009 27 (34) 5800-7

[62]  Carden CP, Lim ES, Jones RL et al: Phase I study of intermittent dosing of OSI-906, a dual tyrosine kinase inhibitor of insulin-like growth factor-1 receptor (IGF- 1R) and insulin receptor (IR) in patients with advanced solid tumors. J Clin Oncol 2010 28:15s (suppl; abstr 2530)

[63]  Mulholland DJ, Dedhar S, Wu H et al: PTEN & GSK3beta: key regulators of progression to androgen-independent prostate cancer. Oncogene 2006 25(3) 329-337

[64]  Jia S, Liu Z, Zhang S et al: Essential roles of PI(3)K-p110b * in cell growth, metabolism and tumourigenesis. Nature 2008 454 776-9

[65]  Edelmann G, Bedell C, Shapiro G et al: A phase I dose escalation study of XL147 (SAR205408), a PI3K inhibitor administered orally to patients with advanced malignancies. J Clin Oncol 2010 28 15s (suppl;abstrc 3004)

[66]  Von Hoff DD, LoRusso P, Tibes R et al: A first in human phase I study to evaluate the pan-PI3K inhibitor GDC-0941 administered QD or BID in patients with advanced solid tumours. J Clin Oncol 2010 28:15s (suppl;abstr 2541)

[67]  Baselga J, De Jonge MJ, Rodon J et al: A first-in-human phase I study of BKM120, an oral pan-class I PI3K inhibitor, in patients (pts) with advanced solid tumours. J Clin Oncol 28:15s 2010 (suppl;abstr 3003)

[68] Kreisberg J I, Malik S N, Prihoda T J et al: Phosphorylation of Akt (ser473) is an excellent predictor of poor clinical outcome in prostate cancer. Cancer Res 2004 64 5232-5236

[69] Ayala G, Thompson t, Yang G et al: High levels of phosphorylated form of Akt-1 in prostate cancer and non-neoplastic prostate tissues are strong predictors of biochemical recurrence. Clin Cancer Res 2004 10 6572-6578

[70] Chee K G, Longmate J, Quinn D I et al: The AKT inhibitor perifosine in biochemically recurrent prostate cancer: a phase II California/Pittsburgh cancer consortium trial. Clin Genitourin Cancer 2007 5(7) 433-7

[71] Tolcher AW, Yap TA, Fearen I et al: A phase I study of MK-2206, an oral potent allosteric Akt inhibitor in patients with advanced solid tumours. J Clin Oncol 2009 27 15s (suppl;abstrc 3503)

[72] George D J, Armstrong A J, Creel P: A phase II study of RAD001 in men with hormone-refractory metastatic prostate cancer (HRPC). ASCO Genitourinary Cancers Symposium 2008: abstract 181

[73] Ross R W, Manola J, Oh W K et al: Phase I trial of RAD001 and docetaxel in castration resistant prostate cancer with FDG-PET assessment of RAD001 activity. J Clin Oncol 2008 26 abstrc 5069

[74] Pan C, Ghosh P, Lara P et al: Encouraging activity of bicalutamide and everolimus in castration-resistant prostate cancer (CRPC): Early results from a phase II clinical trial. J Clin Oncol 2011 suppl. 11 abstrc 157

[75] Hardie D G. AMP-activated/SNF-1 protein kinases: conserved guardians of cellular energy. Nat Rev Mol Cell Biol 2007 8 774-785

[76] Luo Z, Saha AK, Xiang X et al: AMPK, the metabolic syndrome and cancer. Trends Pharmacol Sci 2005 26 69-76

[77] Matsui H, Suzuki K, Ohtake N et al: Genome wide linkage analysis of familial prostate cancer in the Japanese population. J Hum Genet 2004 49 9-15

[78] Xiang X, Saha A K, Wen R et al: AMP-activated protein kinase activators can inhibit the growth of prostate cancer cells by multiple mechanisms. Biochem Biophys Res Commun 2004 321 161-7

[79] Huang X, Wullschleger S, Shapiro N et al: Important role of the LKB1-AMPK pathways in suppressing tumourigenesis in PTEN-deficient mice. Biochem J 2008 412 212-21

[80] Wright J L & Stanford J L: Metformin use and prostate cancer in Caucasian men: results from a population-based case-control study. Cancer Causes Control 2009 20 1617-22

[81] Pollak M: Insulin and insulin-like growth factor signaling in neoplasia. Nat Rev Cancer 2008 8 915-28

[82] Jang M, Cai L, Udeani G O et al: Cancer chemopreventive activity of resveratrol, a natural product derived from grapes. Science 1997 275 218-220

[83] De Marzo AM, De Weese TM, Platz EA et al: Pathological and molecular mechanisms of prostate carcinogenesis: implications for diagnosis, detection, prevention and treatment. J Cell Biochem 2004 91 459-477

[84] De Marzo AM, Marchi VL, Epstein JI & Nelson WG: Proliferative inflammatory atrophy of the prostate: implications for prostate carcinogenesis. Am J Pathol. 1999 59 (22) 1985-1992

[85] Sutcliffe S, Giovanucci E, Alderete JF et al: Plasma antibodies against Trichomonas vaginalis and subsequent risk of prostate cancer. Cancer Epidemiol Biomarkers Prev 2006 15(11) 939-945

[86] Stark JR, Judson G, Alderete JF et al: Prospective study of Trichomonas vaginaslis infection and prostate cancer incidence and mortality: Physicians health study. J Natl Cancer Inst 2009 101 (20) 1406-1411

[87] Nelson WG, De Marzo AM, Isaacs WB et al: Mechanisms of disease: prostate cancer. N Engl J Med 2003 349 366-381

[88] Li H, Kantoff PW, Giovanucci E et al: Manganese superoxide dismutase polymorphism, prediagnostic antioxidant status and risk of clinically significant prostate cancer. Cancer Res 2005 65(6) 2498-2504

[89] Dobrovolskaia MA & Kozlov SV: Inflammation & Cancer:when NFκB amalgamates the perilous partnership. Curr Cancer Drug Targets 2005 5(5) 325-344

[90] Ghosh S, Bhattacharya S, Sirkar M et al: Leishmania donovani suppresses activated protein1 and NF-κB activation in host macrophages via ceramide generation: involovement of extracellular signal-regulated kinase Infect Immun 2002 70(12) 6828-6838

[91] Helbig G, Christopherson KW, Bhat-Nakshatri P et al: NK-κB promotes breast cancer cell migration and metastasis by inducing the expression of the chemokine receptor CXCR4. J Biol Chem 2003 278(24) 21631-21638

[92] Zong WX, Edelstein LC, Chen C et al: The prosurvival Bcl-2 homolog Bfl-1/A1 is a direct transcriptional target of NF-κB that blocks TNF alpha induced apoptosis. Genes Dev 1999 13 (4) 382-387

[93] Dolcet X, Llobet D, Pallares J et al: NF-kB in development and progression of human cancer.Virchows Archiv 2005 446 (5) 475-482

[94] Wang CY, Mayo MW, Baldwin AS: TNF and cancer therapy-induced apoptosis: potentation by inhibition of NF-κB. Science 1996 274: 784-787

[95] Karashima T, Sweeney P, Kamat A et al: Nuclear factor κB mediates angiogenesis and metastasis of human bladder cancer through the regulation of interleukin-8. Clin Cancer Res 2003 9(7) 2786-2797

[96]  Ammirante M, Luo JL, Grivennikov S et al: B-cell derived lymphotoxin promotes cas-
      tration resistant prostate cancer. Nature 2010 464 302-5

[97]  Min J, Zaslavsky A, Fedele G et al: An oncogene-tumor suppressor cascade drives
      metastatic prostate cancer by coordinately activating Ras and nuclear factor-κB. Nat
      Med 2010 16(3) 286-294

[98]  Sweeney C, Li L, Shanmugam R et al: Nuclear factor-kappaB is constitutively activat-
      ed in prostate cancer in vitro and is overexpressed in prostatic intraepithelial neopla-
      sia and adenocarcinoma of the prostate. Clin Cancer Res 2004 10(16) 5501-5507

[99]  Lessard L, Begin LR, Gleave ME et al: Nuclear localization of nuclear factor-κB tran-
      scription factors in prostate cancer: an immunohistochemical study 2005 93(9)
      1019-1023

[100] Lessard L, Mes-Masson AM, Lamarre L et al. NF κB nuclear localization and its prog-
      nostic significant in prostate cancer BJU Int. 2003 91(4) 417-420

[101] Michaelson MD, Oudard S, Ou Y et al: Randomized, placebo-controlled, phase III tri-
      al of sunitinib in combination with prednisone (SU+P) versus prednisone (P) alone in
      men with progressive metastatic castration-resistant prostate cancer (mCRPC). J Clin
      Oncol 2011 29 suppl abstrc 4515

[102] Heidenreich A, Pfister DJ, Thüer D et al: Docetaxel versus docetaxel plus bevacizu-
      mab in progressive castration-resistant prostate cancer following first-line docetaxel.
      J Clin Oncol 2010 28 suppl abstrc e15006

[103] Varkaris A, Corn PG, Gaur S et al: The role of HGF/c-met signaling in prostate cancer
      progression and c-met inhibitors in clinical trials. Exp Opin Investig Drugs 2011 20
      (12) 1677-84

[104] Kurzrock R, Sherman SI, Ball DW et al: Activity of XL-184 (Cabozantinib), an oral ty-
      rosine kinase inhibitor, in patients with medullary thyroid cancer. J Clin Oncol 2011
      29 2660-2666

[105] Hussain M, Sweeney C, Corn PG et al: Cabozantanib (XL184) in metastatic castra-
      tion-resistant prostate cancer (mCRPC): Results from a phase II randomized discon-
      tinuation trial. J Clin Oncol 2011 29 (Suppl) abstrc 4516

[106] Humphrey PA, Zhu X, Zarnegar R et al: Hepatocyte growth factor and its receptor
      (c-MET) in prostatic carcinoma. Am J Pathol. 1995 147 (2) 386-396

[107] Verras M, Lee J, Xue H et al: the androgen receptor negatively regulates the expres-
      sion of c-Met: implications for a novel mechanism of prostate cancer progression.
      Cancer Res 2007 67 (3) 967-975

[108] Tu WH, Zhu C, Clark C et al: Efficacy of c-Met inhibitor fpr advanced prostate can-
      cer. BMC Cancer 2010 10 556

[109] Del Bravo J, Catizone A, Ricci G et al: Hepatocyte growth factor-modulated rat Ley-
      dig cell functions. J Androl. 2007 28(6) 866-874

[110] Knudsen BS, Gmyrek GA, Inra J et al: High expression of the Met receptor in prostate cancer metastasis to bone. Urology 2002 60(6) 1113-1117

[111] Humphrey PA, Halabi S, Picus J et al: Prognostic significance of plasma scatter/hepatocyte growth factor levels in patients with metastatic hormone refractory prostate cancer: results from Cancer & Leukaemia group B 150005/9480. Clin Genitourin Cancer 2006 4(4) 269-274

[112] Grano M, Galimi F, Zambonin G et al: Hepatocyte growth factor is a coupling factor for osteoclasts and osteoblasts in vitro. Proceedings of the National Academy of Sciences of the United States of America. 1996 93(15) 7644-7648

[113] Bruno RD, Vasaitis TS, Gediya LK et al: Synthesis and biological evaluations of putative metabolic stable analogs of TOK-001: head to head anti-tumour efficacy evaluation of TOK-001 and Abiraterone in LAPC-4 human prostate cancer xenograft model. Steroids 2011 76(12) 1268-1279

[114] Yong W, Goh B, Toh H et al: Phase I study of SB939 three times weekly for 3 weeks every 4 weeks in patients with advanced solid malignancies. J Clin Oncol 27:15s, 2009 (suppl; abstr 2560)

[115] Molife LR, Attard G, Fong PC et al: Phase II, two-stage, single arm trial of the histone deacetylase inhibitor (HDAC) romidepsin in metastatic castration-resistant prostate cancer (CRPC). Ann Oncol 2010 21: 109-113

[116] Evans T, Lindsay CR, Chan E et al: Phase I dose-escalation study of continuous oral dosing of OSI-906, a dual tyrosine kinase inhibitor of insulin-like growth factor-1 receptor (IGF-1R) and insulin receptor (IR), in patients with advanced solid tumors. J Clin Oncol 28:15s, 2010 (suppl; abstr 2531).

[117] Ben Sahra I, Laurent K, Loubat A et al: The antidiabetic drug metformin exerts an anti-tumoural effect in vitro and in vivo through a decrease in cyclin D1 level. Oncogene 2008 27 2576-3586

[118] Emmenegger U, Berry SR, Booth C et al: Phase II study of maintenance therapy with temsirolimus (TEM) after response to first-line docetaxel (TAX) chemotherapy in castration-resistant prostate cancer (CRPC). J Clin Oncol 2011 29 Suppl 7 Abstrc 160

[119] Lu J, Me ML, Wang L et al: MiR-26a inhibits cell growth and tumorigenesis of nasopharyngeal carcinoma through repression of EZH2.Cancer Res 2011 71(1) 225-233

[120] Saad F, Hotte S, North S et al: Randomized Phase 2 Trial of Custirsen (OGX-011) with Docetaxel or Mitoxantrone in Patients with Metastatic Castrate-Resistant Prostate Cancer: CUOG Trial P06c. Clin Cancer Res 2011 Epub ahead of print.

[121] Hainsworth JD, Meluch AA, Spigel DR et al; Weekly docetaxel and bortezomib as first-line treatment for patients with hormone-refractory prostate cancer: a Minnie Pearl Cancer Research Network phase II trial. Clin Genitorurin Cancer 2007 5(4) 278-283

[122]  Cresta S Cessa C, Catapano CV et al: Phase I study of bortezomib with weekly paclitaxel in patients with advanced solid tumours. Eur J Cancer 2008 44 (13) 1829-1834

[123]  Kraft AS, Garrett-Mayer E, Wahlquist AE et al: Combination therapy of recurrent
prostate cancer with the proteosome inhibitor Bortezomib plus hormone blockade.
Cancer Biol Ther 2011 12(2) 119-124

[124]  O'Connor OA, Stewart AK, Vallone M et al: A phase I dose escalation study of the
safety and pharmacokinetics of the novel proteosome inhibitor carfilzomib in patients with haematological malignancies. Clin Cancer Res 15 (22) 7085-91

[125]  Fizazi K, Carducci M, Smith M et al: Denosumab versus zoledronic acid for treatment of bone metastases in men with castrate-resistant prostate cancer: a randomized
double blind study. Lancet 2011 377 813-822

[126]  Flaig TW, Glode M, Gustafson D et al: A study of high-dose oral silybin-phytosome
followed by prostatectomy in patients with localized prostate cancer. Prostate 2010
70(8) 848-855

[127]  Liu G, Gandara DR, Lara PN et al: A phase II trial of flavopiridol in patients with
previously untreated metastatic androgen-independent prostate cancer. Clin Cancer
Res 2004 10(3) 924-928

[128]  Ning Y-M, Gulley JL, Arlen PM et al: Phase II trial of bevacizumab, thalidomide, docetaxel and prednisone in patients with metastatic castration resistant prostate cancer. J Clin Oncol 2010 28(12) 2070-2076

[129]  Dahut WL, Gulley JL, Arlen PM et al: Randomised phase II trial of docetaxel plus
thalidominde in androgen-independent prostate cancer. J Clin Oncol 2004 22
2532-2539

[130]  Figg WD, Huassain MH, Gulley JL et al: A double blind randomized crossover study
of oral thalidomide versus placebo for androgen dependent prostate cancer treated
with intermittent androgen ablation. J Urol 2009 181(3) 1104-1113

[131]  Keizman D, Zahurak M, Sinibaldi V et al: Lenolidamide in non-metastatic biochemically relapsed prostate cancer: results of a phase I/II double-blinded randomized
study. Clin Cancer Res 2010 16(21) 5269-5276

[132]  Shanmugam R, Kusumanchi P, Cheng L et al: A water soluble parthenolide analogue
suppresses in vivo prostate cancer growth by targeting NFkB & generating reactive
oxygen species. Prostate 2010 70(10) 1074-1086

[133]  Dorff TB, Goldman B, Pinski JB et al: Clinical and correlative results of SWOG S0354:
a phase II trial of CNTO 328 (Siltuximab), a monoclonal antibody against interleu-
kin-6, in chemotherapy pre-treated patients with castration resistant prostate cancer.
Clin Cancer Res 2010 16(11) 3028-3034

[134]  Loberg RD, Ying C, Craig M et al: Targeting CCL-2 with systemic delivery of neutralizing antibodies induced prostate cancer tumour regression in vivo. Cancer Res 2007
67(19) 9417-9424

# Steroidal CYP17 Inhibitors for Prostate Cancer Treatment: From Concept to Clinic

Jorge A. R. Salvador, Vânia M. Moreira and
Samuel M. Silvestre

Additional information is available at the end of the chapter

## 1. Introduction

The successful application of therapeutic strategies to block the known growth stimulation property of estrogen in breast cancer, namely the aromatase (CYP19) inhibitors formestane (4-OH) and exemestane (Aromasin) [1], has paved the way for the investigation of inhibitors of other P450 enzymes that might impart the growth of hormone-dependent cancers [2]. Cytochrome P450 17α-hydroxylase,$C_{17,20}$-lyase (CYP17) is at the crossroads of androgen and corticoid biosynthesis and has become a valuable target in prostate cancer (PC) treatment [3-8]. Androgens, which are produced in steroidogenic tissues, bind to the androgen receptor (AR) and initiate transcription which in turn results in the synthesis of prostate-specific proteins, as well as in cell proliferation. Systemic ablation of androgen by castration, either surgical or chemical, is highly effective in treating PC when the disease is hormone-dependent [3]. However, within 18-24 months following the onset of primary hormonal therapies, the disease becomes androgen-refractory by mechanisms in which AR-mediated signaling and gene expression is still active despite castrate androgen levels [9]. The FDA approved the combination of docetaxel (Taxotere) *1* and prednisone for the treatment of castrate-resistant PC (CRPC) which improves survival time in about 18 months [10, 11], and cabazitaxel (Jevtana) *2* [12], a novel taxane derivative, for metastatic CRPC (mCRPC) which has progressed following docetaxel therapy (Fig. 1). The immunotherapy Sipuleucel-T (Provenge) is also approved for the treatment of asymptomatic or minimally symptomatic mCPRC. In April 2011, abiraterone acetate (Zytiga) *3* became the first steroidal CYP17 inhibitor to be approved by the FDA for the treatment of docetaxel-resistant mCRPC (Fig. 1) [13, 14]. Following abirateroneacetate *3*, galeterone (TOK-001) *4* (Fig. 1), another steroidal CYP17 inhibitor, with AR antagonistic and ablative activities, is currently undergoing Phase I/II clinical trials for the treatment of chemotherapy-naive CRPC [15, 16].

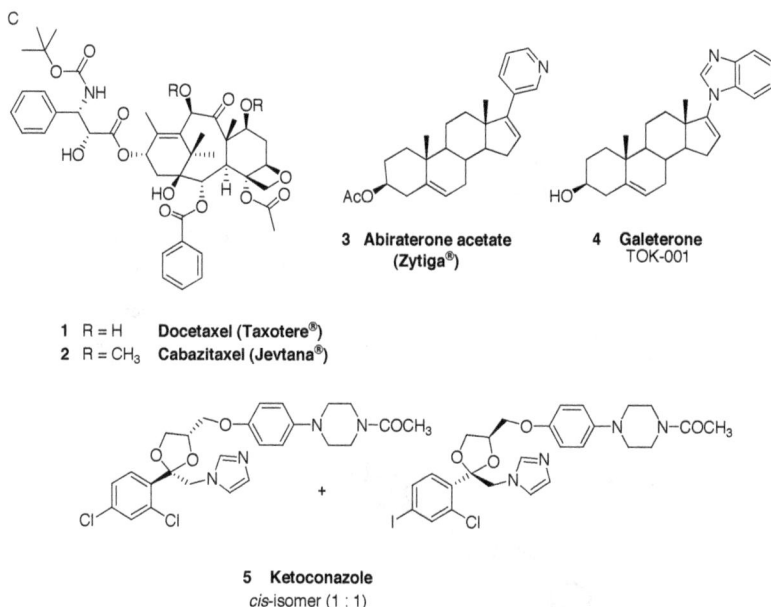

**3  Abiraterone acetate**
(Zytiga®)

**4  Galeterone**
TOK-001

**1  R = H      Docetaxel (Taxotere®)**
**2  R = CH₃  Cabazitaxel (Jevtana®)**

**5  Ketoconazole**
cis-isomer (1 : 1)

**Figure 1.** Compounds used in the clinical practice for PC treatment, and galeterone4, currently undergoing clinical trials for the treatment of chemotherapy-naive CRPC.

The first reports on steroidal CYP17 inhibitors date back to about 40 years ago [3, 8, 17-20]. Many different chemistries have been exploited in their development which has been complicated by the fact that no 3D structure of the enzyme is available. Nonetheless, structure-activity analysis has revealed the general features of a good inhibitor and recent docking and modeling studies have further shed some light on the way these molecules interact with the enzyme's active site [21, 22]. Moreover, additional effects of these compounds on other PC-related targets have been studied and disclosed. This chapter will tell the success story of the development of steroidal CYP17 inhibitors from their early discovery days to their very recent introduction into the clinics for the treatment of advanced PC.

## 2. The CYP17 enzyme: One active site, two activities

The eukaryotic class II cytochrome P450 enzyme CYP17 is an endoplasmic reticulum membrane bound multifunctional protein with 17α-hydroxylase and $C_{17,20}$-lyase activities, both engaged on a single active site (Fig. 2) [23-28].

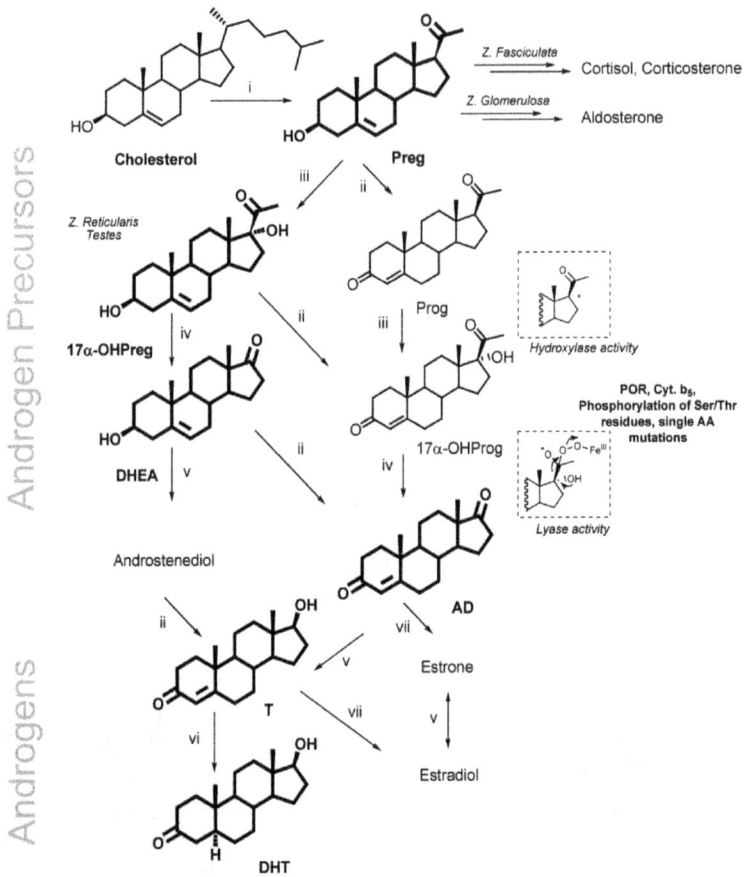

**Figure 2.** CYP17 and androgen physiology. i. P450 cholesterol side-chain cleavage (P450$_{scc}$); ii. 3β-Hydroxysteroid dehydrogenase, Δ$^{4,5}$-isomerase; iii. CYP17 (OHase); iv. CYP17 (lyase); v. 17β-Hydroxysteroid dehydrogenase; vi. 5α-Reductase; vii. Aromatase (CYP19).

Alike other cytochrome P450 enzymes, this cysteinato-heme enzyme functions as a monooxygenase by activating and cleaving molecular dioxygen so that one of the atoms is inserted into its substrate while the other gives rise to a water molecule [29, 30]. P450 reductase transfer of electrons in the presence of nicotinamide adenine dinucleotide phosphate (NADPH) is a requisite for both catalytic activities [29, 30]. Its natural substrates are pregnenolone (Preg) and progesterone (Prog) which are first hydroxylated at the 17 position and then their side chain is cleaved to afford 17-keto derivatives (dehydroepiandrosterone, DHEA and androstenedione, AD respectively), which are androgen precursors. The androgens (testosterone, T and dihydrotestosterone, DHT) that result from further metabolization of both DHEA and AD, bind to the AR and initiate transcription, triggering the synthesis of specific proteins and also cell proliferation [31, 32]. Apart from male physiology, androgens are involved in PC development and progression, as at least 80% of human PCs respond favorably to androgen ablation therapy [33-35]. This dependence of PC on androgen signalling has been known for about 70 years [36, 37] and the use of strategies that effectively lower the levels of circulating androgens in PC patients has been the mainstay of PC therapy for several decades.

CYP17 is localized to the adrenals, testes, placenta and ovaries and plays a fundamental role in the synthesis of not only sex steroids but also corticosteroids. The testes are responsible for about 90-95% of the circulating androgens and the adrenals for the remaining 5-10% [38]. Human CYP17 is expressed from a single gene mapped to a specific sub-band of chromosome 10 at q24.3, in steroidogenic tissue [39-41]. This bifunctionality of the product of a single gene has been explained by modulation of the enzyme's $C_{17,20}$-lyase activity by several factors such as the presence of the electron carrier P450 oxidoreductase (POR) [42, 43], cytochrome b5 (cyt. b5) [44-48], the phosphorylation of serine/threonine residues [44, 49-51], and single amino acid mutations [52-55]. The effective ratio of $C_{17,20}$-lyase to $17\alpha$-hydroxylase activities is under tight control during development in the human adrenal cortex, and becomes greatly elevated in adrenarche, where a rise in DHEA body concentrations is observed without concomitant increase in glucocorticoid or mineralocorticoid production [56]. Thus, production of the mineralocorticoid aldosterone occurs in the adrenal *zona glomerulosa* where CYP17 is absent. In the *zona reticularis* and in the gonads, the presence of both activities drives the production of sex steroids, whereas overexpression of $17\alpha$-hydroxylase activity is fundamental for the production of glucorticoids in the *zona fasciculata*.

The crystal structure of CYP17 remains yet to be determined since purification from its membrane environment and subsequent reconstitution of activity *in vitro* has proved to be a difficult task [26, 29, 30]. However, the availability of some cytochrome P450 crystal structures, such as the ones from prokaryotic P450cam [57, 58], P450BM3 [59-61], and P450 CYPeryF [62], as well as the eukaryotic CYP3A4 [63] and AYP2C9 [64] among others [65], has been a valuable tool in building homology models. In addition, the high-resolution crystal structures of mammalian P450s that are significantly homologous to CYP17 and complexed to a variety of ligands [66] have now been uploaded onto the Protein Data Bank (PDB). A very recent model has been developed based on these crystal structures from closely related mammalian cytochrome P450s [21]. In another approach, a truncated, His-tagged version of human CYP17 was generated from a synthetic complimentary DNA and expressed in *E. coli* [22]. These models were used to dock known CYP17 inhibitors to the active site.

# 3. Steroidal CYP17 inhibitors

Clinical practice outcomes with ketoconazole 5 (Fig. 1), an orally administered non-steroidal imidazole antifungal agent that was first reported to cause gynecomastia in male patients [67-69], have further evidenced the value of inhibition of the steroid synthesis pathway as a therapeutic strategy for advanced PC. This compound is used clinically as the racemate of the cis-isomer [17, 70], and is offered as secondary hormonal therapy to patients with CRPC, despite some significant gastrointestinal and hepatic side-effects when administered in high doses [71-73]. Following ketoconazole 5, several non-steroidal compounds have been synthesized which displayed better inhibitory properties. In addition, modification of the original core of the enzyme's natural substrates has also afforded very potent steroidal inhibitors [3, 8, 17-20]. Based on the knowledge that was generated by this approach which was recently validated by computational studies, common features were established for optimal interaction between enzyme and substrate. Thus, a good inhibitor should possess a sufficiently large hydrophobic core, comparable to a steroid molecule, and bear electronegative groups at its external positions [74]. The presence of a heteroatom-containing group capable of coordination to the heme iron of CYP17, ofa planar $\alpha$-face to pack against the I helix; and in addition of hydrogen bonding groups such as the 3$\beta$-hydroxylto interact with conserved polar residues in a hydrogen binding network, has proved invaluable for optimal inhibition, as is the case of both abiraterone acetate 3 and galeterone 4 [22].

### 3.1. Androstanes

The first reports on CYP17 steroidal inhibitors date back to 1971 when Arth et al. synthesized and evaluated testosterone derivatives against rat testicular CYP17, following the observation that testosterone acetate 6 (Fig. 3, Table 1, entry 1) was a potent inhibitor of the enzyme [75]. Almost total abrogation of the enzyme's activity was observed after treatment with 1.5 µM of compounds 7, 8, and 10 (Table 1, entries 2-3, and 5), with the acetamide derivative 9 being less potent (Table 1, entry 4). Competitive inhibition of pig CYP17 was reported for the anabolic steroids mestanolone 11, stanozolol12, and furazobol 13 (Fig. 3) [76]. Week inhibition in the high µM range was found with compounds 11 and 13 against the $C_{17,20}$-lyase activity whereas stanozolol 12 inhibited both enzyme activities with $IC_{50}$ values of 2.9 µM and 0.74 µM, for the 17$\alpha$-hydroxylase and $C_{17,20}$-lyase activities, respectively.

The irreversible inhibition of CYP17 by compound 14 (Fig. 3, Table 1, entry 6) was reported to occur due to the presence of a cyclopropylamino moiety capable of being activated by the enzyme by one-electron oxidation of the nitrogen atom, which causes ring opening to afford a $\beta$-iminium radical that covalently binds to the enzyme, while the compound is still bound in the active site [77]. Other related irreversible inhibitors reported include compounds 15-18 (Fig. 3, Table 1, entries 7-10) [78-81]. Compounds 15-17 were potent inhibitors of the human CYP17 at 0.8 and 1 µM, after preincubation with the enzyme (Table 1, entries 7-9). The ki values of the 4-amino derivatives 16-17 and of the sulfoxide derivatives 19-20 were determined using cynomolgous monkey and porcine testicular CYP17, respectively (Table 1, entries 8-9 and 11-12) [82]. Compound 18 also potently inhibited the activity of the monkey cynomolgous CYP17 at 0.1 µM, after preincubation with the enzyme (Table 1, entry 10) [80].

The introduction of heterocyclic moieties into molecules is a commonly used strategy in drug discovery and the design of potent steroidal CYP17 inhibitors based on this feature is an example of success. Thus, several androstane derivatives have been synthesized bearing a heterocycle ring at C17 either connected to it by a carbon (Fig. 4, Compounds 21-50) or a nitrogen (Fig. 5, Compounds 53-60) atom. In 1995, Jarman et al. reported the synthesis of abiraterone 21 (Fig. 4), a 17-(3-pyridyl)androstane derivative and a potent irreversible inhibitor of human testicular CYP17 (Table 2, entry 1), about 16- and 9-fold more potent than ketoconazole 5 for the inhibition of the hydroxylase and lyase activities, respectively, with $IC_{50}$ values in the low nM range [86]. Its 3β-acetoxy derivative and prodrug, abiraterone acetate 3 (Table 2, entry 2) has helped to further evidence and establish the utility of specific CYP17 inhibition in metastatic PC (mPC) patients. In 2001, Hartmann et al. reported that the introduction of a pyrimidyl substituent at C17 originated compounds such as 22 and 23 (Fig. 4, Table 2, entries 3-4) which were more potent inhibitors of the human enzyme than both ketoconazole 5 and abiraterone 21, under the same assay conditions, and that compound 23 effectively lowered T plasma concentrations to castrate levels after administration to mice [87, 88]. The thiazole and furan derivatives 24 and 25 were also synthesized and tested on the monkey cynomolgous enzyme (Fig. 4, Table 1, entries 13-14) [83, 85].

| Entry | Compound | Inhibitor concentration (µM) | % Inhibition[a] | Ki (nM) | $IC_{50}$ (µM) | Ref. |
|-------|----------|------------------------------|-----------------|---------|----------------|------|
| 1 | 6 | 1.5 | 65 | — | — | |
| 2 | 7 | 1.5 | 95 | — | — | |
| 3 | 8 | 1.5 | 100 | — | — | [75] |
| 4 | 9 | 1.5 | 85 | — | — | |
| 5 | 10 | 1.5 | 90 | — | — | |
| 6 | 14 | — | — | 90[b] | 4.6[c] | [77] |
| 7 | 15 | 0.8 | 64 | — | — | [78,79] |
| 8 | 16 | 1 | 84 | 339[b] | — | [80,81] |
| 9 | 17 | 1 | 86 | 286[b] | — | |
| 10 | 18 | 0.1 | 79[b] | — | — | [80] |
| 11 | 19 | — | — | 380[c, d] | 1.9[c] | [82] |
| 12 | 20 | — | — | 380[c, d] | 1.9[c] | |
| 13 | 24 | 0.1 | 58[b] | — | 0.063[b] | [83-85] |
| 14 | 25 | 0.1 | 53[b] | — | — | |

**Table 1.** Inhibition of CYP17 by androstane derivatives. [a]Human CYP17; [b]Determined on cynomolgous monkey testis enzyme; [c]Porcine testicular CYP17; [d]ki for compound 14 under the same assay conditions was 3620 nM.

A series of interesting effects on PC cells other than just CYP17 inhibition was reported by Brodie et al. for the imidazolyl, pyrazolyl, and isoxazolylandrostane derivatives 26-32 (Fig. 4, Table 2, entries 5-11). The isoxazolyl compound 32 was not only a non-competitive inhibitor of human CYP17 but also a competitive inhibitor of 5α-reductase, with potency similar to finasteride, while in addition bearing antiandrogenic activity [89-93]. Its effects were confirmed using PC xenograftmodels, however, its short half-life and relatively low bioavailability were reasoned to limit its efficacy *in vivo* [93-95]. Less success-ful attempts of CYP17 inhibitors design include the 5'-methyl-2'-thiazolyl androstane *33* (Fig. 4) which was a weak inhibitor of human CYP17 expressed in *E. coli* when com-pared to ketoconazole *5* [3]. In 2006, Wolfling et al. reported the synthesis of a series of dihydrooxazine derivatives *34-45* (Fig. 4) which low inhibitory activity of CYP17 is most likely due to the bulkiness of the C17 moieties and the absence of a double bond at C16 [96]. The same group later reported the synthesis of the oxazolidone derivative *46* (Fig. 4, Table 2, entry 12) which inhibited the activity of rat testicular $C_{17,20}$-lyase with an $IC_{50}$ value of 3 μM [97]. Similar inhibition of the enzyme was observed with the halogenated oxazoline derivatives *47* and *48* [98], and with the D-ring fused arylpyrazoline *51* (Fig. 4, Table 2, entries 13-14, and 17) [99]. The *N*-phenylpyrazolyl derivatives *49* and *50* were however much less active, with $IC_{50}$ values in the high μM range [100], as was the steroi-dal D-ring fused oxazolidine *52* (Fig. 4, Table 2, entries 15-16, and 18) [99].

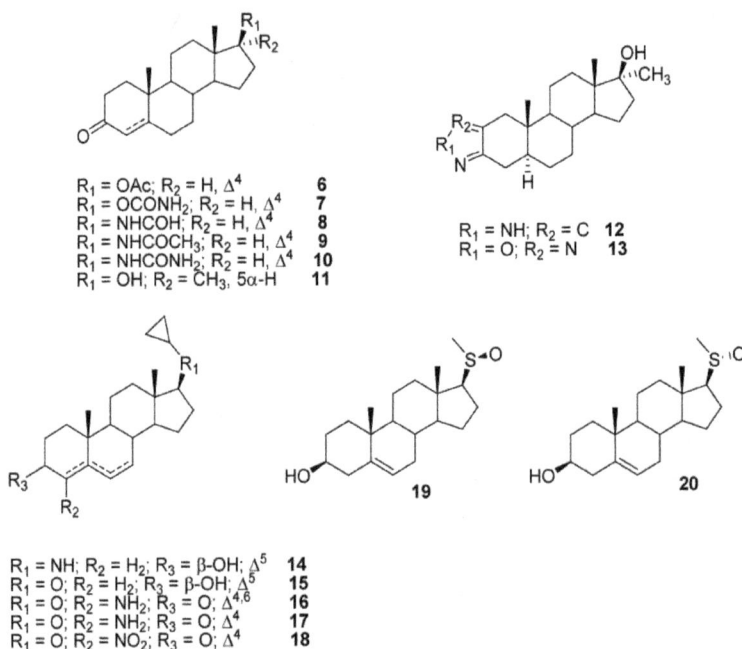

$R_1$ = OAc; $R_2$ = H, $\Delta^4$    **6**
$R_1$ = OCONH$_2$; $R_2$ = H, $\Delta^4$    **7**
$R_1$ = NHCOH; $R_2$ = H, $\Delta^4$    **8**
$R_1$ = NHCOCH$_3$; $R_2$ = H, $\Delta^4$    **9**
$R_1$ = NHCONH$_2$; $R_2$ = H, $\Delta^4$    **10**
$R_1$ = OH; $R_2$ = CH$_3$, 5α-H    **11**

$R_1$ = NH; $R_2$ = C    **12**
$R_1$ = O; $R_2$ = N    **13**

$R_1$ = NH; $R_2$ = H$_2$; $R_3$ = β-OH; $\Delta^5$    **14**
$R_1$ = O; $R_2$ = H$_2$; $R_3$ = β-OH; $\Delta^5$    **15**
$R_1$ = O; $R_2$ = NH$_2$; $R_3$ = O; $\Delta^{4,6}$    **16**
$R_1$ = O; $R_2$ = NH$_2$; $R_3$ = O; $\Delta^4$    **17**
$R_1$ = O; $R_2$ = NO$_2$; $R_3$ = O; $\Delta^4$    **18**

**Figure 3.** Androstane based CYP17 inhibitors.

In 1996, Njar et al. reported the first steroidal inhibitors of CYP17 bearing a heterocyclic moi-ety bound to C17 by a nitrogen atom [101], which included compounds *53-55* (Fig. 5, Table 2, entries 19-21), among which the imidazolyl derivative *53* was found to be the most prom-ising [101-104]. Later, in 2005, the same group reported the synthesis of galeterone *4* and its $\Delta^4$-3-keto derivative *56* (Fig. 5, Table 2, entries 22-23) [104-106].

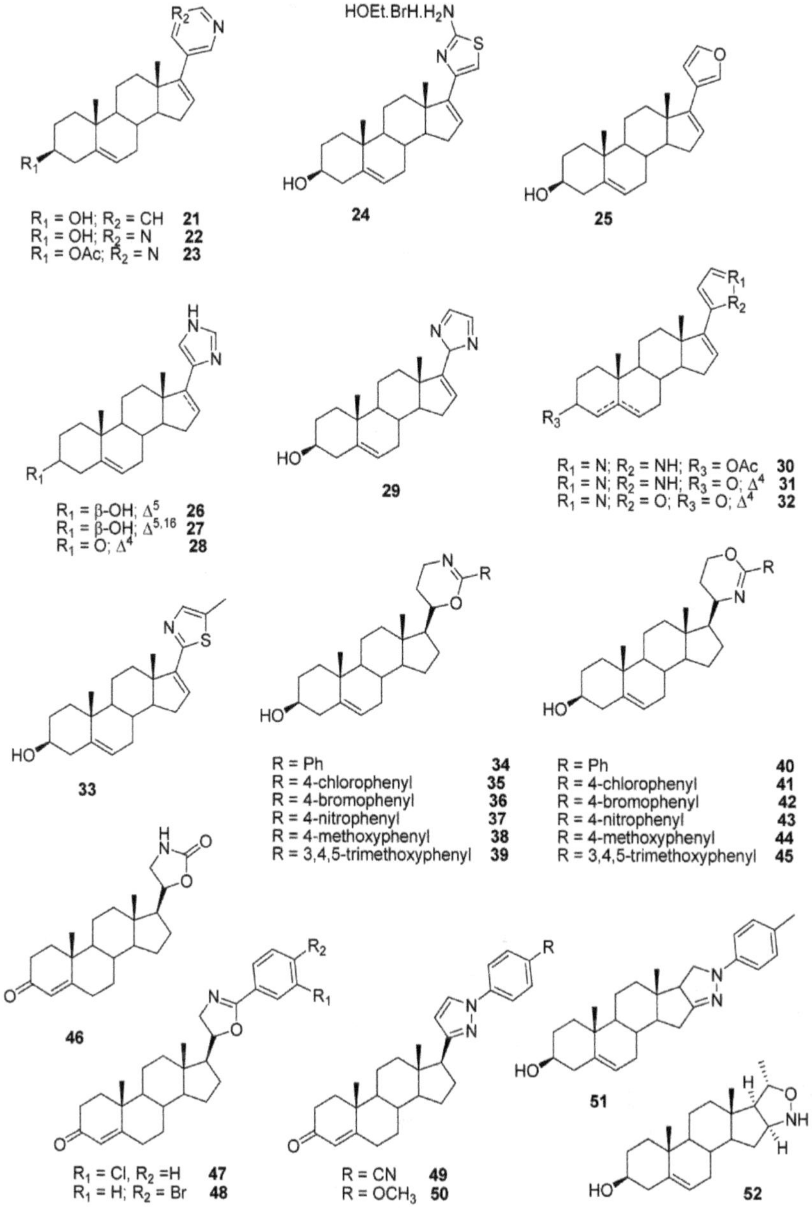
R1 = OH; R2 = CH 21
R1 = OH; R2 = N 22
R1 = OAc; R2 = N 23
HOEt.BrH.H2N
24
25
R1 = β-OH; Δ5 26
R1 = β-OH; Δ5,16 27
R1 = O; Δ4 28
29
R1 = N; R2 = NH; R3 = OAc 30
R1 = N; R2 = NH; R3 = O; Δ4 31
R1 = N; R2 = O; R3 = O; Δ4 32
33
R = Ph 34
R = 4-chlorophenyl 35
R = 4-bromophenyl 36
R = 4-nitrophenyl 37
R = 4-methoxyphenyl 38
R = 3,4,5-trimethoxyphenyl 39
R = Ph 40
R = 4-chlorophenyl 41
R = 4-bromophenyl 42
R = 4-nitrophenyl 43
R = 4-methoxyphenyl 44
R = 3,4,5-trimethoxyphenyl 45
46
R1 = Cl, R2 =H 47
R1 = H; R2 = Br 48
R = CN 49
R = OCH3 50
51
52

**Figure 4.** Androstane based CYP17 inhibitors.

| Entry | Compound | CYP17 inhibition (nM) | Ref. |
|-------|----------|----------------------|------|
| 1 | 21 | Human (OHase): 4<br>Human (lyase): 2.9 | [86,107] |
| 2 | 3 | Human (OHase): 18<br>Human (lyase): 17 | |
| 3 | 22 | Rat: 220<br>Human: 24<br>E.coli [a]: 30 | [87, 88] |
| 4 | 23 | Rat: 1460<br>Human: 38<br>E.coli [a]: 2500 | |
| 5 | 26 | Rat: 91<br>Human: 66 | |
| 6 | 27 | Rat: 49<br>Human: 24 | |
| 7 | 28 | Rat: 79<br>Human: 58 | |
| 8 | 29 | ND[b]<br>Human: 21 | [89, 90] |
| 9 | 30 | Rat: 28<br>Human: 42 | |
| 10 | 31 | Rat: 76<br>Human: 59 | |
| 11 | 32 | Rat: 32<br>Human: 39 | |
| 12 | 46 | Rat: 3000 | [97] |
| 13 | 47 | Rat: 4800 | [98] |
| 14 | 48 | Rat: 5000 | |
| 15 | 49 | Rat: 22000 | [100] |
| 16 | 50 | Rat: 59000 | |
| 17 | 51 | Rat: 5800 | [99] |
| 18 | 52 | Rat: 26000 | |
| 19 | 53 | Rat: 9<br>Human: 8<br>LNCaP-CYP17 cells[c]: 1.25 | [102, 103] |
| 20 | 54 | Rat: 8<br>Human: 7<br>LNCaP-CYP17 cells[c]: 2.96 | |
| 21 | 55 | Rat: 10<br>Human: 13 | |

| Entry | Compound | CYP17 inhibition (nM) | Ref. |
|-------|----------|----------------------|------|
| | | LNCaP-CYP17 cells[c]: 7.97 | |
| 22 | 4 | E.coli[a]: 300 | [105, 106] |
| 23 | 56 | E.coli[a]: 915 | |
| 24 | 61 | LNCaP-CYP17 cells[c]: 11500 | [4] |
| 25 | 62 | LNCaP-CYP17 cells[c]: 17100 | |

**Table 2.** IC$_{50}$ values for androstane CYP17 inhibitors. [a]Recombinant human CYP17 expressed in E.coli; [b]ND = Not Determined; [c]Recombinant human CYP17 expressed in LNCaP cells.

Thus, *in vitro* results with compounds *53-55* revealed a high inhibitory potential of the human enzyme expressed in LNCaP cells. In addition, compounds *53* and *55* completely suppressed T and DHT stimulated growth of LNCaP cells below 5 µM, and displayed antiandrogenic activity [102, 108]. *In vivo* experiments confirmed these results and showed that the compounds were however less effective than castration [109]. The C17-benzimidazole derivative 4 became the first example of a CYP17 inhibitor and antiandrogen that could effectively suppress androgen-dependent tumor growth better than castration [105]. In 2007, our group reported the synthesis of the 1*H*- and 2*H*-indazole androstanes *57-60* which despite being poor inhibitors of human CYP17 displayed selective inhibition of PC-3 cells suggesting that mechanisms other than interference with the AR could be involved in their cytotoxicity [5]. We also synthesized a series of steroidal carbamates out of which compounds *61* and *62* (Fig. 5, Table 2, entries 24-25) were inhibitors of human CYP17 with IC$_{50}$ values of 11.5 and 17.1 µM, respectively [4].

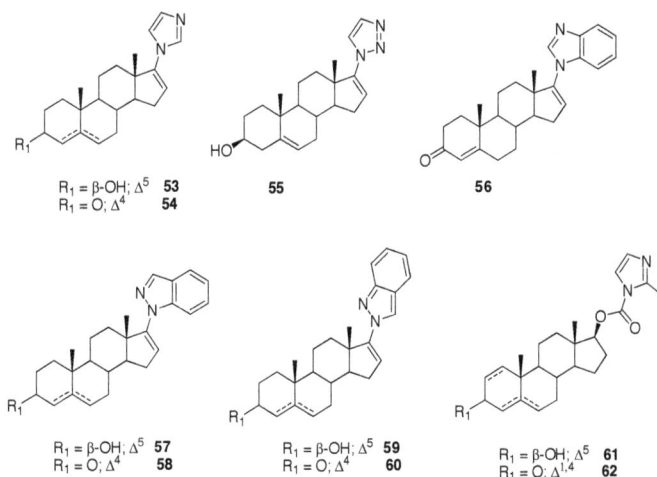

R$_1$ = β-OH; Δ$^5$  **53**
R$_1$ = O; Δ$^4$  **54**

**55**

**56**

R$_1$ = β-OH; Δ$^5$  **57**
R$_1$ = O; Δ$^4$  **58**

R$_1$ = β-OH; Δ$^5$  **59**
R$_1$ = O; Δ$^4$  **60**

R$_1$ = β-OH; Δ$^5$  **61**
R$_1$ = O; Δ$^{1,4}$  **62**

**Figure 5.** Androstane based CYP17 inhibitors.

## 3.2. Pregnanes

Among the pregnane CYP17 inhibitors, compounds *63-65* (Fig. 6, Table 3, entries 1-3) bearing 20-substituents with moderate to strong dipole properties were more active than ketoconazole in inhibiting human CYP17, displaying $IC_{50}$ values of 16 to 230 nM and 16 to 190 nM for the hydroxylase and lyase activities, respectively [90, 110, 111]. In 2000, Hartman et al. tested several pregneneoximes *66-76* among which some were potent inhibitors of both rat and human CYP17 (Fig. 6, Table 3, entries 4-11) [112]. Compound *66* was effective *in vivo* and suppressed plasma T concentrations more potently than ketoconazole. The hydroxamic acid derivative *77* (Fig. 6) was not a CYP17 inhibitor [113].

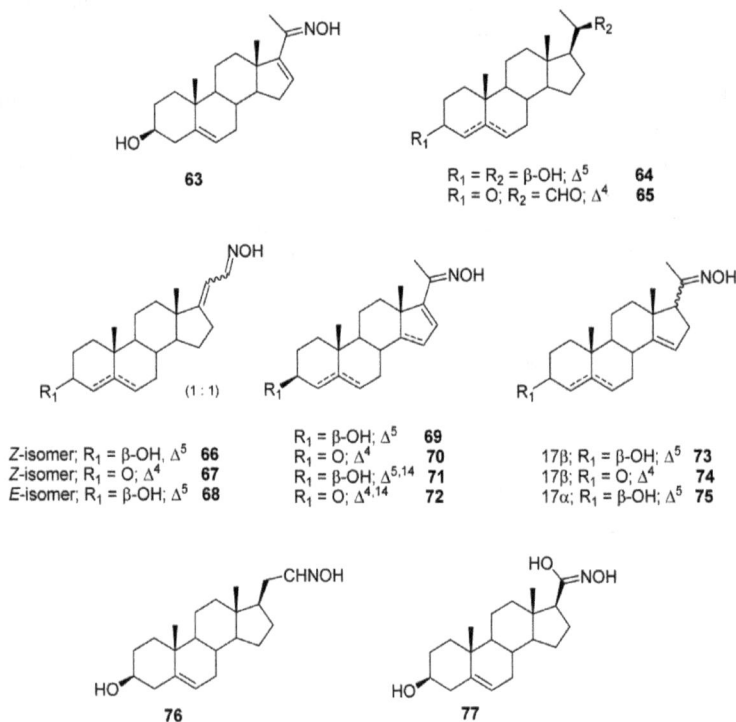

**63**

$R_1 = R_2 = \beta$-OH; $\Delta^5$    **64**
$R_1 = O$; $R_2 = CHO$; $\Delta^4$    **65**

(1 : 1)

Z-isomer; $R_1 = \beta$-OH, $\Delta^5$    **66**
Z-isomer; $R_1 = O$; $\Delta^4$    **67**
E-isomer; $R_1 = \beta$-OH; $\Delta^5$    **68**

$R_1 = \beta$-OH; $\Delta^5$    **69**
$R_1 = O$; $\Delta^4$    **70**
$R_1 = \beta$-OH; $\Delta^{5,14}$    **71**
$R_1 = O$; $\Delta^{4,14}$    **72**

$17\beta$; $R_1 = \beta$-OH; $\Delta^5$    **73**
$17\beta$; $R_1 = O$; $\Delta^4$    **74**
$17\alpha$; $R_1 = \beta$-OH; $\Delta^5$    **75**

**76**

**77**

**Figure 6.** Pregnane based CYP17 inhibitors.

| Entry | Compound | CYP17 inhibition (nM) | Ref. |
|-------|----------|----------------------|------|
| 1 | 63 | Human (OHase): 16<br>Human (lyase): 16 | [90, 110, 111] |
| 2 | 64 | Human (OHase): 180<br>Human (lyase): 190 | |
| 3 | 65 | Human (OHase): 230<br>Human (lyase): 160 | [90, 110, 111, 114] |
| 4 | 66 | Rat: 520<br>Human: 77<br>E. coli [b]: 230 | |
| 5 | 67 | Rat: 140<br>Human: 180 | |
| 6 | 69 | Rat: [a]<br>Human: 170<br>E. coli [b]: 520 | |
| 7 | 70 | Rat: [a]<br>Human: 100 | [112] |
| 8 | 71 | Rat: [a]<br>Human: 200<br>E. coli [b]: 420 | |
| 9 | 72 | Rat: [a]<br>Human: 200 | |
| 10 | 74 | Rat: 300<br>Human: 300 | |
| 11 | 76 | Rat: 2760<br>Human: 270 | |
| 12 | 78 | Rat: 210<br>Human: 540 | [115, 116] |
| 13 | 79 | Rat: 34000<br>Human: 1520 | |
| 14 | 80 | Rat: 1200 | [115] |
| 15 | 81 | Rat: 36000 | |
| 16 | 82 | Rat: 9670<br>Human: 970 | |
| 17 | 83 | Rat: 430<br>Human: 290 | [116] |
| 18 | 84 | Rat: 530<br>Human: 400 | |

| Entry | Compound | CYP17 inhibition (nM) | Ref. |
|-------|----------|------------------------|------|
| 19 | 85 | Rat (OHase): 75.8 <br> Rat (lyase): 55.8 | [117] |
| 20 | 86 | Rat: 600 | [118] |

**Table 3.** $IC_{50}$ values for pregnane CYP17 inhibitors. [a] $\geq 125$ µM; [b] *E. Coli* cells coexpressing human CYP17 and NADPH reductase

A difference in the inhibitory potential of rat CYP17 of the aziridinylpregnanes *78-81* was observed between the *S*- and *R*-isomers, the *S*-isomers *78* and *80* being 162 and 30-fold more potent than the *R*-isomers, respectively (Fig. 7, Table 3, entries 12-15) [115]. However, this finding was not corroborated by later studies that used the human enzyme [116]. The activity of compounds *82-85* (Fig. 7, Table 2, entries 16-19) was also reported [116, 117]. Several fluorinated pregnanes *86–91* and *93* were synthesized in search of greater metabolic stability (Fig. 7, Table 3, entry 20, Table 4). Inhibition of the cynomolgous monkey enzyme at 1 µM, following preincubation with the enzyme with compounds *87-93*, is depicted on Table 4 [118-122].

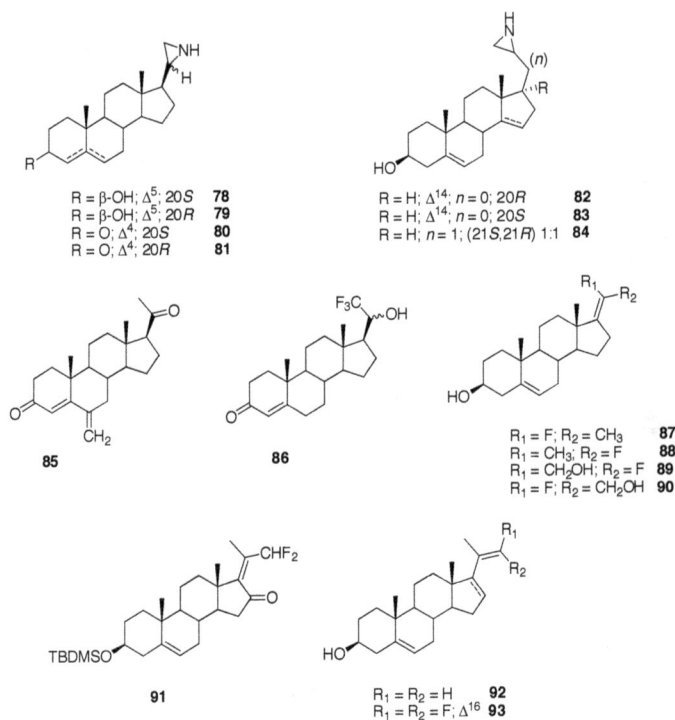

R = β-OH; $\Delta^5$; 20S    78
R = β-OH; $\Delta^5$; 20R    79
R = O; $\Delta^4$; 20S    80
R = O; $\Delta^4$; 20R    81

R = H; $\Delta^{14}$; n = 0; 20R    82
R = H; $\Delta^{14}$; n = 0; 20S    83
R = H; n = 1; (21S,21R) 1:1    84

85

86

$R_1$ = F; $R_2$ = $CH_3$    87
$R_1$ = $CH_3$; $R_2$ = F    88
$R_1$ = $CH_2OH$; $R_2$ = F    89
$R_1$ = F; $R_2$ = $CH_2OH$    90

91

$R_1$ = $R_2$ = H    92
$R_1$ = $R_2$ = F; $\Delta^{16}$    93

**Figure 7.** Pregnane based CYP17 inhibitors.

| Entry | Compound | % Inhibition | Ref. |
|-------|----------|--------------|------|
| 1 | 87 | 61 | |
| 2 | 88 | 60 | [119-121] |
| 3 | 89 | 61 | |
| 4 | 90 | 94 | |
| 5 | 91 | 85 | |
| 6 | 92 | 60 | [122] |
| 7 | 93 | 62 | |

Table 4. Inhibition of cynomolgous monkey testicular CYP17 by pregnane derivatives, at 1 μM, following preincubation with enzyme.

## 3.3. Other steroidal inhibitors

Other reported steroidal inhibitors of CYP17 are depicted on figure 8. The 17-aza derivative 94 inhibited human CYP17 with an $IC_{50}$ value of 4.9 μM [123]. Compound 95 inhibited both 5α-reductase and CYP17 with $k_i$ values of 27 and 14 nM, respectively [124]. The oxime 96 was also a dual inhibitor with the ability to reduce serum and prostatic T and DHT concentrations *in vivo* [125].

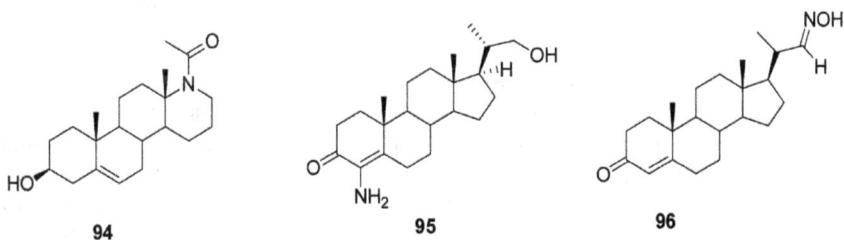

**94**    **95**    **96**

Figure 8. Other steroidal inhibitors of CYP17.

## 4. Abiraterone and galeterone

As previously mentioned, abiraterone acetate 3 (Fig. 1) constitutes the first and still the only steroidal CYP17 inhibitor approved by the FDA in 2011, being indicated for the treatment of mCRPC after chemotherapy [14].

This drug was developed at the Institute of Cancer Research (UK) considering the known efficacy and limitations of ketoconazole in this field and following the observation that non-steroidal 3-pyridyl esters had improved selectivity for the inhibition of CYP17. This led to the preparation of abiraterone 21 (Fig. 4), a $\Delta^{5,16}$-steroid with a 3-pyridyl group bound to C17, which revealed to be a potent and selective irreversible inhibitor of both 17α-hydroxy-lase and $C_{17,20}$-lyase activities of CYP17 [86, 126, 127]. In fact, it was observed that abirater-one 21 is not only a more potent CYP17 inhibitor than ketoconazole but also is a less effective inhibitor of other CYP450 enzymes, responsible for the significant side effects and potential pharmacological interactions of ketoconazole in PC therapy [14, 128]. Accordingly, preclinical studies in mice demonstrated that abiraterone 21 reduced serumT to castrate lev-els, in spite of a compensatory significant increase in luteinizing hormone (LH) [126]. How-ever, when abiraterone acetate 3was tested in human PC patients for the first time as a substitute to gonadotropin-releasing hormone (GnRH) analogues, sustained suppression of T production was not observed due to an increase in LH levels [129]. For this reason, abira-terone 21was developed to be concomitantly used with GnRH analogues in mCRPC [130]. Studies in xenograft models devoid of testicular and adrenal androgens further evidenced that abiraterone 21 inhibited CRPC growth and thus also seem to suppress androgen pro-duction in PC tumors [128].

Several Phase I clinical studies [131, 132] revealed that abiraterone acetate 3 is safe and effec-tive on lowering serum androgen levels in both ketoconazole naïve and exposed patients. In addition, its antitumor activity was nearly equivalent in both groups. However, a significant increase in adrenocorticotrophic hormone (ACTH) was developed leading to hypokalemia and hypertension as the predominant toxicities. In order to reduce these side effects eplere-none, a mineralocorticoid antagonist, was introduced. As the highest studied dosage of abir-aterone acetate 3 (1000mg) did not lead to limiting toxicities, the useof 1000mg daily was chosen in additional trials [8, 131, 133 135].

The concomitant use of the corticosteroids dexamethasone or prednisone in the efficacy of abiraterone acetate 3in several conditions was studied in Phase II trials [133-135]. A signifi-cant decrease in hyperaldosteronism-related symptoms was observed and therefore predni-sone 5mg b.i.d. was included in all subsequent studies, as well as in the FDA label indication. Other Phase II studies evaluated the efficacy of abiraterone in docetaxel-treated CRPC patients, and continued to evidence the importance of this steroidal drug in this stage of the pathology [135].

A Phase III study compared the use of abiraterone acetate 3and prednisone versus predni-sone alone in 1195 ketoconazole-naïve men with mCRPCshowing disease progression during or after therapy withdocetaxel. The primary endpoint was overall survival and the secondary endpoints were PSA decline, time to PSA progression and progression-free survival. In this study an increased median overall survival in the abiraterone acetate 3+ predisone group was observed when compared to that of patients treated with prednisone alone (14.8 vs 10.9 months; hazard ratio of 0.65). In addition, all the other endpoints were met and as expected the toxicities caused by CYP17 blockage occurred mostly in the abiraterone acetate 3+ prednisone group. Another Phase III study set to be completed in 2014 is evaluating the use of abiraterone acetate 3 and prednisone versus prednisone alone in CRPC prior to chemotherapy [136].

Due to all these beneficial results and after the first Phase III studies, in April 2011, abiraterone acetate 3was approved by the FDA for the treatment of mCRPC after chemotherapy [14].

Abiraterone 3 is being used in the form of its 3β-acetyl prodrug in order to increase its oral bioavailability, and is quickly deacetylated to the active drug once absorbed. In spite of the fact that high-fat meals increase its oral absorption, it is recommended that this drug should be taken on an empty stomach. Other pharmacokinetic studies revealed that this drug is highly bound to plasma proteins and has a plasma half-life of 10-14h [131, 132]. At present, several other clinical trials are ongoing, mainly for the study of the combination of abiraterone acetate 3 with other relevant drugs in PC treatment [137].

Galeterone 4 (Fig. 1) is structurally similar to abiraterone 21 and was rationally designed as an androgen biosynthesis inhibitor via CYP17 inhibition [8]. In fact, as previously mentioned, several research works evidenced that modification of the C17 substituent of $\Delta^{16}$-steroids, particularly by attachment of nitrogen heterocycles, was a relevant strategy to produce potent inhibitors of the enzyme. Following these considerations, Handratta et al. designed and prepared several $\Delta^{16}$-steroidal C17 benzoazoles and pyrazines and evaluated their CYP17 and 5α-reductase inhibitory activities, binding to and transactivation of the AR, as well as their antiproliferative effects against two human PC cell lines (LNCaP and LAPC4). Some of the compounds including 4 and its $\Delta^4$-3-ketone derivative 56 (Fig. 5) were potent CYP17 inhibitors and antagonists of both wild type and mutant AR. These compounds were the first reported examplesbearing such a dual activity. In addition, these steroids inhibited the growth of DHT-stimulated LNCaP and LACP4 PC cells with $IC_{50}$ values in the low micromolar range. Galeterone 4 and compound 56 were further studied for pharmacokinetic properties and antitumor activities against androgen-dependent LAPC4 human prostate tumor xenografts in severe combined immunodeficient (SCID) mice. Galeterone 4 was more effective than castration in its *in vivo* antitumor activity [104]. Taking this into account, Vasaitis et al. demonstrated by *in vitro* and *in vivo* studies that unlike bicalutamide and castration, galeterone 4 also caused down-regulation of AR protein expression, which appears to contribute to its antitumor efficacy. The authors also evidenced that this compound caused a significant regression of LAPC4 tumors in xenograft models, being more potent than castration, and that treatment with galeterone 4 was also very effective in preventing the formation of LAPC4 tumors [138].

An *in vitro* study using high-passage LNCaP cells demonstrated that galeterone 4 inhibited the proliferation of these cells that were no longer sensitive to bicalutamide and had increased AR expression. In addition, the combination of galeterone 4with inhibitors of signal transduction pathways such as gefitinib and everolimus, was proven to be synergistic when compared to either agent alone and superior to their combination with bicalutamide [139]. Later, *in vivo* studies with LNCaP and high-passage LNCaP tumor xenografts in SCID mice indicated that dual inhibition of AR and mammalian target of rapamycin (mTOR) in castration-resistant models can restore the sensitivity of tumours to anti-androgen therapy. The results observed in this study also indicated that the CYP17 and AR inhibitor galeterone 4 combined with the mTOR inhibitor everolimus may be effective in resistant PC [140].

A very recent *in vitro* study with LNCaP and LAPC4 cells demonstrated that both galeterone 4 and abiraterone 21 directly down-regulated the expression and activation of the AR via multiple mechanisms, in addition to their CYP17 inhibitory activities [141].

Due to the impressive biological activities observed, galeterone 4 is currently being evaluated in a phase I/II open label clinical trial (ARMOR1 study) as a potential drug for the treatment of castration resistant prostate cancer. This study began in 2009 and has as primary outcomes the incidence of adverse effects (phase I) and the proportion of patients with 50% or greater decrease in PSA from baseline (phase II) [137].

Recently, in a continuing study of the clinical candidate 4 and analogues as potential agents for PC treatment, putative metabolites of 4 and metabolically stable derivatives were prepared. Putative metabolites included compounds with no double bonds at C16, C5, or both as well as their corresponding 3-oxo derivatives. Metabolically stable analogues of 4, developed to optimize its potency and to increase its stability and oral bioavailability, included their 3α-azido, 3ξ-fluoro, 3β-mesylate and 3β-O-sulfamoyl derivatives. Several *in vitro* studies, including CYP17 inhibitory activity, binding to and transactivation of AR, as well as antiproliferative effects against LNCaP and LAPC4 cell lines, demonstrated that none of the compounds were superior to 4 in the observed effects. The 3ξ-fluoro analogue was, however, nearly 2-fold more efficacious *vs* LAPC4 xenografts than 4. Nonetheless, the toxicity observed with this halogenated compound was of concern [142].

## 5. Conclusion

PC is one of the most prevalent causes of death in Europe and USA. In spite of important advances in the treatment of localized disease, advanced PC is still incurable. One of the most relevant PC therapeutic strategies involves the inhibition of androgen biosynthesis by

CYP17 inhibition. In fact, starting from the structure of the natural substrates of this enzyme, several steroids, mainly with a heterocyclic ring bound to C17, have been developed over the years as CYP17 inhibitors. All these studies successfully led to the approval of abiraterone acetate 3 by the FDA in 2011 for the treatment of mCRPC after chemotherapy. In addition, other clinical trials involving this drug are being performed in order to expand its clinical usefulness, namely in CRPC prior to chemotherapy and in combination with other drugs. Another steroid that is in Phase I/II clinical trials for CRPC is galeterone 4, which is structurally similar to abiraterone 21. However, in addition to bearing a potent and selective CYP17 inhibitory activity, this compound also modulates AR activity. As it is now clear that function of the AR axis remains crucial to a majority of patients with CRPC, its mechanism of action can be of great advantage in PC therapy, either alone or in combination with other AR-modulating agents.In the future it is expected that the invaluable knowledge provided by the use of CYP17 inhibitors in PC treatment will shed more light on the most significant biological pathways involved in this disease. The establishment of a possible role for combination regimens including CYP17 inhibitors in earlier stages of PC as a means to prevent surgery and classical chemotherapy drugs would undoubtedly contribute to improving the quality of life of PC patients.

# Acknowledgments

Jorge A. R. Salvador thanks Universidade de Coimbra and Centro de Neurociências e Biologia Celular for financial support. Vânia M. Moreira acknowledges Fundação para a Ciência e a Tecnologia for financial support (SFRH/BPD/45037/2008).

# Author details

Jorge A. R. Salvador[1,2], Vânia M. Moreira[3] and Samuel M. Silvestre[4]

*Address all correspondence to: salvador@ci.uc.pt

1 Laboratório de Química Farmacêutica, Faculdade de Farmácia, Universidade de Coimbra,Pólo das Ciências da Saúde, Azinhaga de Santa Comba, Coimbra, Portugal

2 Centro de Neurociências e Biologia Celular, Universidade de Coimbra, Coimbra, Portugal

3 Division of Pharmaceutical Chemistry, Faculty of Pharmacy, Viikinkaari, University of Helsinki, Helsinki, Finland

4 Health Sciences Research Centre, Faculdade de Ciências da Saúde,Universidade da Beira Interior,Covilhã, Portugal

# References

[1] Jordan V C and Brodie A M H. Development and evolution of therapies targeted to the estrogen receptor for the treatment and prevention of breast cancer. Steroids 2007;72(1): 7-25.

[2] Brodie A, Njar V, Macedo L F, Vasaitis T S and Sabnis G. The Coffey Lecture: Steroidogenic enzyme inhibitors and hormone dependent cancer. Urologic Oncology: Seminars and Original Investigations 2009;27(1): 53-63.

[3] Moreira V M, Salvador J A R, Vasaitis T S and Njar V C. CYP17 Inhibitors for Prostate Cancer Treatment - An Update. Current Medicinal Chemistry 2008;15(9): 868-899.

[4] Moreira V M A, Vasaitis T S, Guo Z, Njar V C O and Salvador J A R. Synthesis of Novel C17 Steroidal Carbamates. Studies on CYP17 Action, Androgen Receptor Binding and Function, and Prostate Cancer Cell Growth. Steroids 2008;73(12): 1217-1227.

[5] Moreira V M A, Vasaitis T S, Njar V C O, and Salvador J A R. Synthesis and evaluation of novel 17-indazole androstene derivatives designed as CYP17 inhibitors. Steroids 2007;72(14): 939-948.

[6] Owen C P. $17\alpha$-Hydroxylase/17,20-Lyase (P450$_{17\alpha}$) Inhibitors in the Treatment of Prostate Cancer: A Review. Anti-Cancer Agents in Medicinal Chemistry 2009;9(6): 613-626.

[7] Pezaro C J, Mukherji D and De Bono J S. Abiraterone acetate: redefining hormone treatment for advanced prostate cancer. Drug Discovery Today 2012;17(5-6): 221-226.

[8] Vasaitis T S, Bruno R D and Njar V C O. CYP17 inhibitors for prostate cancer therapy. Journal of Steroid Biochemistry and Molecular Biology 2011;125(1-2): 23-31.

[9] Ang J E, Olmos D and Bono J S. CYP17 blockade by abiraterone: further evidence for frequent continued hormone-dependence in castration-resistant prostate cancer. British Journal of Cancer 2009;100(5): 671-675.

[10] Mancuso A, Oudard S and Sternberg C N. Effective chemotherapy for hormone-refractory prostate cancer (HRPC): Present status and perspectives with taxane-based treatments. Critical Reviews in Oncology/Hematology 2007;61(2): 176-185.

[11] Harzstark A L and Small E J. Castrate-resistant prostate cancer: therapeutic strategies. Expert Opinion on Pharmacotherapy 2010;11(6): 937-945.

[12] Sartor A O. Progression of metastatic castrate-resistant prostate cancer: impact of therapeutic intervention in the post-docetaxel space. Journal of Hematology & Oncology 2011;4: 18.

[13] Logothetis C J, Efstathiou E, Manuguid F and Kirkpatrick P. Abiraterone acetate. Nature Reviews Drug Discovery 2011;10: 573-574.

[14] Bryce A and Ryan C J. Development and Clinical Utility of Abiraterone Acetate as an Androgen Synthesis Inhibitor. Clinical Pharmacology & Therapeutics 2012;91(1): 101-108.

[15] Vasaitis T S and Njar V C O. Novel, potent anti-androgens of therapeutic potential: recent advances and promising developments. Future Medicinal Chemistry 2010;2(4): 667-680.

[16] Molina A and Belldegrun A. Novel Therapeutic Strategies for Castration Resistant Prostate Cancer: Inhibition of Persistent Androgen Production and Androgen Receptor Mediated Signaling. Journal of Urology 2011;185(3): 787-794.

[17] Jarman M, Smith H J, Nicholls P J and Simons C. Inhibitors of Enzymes of Androgen Biosynthesis: Cytochrome $P450_{17\alpha}$ and $5\alpha$-Steroid Reductase. Natural Product Reports 1998;15(5): 495-512.

[18] Baston E and Leroux F. Inhibitors of Steroidal Cytochrome P450 Enzymes as Targets For Drug Development. Recent Patents on Anti-cancer Drug Discovery 2007;2(1): 31-58.

[19] Hartmann R W, Ehmer P B, Haidar S, Hector M, Jose J, Klein C D, Seidel S B, Sergejew T F, Wachall B G, Wächter G A, and Zhuang Y. Inhibition of CYP 17, a New Strategy for the Treatment of Prostate Cancer. Archiv der Pharmazie (Weinheim) 2002;335(4): 119-128.

[20] Schneider G and Wolfling J. Synthetic Cardenolides and Related Compounds. Current Organic Chemistry 2004;8(14): 1381-1403.

[21] Haider S M, Patel J S, Poojari C S, and Neidle S. Molecular Modeling on Inhibitor Complexes and Active-Site Dynamics of Cytochrome P450 C17, a Target for Prostate Cancer Therapy. Journal of Molecular Biology 2010;400(5): 1078-1098.

[22] DeVore N M and Scott E E. Structures of cytochrome P450 17A1 with prostate cancer drugs abiraterone and TOK-001. Nature 2012;482: 116-119.

[23] Nakajin S, Hall P F and Onoda M. Testicular Microsomal Cytochrome P-450 for $C_{21}$ Steroid Side Chain Cleavage. Spectral and Binding Studies. Journal of Biological Chemistry 1981;256(12): 6134-6139.

[24] Nakajin S and Hall P F. Microsomal Cytochrome P-450 from Neonatal Pig Testis. Purification and Properties of a $C_{21}$ Steroid Side-chain Cleavage System ($17\alpha$-hydroxylase-$C_{17,20}$ lyase). Journal of Biological Chemistry 1981;256(8): 3871-3876.

[25] Nakajin S, Shively J E, Yuan P M and Hall P F. Microsomal Cytochrome P-450 from Neonatal Pig Testis: Two Enzymatic Activities ($17\alpha$-Hydroxylase and $C_{17,20}$-Lyase) Associated with One Protein. Biochemistry 1981;20(14): 4037-4042.

[26] Zuber M X, Simpson E R and Waterman M R. Expression of Bovine $17\alpha$-Hydroxylase Cytochrome P-450 cDNA in Nonsteroidogenic (COS 1) Cells. Science 1986;234(4781): 1258-1261.

[27] Onoda M, Haniu M, Yanagibashi K, Sweet F, Shively J E and Hall P F. Affinity Alkylation of the Active Site of $C_{21}$ Steroid Side-chain Cleavage Cytochrome P-450 from Neonatal Porcine Testis: a Unique Cysteine Residue Alkylated by 17-(Bromoacetoxy)progesterone. Biochemistry 1987;26(2): 657-662.

[28] Hall P F. Cytochrome P-450 $C_{21scc}$: One Enzyme with Two Actions: Hydroxylase and Lyase. Journal of Steroid Biochemistry and Molecular Biology 1991;40(4-6): 527-532.

[29] Meunier B, Visser S P and Shaik S. Mechanism of Oxidation Reactions Catalyzed by Cytochrome P450 Enzymes. Chemical Reviews 2004;104(9): 3947-3980.

[30] Denisov I G, Makris T M, Sligar S G and Schlichting I. Structure and Chemistry of Cytochrome P450. Chemical Reviews 2005;105(6): 2253-2277.

[31] Gao W, Bohl C E and Dalton J T. Chemistry and Structural Biology of Androgen Receptor. Chemical Reviews 2005;105(9): 3352-3370.

[32] Guyton A C and Hall J E. Textbook of Medical Physiology. Philadelphia: WB Saunders Company; 2000.

[33] Koivisto P, Kolmer M, Visakorpi T and Kallioniemi O P. Androgen Receptor Gene and Hormonal Therapy Failure of Prostate Cancer. American Journal of Pathology 1998;152(1): 1-9.

[34] Isaacs J T and Isaacs W B. Androgen Receptor Outwits Prostate Cancer Drugs. Nature Medicine 2004;10(1): 26-27.

[35] Chatterjee B. The Role of the Androgen Receptor in the Development of Prostatic Hyperplasia and Prostate Cancer. Molecular and Cellular Biochemistry 2003;253(1-2): 89-101.

[36] Huggins C and Hodges C V. Studies on Prostatic Cancer. I. The Effect of Castration, of Estrogen and of Androgen Injection on Serum Phosphatases in Metastatic Carcinoma of the Prostate. Cancer Research 1941;1: 293-297.

[37] Huggins C, Stevens R E and Hodges C V. Studies on Prostatic Cancer. II. The Effect of Castration on Clinical Patients with Carcinoma of the Prostate. Archives of Surgery 1941;43: 209-223.

[38] Denis L J and Griffiths K. Endocrine Treatment in Prostate Cancer. Seminars in Surgical Oncology 2000;18(1): 52-74.

[39] Chung B C, Picado-Leonard J, Haniu M, Bienkowski M, Hall P F, Shively J E and Miller W L. Cytochrome P450c17 (Steroid 17α-Hydroxylase/17,20 Lyase): Cloning of Human Adrenal and Testis cDNAs Indicates the Same Gene is Expressed in Both Tissues. Proceedings of the National Academy of Sciences of the United States of America 1987;84(2): 407-411.

[40] Sparkes R S, Klisak I and Miller W L. Regional Mapping of Genes Encoding Human Steroidogenic Enzymes: $P450_{scc}$ to 15q23-q24, Adrenodoxin to 11q22; Adrenodoxin

Reductase to 17q24-q25; and P450c17 to 10q24-q25.DNA and Cell Biology 1991;10(5): 359-365.

[41] Fan Y S, Sasi R, Lee C, Winter J S, Waterman M R and Lin C C. Localization of the Human CYP17 gene (cytochrome P450$_{17\alpha}$) to 10q24.3 by Fluorescence *in situ* Hybridization and Simultaneous Chromosome Banding. Genomics 1992;14(4): 1110-1111.

[42] Yanagibashi K and Hall P F. Role of Electron Transport in the Regulation of the Lyase Activity of C21 Side-chain Cleavage P-450 From Porcine Adrenal and Testicular Microsomes. Journal of Biological Chemistry 1986;261(18): 8429-8433.

[43] Lin D, Black S M, Nagahama Y and Miller W L. Steroid 17$\alpha$-Hydroxylase and 17,20-Lyase Activities of P450c17: Contributions of Serine106 and P450 Reductase. Endocrinology 1993;132(6): 2498-2506.

[44] Pandey A V and Miller W L. Regulation of 17,20-Lyase Activity by Cytochrome $b_5$ and by Serine Phosphorylation of P450c17. Journal of Biological Chemistry 2005;280(14): 13265-13271.

[45] Dharia S, Slane A, Jian M, Conner M, Conley A J and Parker C R. Colocalization of P450c17 and Cytochrome $b_5$ in Androgen-synthesizing Tissues of the Human. Biology of the Reproduction 2004;71(1): 83-88.

[46] Akhtar M K, Kelly S L, and Kaderbhai M A. Cytochrome $b_5$ Modulation of 17$\alpha$-Hydroxylase and 17,20-lyase (CYP17) Activities in Steroidogenesis. Journal of Endocrinology 2005;187(2): 267-274.

[47] Naffin-Olivos J L and Auchus R J. Human Cytochrome $b_5$ Requires Residues E48 and E49 to Stimulate the 17,20-Lyase Activity of Cytochrome P450c17. Biochemistry 2006;45(3): 755-762.

[48] Akhtar M, Wright J N and Lee-Robichaud P. A review of mechanistic studies on aromatase (CYP19) and 17$\alpha$-hydroxylase-17,20-lyase (CYP17). Journal of Steroid Biochemistry and Molecular Biology 2011;125(1-2): 2-12.

[49] Zhang L H, Rodriguez H, Ohno S and Miller W L. Serine Phosphorylation of Human P450c17 Increases 17,20-Lyase Activity: Implications for Adrenarche and the Polycystic Ovary Syndrome. Proceedings of the National Academy of Sciences of the United States of America 1995;92(23): 10619-10623.

[50] Pandey A V, Mellon S H and Miller W L. Protein Phosphatase 2A and Phosphoprotein SET Regulate Androgen Production by P450c17. Journal of Biological Chemistry 2003;278(5): 2837-2844.

[51] Souter I, Munir I, Mallick P, Weitsman S R, Geller D H and Magoffin D A. Mutagenesis of Putative Serine-threonine Phosphorylation Sites Proximal to Arg255 of Human Cytochrome P450c17 Does Not Selectively Promote Its 17,20-Lyase Activity.Fertility and Sterility 2006;85: 1290-1299.

[52]  Geller D H, Auchus R J, Mendonca B B and Miller W L. The Genetic and Functional Basis of Isolated 17,20-Lyase Deficiency. Nature Genetics 1997;17(2): 201-205.

[53]  Lee-Robichaud P, Akhtar M E and Akhtar M. Lysine Mutagenesis Identifies Cationic Charges of Human CYP17 That Interact With Cytochrome $b_5$ to Promote Male Sex-hormone Biosynthesis. Biochemical Journal 1999;342: 309-312.

[54]  Van Den Akker E L, Koper J W, Boehmer A L, Themmen A P, Verhoef-Post M, Timmerman M A, Otten B J, Drop S L and De Jong F H. Differential Inhibition of 17α-Hydroxylase and 17,20-Lyase Activities by Three Novel Missense CYP17 Mutations Identified in Patients With P450c17 Deficiency. Journal of Clinical Endocrinology & Metabolism 2002;87(12): 5714-5721.

[55]  Sherbet D P, Tiosano D, Kwist K M, Hochberg Z and Auchus R J. CYP17 Mutation E305G Causes Isolated 17,20-Lyase Deficiency by Selectively Altering Substrate Binding. Journal of Biological Chemistry 2003;278(49): 48563-48569.

[56]  Miller W L, Auchus R J and Geller D H. The Regulation of 17,20-Lyase Activity. Steroids 1997;62(1): 133-142.

[57]  Laughton C A, Neidle S, Zvelebil M J and Sternberg M J. A Molecular Model for The Enzyme Cytochrome P450$_{17α}$, a Major Target for The Chemotherapy of Prostatic Cancer.Biochemical and Biophysical Research Communications 1990;171(3): 1160-1167.

[58]  Lin D, Zhang L H, Chiao E and Miller W L. Modeling and Mutagenesis of the Active Site of Human P450c17. Molecular Endocrinology 1994;8(3): 392-402.

[59]  Burke D F, Laughton C A and Neidle S. Homology Modelling of the Enzyme P450 17α-Hydroxylase/17,20-Lyase - A Target For Prostate Cancer Chemotherapy - From the Crystal Structure of P450BM-3. Anticancer Drug Design 1997;12(2): 113-123.

[60]  Lewis D F and Lee-Robichaud P. Molecular Modelling of Steroidogenic Cytochromes P450 From Families CYP11, CYP17, CYP19 and CYP21 Based on the CYP102 Crystal Structure. Journal of Steroid Biochemistry and Molecular Biology 1998;66(4): 217-233.

[61]  Auchus R J and Miller W L. Molecular Modeling of Human P450c17 (17α-Hydroxylase/17,20-Lyase): Insights into Reaction Mechanisms and Effects of Mutations. Molecular Endocrinology 1999;13(7): 1169-1182.

[62]  Schappach A and Holtje H D. Molecular Modelling of 17α-Hydroxylase-17,20-Lyase. Pharmazie 2001;56(6): 435-442.

[63]  Yang J, Cui B, Sun S, Shi T, Zheng S, Bi Y, Liu J, Zhao Y, Chen J, Ning G and Li X. Phenotype–genotype correlation in eight Chinese 17α-hydroxylase/17,20 lyase-deficiency patients with five novel mutations of CYP17A1 gene. Journal of Clinical Endocrinology & Metabolism 2006;91(9): 3619–3625.

[64]  Mendieta M A E P B, Negri M, Jagusch C, Muller-Vieira U, Lauterbach T and Hartmann R W. Synthesis, biological evaluation, and molecular modeling of abiraterone

analogues: novel CYP17 inhibitors for the treatment of prostate cancer. Journal of Medicinal Chemistry 2008;51(16): 5009–5018.

[65] Swart A C, Storbeck K H and Swart P. A single amino acid residue, Ala 105, confers 16α-hydroxylase activity to human cytochrome P450 17α-hydroxylase/17,20 lyase. Journal of Steroid Biochemistry and Molecular Biology 2010;119(3-5): 112–120.

[66] Wang J F, Zhang C C, Chou K C and Wei D Q. Structure of cytochrome P450s and personalized drug. Current Medicinal Chemistry 2009;16(2): 232–244.

[67] Moncada B and Baranda L. Ketoconazole and gynecomastia. Journal of the American Academy of Dermatology 1982;7(4): 557-558.

[68] Pont A, Williams P L, Azhar S, Reitz R E, Bochra C, Smith E R and Stevens D A. Ketoconazole Blocks Testosterone Synthesis. Archives of Internal Medicine 1982;142(12): 2137-2140.

[69] De Felice R, Johnson D G and Galgiani J N. Gynecomastia With Ketoconazole. Antimicrobial Agents and Chemotherapy 1981;19(6): 1073-1074.

[70] Heeres J, Backx L J, Mostmans J H and Cutsem J V. Antimycotic Imidazoles. Part 4. Synthesis and Antifungal Activity of Ketoconazole, a New Potent Orally Active Broad-spectrum Antifungal Agent. Journal of Medicinal Chemistry 1979;22(8): 1003-1005.

[71] Moffat L E, Kirk D, Tolley D A, Smith M F and Beastall G. Ketoconazole as Primary Treatment of Prostatic Cancer. British Journal of Urology 1988;61(5): 439-440.

[72] Mahler C, Verhelst J and Denis L. Ketoconazole and Liarozole in the Treatment of Advanced Prostatic Cancer. Cancer 1993;71(3 Suppl): 1068-1073.

[73] Lake-Bakaar G, Scheuer P J and Sherlock S. Hepatic Reactions Associated With Ketoconazole in the United Kingdom. British Medical Journal 1987;294: 419-422.

[74] Schappach A and Holtje H D. Investigations on Inhibitors of Human 17α-Hydroxylase-17,20-Lyase and Their Interactions With the Enzyme. Molecular Modelling of 17α-Hydroxylase-17,20-Lyase, Part II. Pharmazie 2001;56(11): 835-842.

[75] Arth G E, Patchett A A, Jefopoulus T, Bugianesi R L, Peterson L H, Ham E A, Kuehl F A and Brink N G. Steroidal Androgen Biosynthesis Inhibitors. Journal of Medicinal Chemistry 1971;14(8): 675-679.

[76] Nakajin S, Takahashi K and Shinoda M. Inhibitory Effect and Interaction of Stanozolol With Pig Testicular Cytochrome P-450 (17α-hydroxylase/C$_{17,20}$-lyase). Chemical & Pharmaceutical Bulletin (Tokyo) 1989;37(7): 1855-1858.

[77] Angelastro M R, Laughlin M E, Schatzman G L, Bey P and Blohm T R. 17β-(Cyclopropylamino)-androst-5-en-3β-ol, A Selective Mechanism-based Inhibitor of Cytochrome P450$_{17α}$ (Steroid 17α-Hydroxylase/C$_{17,20}$-Lyase). Biochemical and Biophysical Research Communications 1989;162(3): 1571-1577.

[78]  Angelastro M R and Blohm T R. 4-Substituted 17β-(cyclopropyloxy)androst-5-en-3β-ol and Related Compounds Useful as $C_{17,20}$-Lyase Inhibitors. *US Patent* 4,966,897; 1990.

[79]  Angelastro M R, Marquart A L, Weintraub P M, Gates C A, Laughlin M E, Blohm T R and Peet N P. Time-dependent Inactivation of Steroid $C_{17(20)}$-Lyase by 17β-Cyclopropyl Ether-substituted Steroids. Bioorganic & Medicinal Chemistry Letters 1996;6(1): 97-100.

[80]  Weintraub P M, Gates C, Angelastro M R and Flynn G A. Process For the Preparation of 4-Amino-$\Delta^4$-3-ketosteroids Via Nitro-$\Delta^4$-3-ketosteroids. *WO Patent* 95/29932; 1995.

[81]  Weintraub P M, Gates C A, Angelastro M R, Curran T T and Johnston J O. 4-Amino-17β- (Cyclopropyloxy)androst-4-en-3-one, 4-Amino-17β-(Cyclopropylamino)androst-4-en-3-one and Related Compounds as $C_{17,20}$-Lyase and 5α-Reductase Inhibitors. *US Patent* 5,486,511; 1996.

[82]  Wilson S R and Miao E. Anti-testosterone compounds and Method of Use Thereof. *WO Patent* 92/15604; 1992.

[83]  Burkhart J P, Gates C A, Laughlin M E, Resvick R J and Peet N P. Inhibition of Steroid $C_{17(20)}$-Lyase With C17-Heteroaryl Steroids. Bioorganic & Medicinal Chemistry 1996;4(9): 1411-1420.

[84]  Peet N P, Burkhart J P and Gates C. 16-Unsaturated C17 Heterocyclic Steroids Useful as Steroid $C_{17,20}$-Lyase Inhibitors. *US Patent* 5,677,293; 1997.

[85]  Peet N P, Burkhart J P and Gates C. Methods and Compositions using $\Delta^{16}$-Unsaturated C17-Heterocyclic Steroids Useful as $C_{17,20}$-Lyase Inhibitors. *US Patent* 5,977,094; 1999.

[86]  Potter G A, Barrie S E, Jarman M and Rowlands M G. Novel Steroidal Inhibitors of Human Cytochrome P450$_{17\alpha}$ (17α-Hydroxylase-$C_{17,20}$-Lyase): Potential Agents For the Treatment of Prostatic Cancer. Journal of Medicinal Chemistry 1995;38(13): 2463-2471.

[87]  Haidar S, Ehmer P B and Hartmann R W. Novel Steroidal Pyrimidyl Inhibitors of P450 17 (17α-Hydroxylase/$C_{17,20}$-Lyase). Archiv der Pharmazie (Weinheim) 2001;334(12): 373-374.

[88]  Haidar S, Ehmer P B, Barassin S, Batzl-Hartmann C and Hartmann R W. Effects of Novel 17α-Hydroxylase/$C_{17, 20}$-Lyase (P450 17, CYP 17) Inhibitors on Androgen Biosynthesis *in vitro* and *in vivo*. Journal of Steroid Biochemistry and Molecular Biology 2003;84(5): 555-562.

[89]  Ling Y Z, Li J S, Liu Y, Kato K, Klus G T and Brodie A. 17-Imidazolyl, Pyrazolyl, and Isoxazolyl Androstene Derivatives. Novel Steroidal Inhibitors of Human Cytochrome $C_{17,20}$-Lyase (P450$_{17\alpha}$). Journal of Medicinal Chemistry 1997;40(20): 3297-3304.

[90]  Brodie A and Yangzhi L. Androgen Synthesis Inhibitors. *US Patent* 6,133,280; 2000.

[91]  Nnane I P, Kato K, Liu Y, Lu Q, Wang X, Ling Y Z and Brodie A. Effects of Some Novel Inhibitors of $C_{17,20}$-Lyase and 5α-Reductase *in vitro* and *in vivo* and Their Potential Role in the Treatment of Prostate Cancer. Cancer Research 1998;58(17): 3826-3832.

[92]  Klus G T, Nakamura J, Li J S, Ling Y Z, Son C, Kemppainen J A, Wilson E M and Brodie A M. Growth Inhibition of Human Prostate Cells *in vitro* by Novel Inhibitors of Androgen Synthesis. Cancer Research 1996;56(21): 4956-4964.

[93]  Long B J, Grigoryev D N, Nnane I P, Liu Y, Ling Y Z and Brodie A M. Antiandrogenic Effects of Novel Androgen Synthesis Inhibitors on Hormone-dependent Prostate Cancer. Cancer Research 2000;60(23): 6630-6640.

[94]  Nnane I P, Long B J, Ling Y Z, Grigoryev D N and Brodie A M. Anti-tumour Effects and Pharmacokinetic Profile of 17-(5'-Isoxazolyl)androsta-4,16-dien-3-one (L-39) in Mice: An Inhibitor of Androgen Synthesis. British Journal of Cancer 2000;83(1): 74-82.

[95]  Nnane I P, Njar V C O and Brodie A M H. Pharmacokinetics of Novel Inhibitors of Androgen Synthesis After Intravenous Administration in Mice. Cancer Chemotherapy and Pharmacology 2003;51(6): 519-524.

[96]  Wolfling J, Oravecz E A, Ondre D, Mernyak E, Schneider G, Toth I, Szecsi M and Julesz J. Stereoselective Synthesis of Some 17β-Dihydrooxazinyl Steroids, as Novel Presumed Inhibitors of 17α-Hydroxylase-$C_{17,20}$-Lyase. Steroids 2006;71: 809-816.

[97]  Ondre D, Wölfling J, Iványi Z, Schneider G, Tóth I, Szécsi M and Julesz J. Neighboring group participation. Part 17 Stereoselective synthesis of some steroidal 2-oxazolidones, as novel potential inhibitors of 17α-hydroxylase-C17,20-lyase. Steroids 2008;73: 1375-1384.

[98]  Ondre D, Wölfling J, Tóth I, Szécsi M, Julesz J and Schneider G. Steroselective synthesis of some steroidal oxazolines, as novel potential inhibitors of 17α-hydroxylase-C17,20-lyase. Steroids 2009;74: 1025-1032.

[99]  Frank E, Mucsi Z, Szecsi M, Zupko I, Wolfling J and Schneider G. Intramolecular approach to some new D-ring-fused steroidal isoxazolidines by 1,3-dipolar cycloaddition: synthesis, theoretical and *in vitro* pharmacological studies. New Journal of Chemistry 2010;34: 2671-2681.

[100] Iványi Z, Wölfling J, Görbe T, Szécsi M, Wittmann T and Schneider G. Synthesis of regioisomeric 17-N-phenylpyrazolyl steroid derivatives and their inhibitory effect on 17α-hydroxylase/C17,20-lyase. Steroids 2010;75: 450-456.

[101] Njar V C, Klus G T and Brodie A M H. Nucleophilic Vinylic "Addition-elimination" Substitution Reaction of 3β-Acetoxy-17-chloro-16-formylandrosta-5,16-diene: A Novel and General Route to 17-Substituted Steroids. Part 1 - Synthesis of Novel 17-Azolyl-$\Delta^{16}$-steroids; Inhibitors of 17α-Hydroxylase/17,20-Lyase (17α-Lyase). Bioorganic & Medicinal Chemistry Letters 1996;6(22): 2777-2782.

[102] Njar V C, Kato K, Nnane I P, Grigoryev D N, Long B J and Brodie A M. Novel 17-Azolyl Steroids, Potent Inhibitors of Human Cytochrome $17\alpha$-Hydroxylase-$C_{17,20}$-Lyase (P450$_{17}\alpha$): Potential Agents for the Treatment of Prostate Cancer. Journal of Medicinal Chemistry 1998;41(6): 902-912.

[103] Brodie A and Njar V C. 17-Azolyl Steroids Useful as Androgen Synthesis Inhibitors. US Patent 6,200,965 B1; 2001.

[104] Handratta V D, Jelovac D, Long B J, Kataria R, Nnane I P, Njar V C and Brodie A M. Potent CYP17 Inhibitors: Improved Syntheses, Pharmacokinetics and Anti-tumor Activity in the LNCaP Human Prostate Cancer Model. Journal of Steroid Biochemistry and Molecular Biology 2004;92(3): 155-165.

[105] Handratta V D, Vasaitis T S, Njar V C, Gediya L K, Kataria R, Chopra P, Newman D, Farquhar R, Guo Z, Qiu Y and Brodie A M. Novel C17-Heteroaryl Steroidal CYP17 Inhibitors/Antiandrogens: Synthesis, in vitro Biological Activity, Pharmacokinetics, and Antitumor Activity in the LAPC4 Human Prostate Cancer Xenograft Model. Journal of Medicinal Chemistry 2005;48(8): 2972-2984.

[106] Brodie A and Njar V C. Novel C-17-Heteroaryl Steroidal CYP17 Inhibitors/Antiandrogens: Synthesis, in vitro Biological Activities, Pharmacokinetics and Antitumor Activity. WO Patent 2006/093993; 2006.

[107] Barrie S E, Jarman M, Potter G A and Hardcastle I R. 17-Substituted Steroids Useful in Cancer Treatment. US Patent 5,604, 213; 1997.

[108] Grigoryev D N, Long B J, Nnane I P, Njar V C, Liu Y and Brodie A M. Effects of New $17\alpha$-Hydroxylase/C17,20-Lyase Inhibitors on LNCaP Prostate Cancer Cell Growth in vitro and in vivo. British Journal of Cancer 1999;81(4): 622-630.

[109] Nnane I P, Njar V C, Liu Y, Lu Q and Brodie A M. Effects of Novel 17-Azolyl Compounds on Androgen Synthesis in vitro and in vivo. Journal of Steroid Biochemistry and Molecular Biology 1999;71(3-4): 145-152.

[110] Brodie A and Jisong L. 20-Substituted Pregnene Derivatives and Their Use as Androgen Inhibitors. US Patent 5,264,427; 1993.

[111] Li J S, Li Y, Son C and Brodie A M. Synthesis and Evaluation of Pregnane Derivatives as Inhibitors of Human Testicular $17\alpha$-Hydroxylase/$C_{17,20}$-Lyase. Journal of Medicinal Chemistry 1996;39(21): 4335-4339.

[112] Hartmann R W, Hector M, Haidar S, Ehmer P B, Reichert W and Jose J. Synthesis and Evaluation of Novel Steroidal Oxime Inhibitors of P450 17 ($17\alpha$-Hydroxylase/$C_{17,20}$-Lyase) and $5\alpha$-Reductase Types 1 and 2. Journal of Medicinal Chemistry 2000;43(22): 4266-4277.

[113] Haidar S, Klein C D and Hartmann R W. Synthesis and Evaluation of Steroidal Hydroxamic Acids as Inhibitors of P450 17 ($17\alpha$-Hydroxylase/$C_{17,20}$-Lyase). Archiv der Pharmazie (Weinheim) 2001;334(4): 138-140.

[114] Li J, Li Y, Son C, Banks P and Brodie A. 4-Pregnene-3-one-20β-carboxaldehyde: A Potent Inhibitor of 17α-Hydroxylase/$C_{17,20}$-Lyase and of 5α-Reductase. Journal of Steroid Biochemistry and Molecular Biology 1992;42(3-4): 313-320.

[115] Njar V C, Hector M and Hartmann R W. 20-Amino and 20,21-Aziridinyl Pregnene Steroids: Development of Potent Inhibitors of 17α-Hydroxylase/$C_{17,20}$-Lyase (P450 17). Bioorganic & Medicinal Chemistry 1996;4(9): 1447-1453.

[116] Hartmann R W, Hector M, Wachall B G, Palusczak A, Palzer M, Huch V and Veith M. Synthesis and Evaluation of 17-Aliphatic Heterocycle-substituted Steroidal Inhibitors of 17α-Hydroxylase/$C_{17,20}$-Lyase (P450 17). Journal of Medicinal Chemistry 2000;43(23): 4437-4445.

[117] Neubauer B L, Best K L, Blohm T R, Gates C, Goode R L, Hirsch K S, Laughlin M E, Petrow V, Smalstig E B, Stamm N B, Toomey R E and Hoover D M. LY207320 (6-Methylene-4-pregnene-3,20-dione) Inhibits Testosterone Biosynthesis, Androgen Uptake, 5α-Reductase, and Produces Prostatic Regression in Male-Rats. Prostate 1993;23(3): 181-199.

[118] Njar V C, Klus G T, Johnson H H and Brodie A M. Synthesis of Novel 21-Trifluoropregnane Steroids: Inhibitors of 17α-Hydroxylase/17,20-Lyase (17α-Lyase). Steroids 1997;62(6): 468-473.

[119] Burkhart J P, Weintraub P M, Gates C A, Resvick R J, Vaz R J, Friedrich D, Angelastro M R, Bey P and Peet N P. Novel Steroidal Vinyl Fluorides as Inhibitors of Steroid $C_{17(20)}$-Lyase. Bioorganic & Medicinal Chemistry 2002;10(4): 929-934.

[120] Peet N P, Weintraub P M, Burkhart J P and Gates C. 20-Fluoro-17(20)-Vinyl steroids as Inhibitors of $C_{17,20}$-Lyase and 5α-Reductase. WO Patent 02/00681 A1; 2002.

[121] Peet N P, Weintraub P M, Burkhart J P and Gates C. 20-Fluoro-17(20)-Vinyl Steroids. US Patent 6,413,951 B2; 2002.

[122] Weintraub P M, Holland A K, Gates C A, Moore W R, Resvick R J, Bey P and Peet N P. Synthesis of 21,21-Difluoro-3β-hydroxy-20-methylpregna-5,20-diene and 5,16,20-Triene as Potential Inhibitors of Steroid $C_{17(20)}$-Lyase. Bioorganic & Medicinal Chemistry 2003;11(3): 427-431.

[123] Deadman J J, McCague R, and Jarman M. Heptafluoro-p-tolyl as a protecting group in a synthesis of 3-hydroxy-17a-aza-17a-homopregn-5-en-20-one. A potential inhibitor of androgen biosynthesis. Journal of the Chemical Society, Perkin Transactions 1 1991;(10): 2413-2416.

[124] Curran T T, Flynn G A, Rudisill D E and Weintraub P M. A Novel Route to a 4-Amino Steroid - MDL 19687. Tetrahedron Letters 1995;36(27): 4761-4764.

[125] Li J, Li Y, Son C and Brodie A M. Inhibition of Androgen Synthesis by 22-Hydroximino-23,24-Bisnor-4-cholen-3-one. Prostate 1995;26(3): 140-150.

[126]  Barrie S E, Potter G A, Goddard P M, Haynes B P, Dowset M, Jarman M. Pharmacology of novel steroidal inhibitors of cytochrome $P450_{17\alpha}$ ($17\alpha$-hydroxylase C17-20 lyase). Journal of Steroid Biochemistry and Molecular Biology 1994;50(5-6): 267-273.

[127]  Jarman M, Barrie S E and Llera J M. The 16,17-Double Bond Is Needed for Irreversible Inhibition of Human Cytochrome $P450_{17\alpha}$ by Abiraterone (17-(3-Pyridyl)androsta-5,16-dien-3β-ol) andRelated Steroidal Inhibitors. Journal of Medicinal Chemistry 1998;41(27): 5375-5381.

[128]  Molina A and Belldegrun A. Novel Therapeutic Strategies for Castration Resistant Prostate Cancer: Inhibition of Persistent Androgen Production and Androgen Receptor Mediated Signaling. Journal of Urology 2011;185: 787-794.

[129]  O'Donnell A, Judson I, Dowset M, Raynaud F, Dearnaley D, Mason M, Harland S, Robbins A, Halbert G, Nutley B and Jarman M. Hormonal impact of the $17\alpha$-hydroxylase/$C_{17,20}$-lyase inhibitor abiraterone acetate (CB7630) in patients with prostate cancer. British Journal of Cancer 2004;90: 2317–2325.

[130]  Eichholz A, Ferraldeschi R, Attard G and de Bono J S. Putting the brakes on continued androgen receptor signaling in castration-resistant prostate cancer. Molecular and Cellular Endocrinology 2012;360: 68–75.

[131]  Attard G, Reid AH, Yap TA, Raynaud F, Dowsett M, Settatree S, Barrett M, Parker C, Martins V, Folkerd E, Clark J, Cooper CS, Kaye SB, Dearnaley D, Lee G and de Bono JS. Phase I clinical trial of a selective inhibitor of CYP17, abiraterone acetate, confirms that castration-resistant prostate cancer commonly remains hormone driven. Journal of Clinical Oncology 2008;26(28): 4563–4571.

[132]  Ryan CJ, Smith MR, Fong L, Rosenberg JE, Kantoff P, Raynaud F, Martins V, Lee G, Kheoh T, Kim J, Molina A and Small EJ. Phase I clinical trial of the CYP17 inhibitor abiraterone acetate demonstrating clinical activity in patients with castration-resistant prostate cancer who received prior ketoconazole therapy. Journal of Clinical Oncology 2010;28(9): 1481–1488.

[133]  Attard G, Reid AH M, A'Hern R, Parker C, Oommen NB, Folkerd E, Messiou C, Molife LR, Maier G, Thompson E, Olmos D, Sinha R, Lee G, Dowsett M, Kaye SB, Dearnaley D, Kheoh T, Molina A and de Bono JS. Selective inhibition of CYP17 with abiraterone acetate is highly active in the treatment of castration-resistant prostate cancer. Journal of Clinical Oncology 2009;27(23): 3742–3748.

[134]  Danila DC, Morris MJ, de Bono JS, Ryan CJ, Denmeade SR, Smith MR, Taplin ME, Bubley GJ, Kheoh T, Haqq C, Molina A, Anand A, Koscuiszka M, Larson SM, Schwartz L H, Fleisher M and Scher HI. Phase II multicenter study of abiraterone acetate plus prednisone therapy in patients with docetaxel-treated castration-resistant prostate cancer. Journal of Clinical Oncology 2010;28(9): 1496–1501.

[135]  Reid AH, Attard G, Danila DC, Oommen NB, Olmos D, Fong PC, Molife LR, Hunt J, Messiou C, Parker C, Dearnaley D, Swennenhuis JF, Terstappen LW, Lee G, Kheoh T,

Molina A, Ryan CJ, Small E, Scher H I and de Bono JS. Significant and sustained anti-tumor activity in post-docetaxel, castration-resistant prostate cancer with the CYP17 inhibitor abiraterone acetate. Journal of Clinical Oncology 2010;28(9): 1489–1495.

[136]    de Bono JS, Logothetis CJ, Molina A, Fizazi K, North S, Chu L, Chi KN, Jones RJ, Goodman OB Jr, Saad F, Staffurth JN, Mainwaring P, Harland S, Flaig TW, Hutson TE, Cheng T, Patterson H, Hainsworth JD, Ryan CJ, Sternberg CN, Ellard SL, Fléchon A, Saleh M, Scholz M, Efstathiou E, Zivi A, Bianchini D, Loriot Y, Chieffo N, Kheoh T, Haqq C M and Scher HI. Abiraterone and increased survival in metastatic prostate cancer. The New England Journal of Medicine 2011;364(21): 1995–2005.

[137]    ClinicalTrials.gov: US National Institute of Health. www.ClinicalTrials.gov (accessed 27 July 2012).

[138]    Vasaitis T, Belosay A, Schayowitz A, Khandelwal A, Chopra P, Gediya LK, Guo Z, Fang HB, Njar VC O and Brodie AM H. Androgen receptor inactivation contributes to antitumor efficacy of 17α-hydroxylase/17,20-lyase inhibitor 3β-hydroxy-17-(1H-benzimidazole-1-yl)androsta-5,16-diene in prostate cancer. Molecular Cancer Therapeutics 2008;7(8):2348–2357.

[139]    Schayowitz A, Sabnis G, Njar V C O and Brodie A M H. Synergistic effect of a novel antiandrogen, VN/124-1, and signal transduction inhibitors in prostate cancer progression to hormone independence in vitro. Molecular Cancer Therapeutics 2008;7(1): 121–132.

[140]    Schayowitz A, Sabnis G, Goloubeva O, Njar V C O and Brodie A M H. Prolonging hormone sensitivity in prostate cancer xenografts through dual inhibition of AR and mTOR. British Journal ofCancer 2010;103(7): 1001–1007.

[141]    Soifer HS, Souleimanian N, Wu S, Voskresenskiy AM, Collak F K, Cinar B and Stein CA.Direct Regulation of Androgen Receptor Activity by Potent CYP17 Inhibitors in Prostate Cancer Cells. Journal of Biological Chemistry 2012;287(6): 3777-3787.

[142]    Bruno RD, Vasaitis TS, Gediya LK, Purushottamachar P, Godbole AM, Ates-Alagoz Z, Brodie AM H and Njar VC O. Synthesis and biological evaluations of putative metabolically stable analogs of VN/124-1 (TOK-001): Head to head anti-tumor efficacy evaluation of VN/124-1 (TOK-001) and abiraterone in LAPC-4 human prostate cancer xenograft model. Steroids 2011;76(12): 1268–1279.

# Chapter 12

# Novel Therapeutic Settings in the Treatment of Castration-Resistant Prostate Cancer

Miguel Álvarez Múgica, Jesús M. Fernández Gómez,
Antonio Jalón Monzón,
Erasmo Miguelez García and
Francisco Valle González

Additional information is available at the end of the chapter

## 1. Introduction

Prostate cancer is the most common non-dermatological malignant disease in men in western countries. According to the American Cancer Society in 2010, the incidence of prostate cancer was 217,730 cases with 32,050 deaths from the disease [1]. Overall, the actuarial 10 and 15 years survival are 93% and 77% respectively [1]. The rise in incidence and improved survival of prostate cancer over the past decades have often been attributed to prostate cancer screening and early detection. Definite evidence supporting this relationship is, however, still pending. There are also alternative explanations such as improved treatment at advanced stages that could lower prostate cancer mortality. Because of earlier detection, up to 90% of new cases in the post prostate-specific antigen (PSA) era present with clinically localized disease, the majority of which do well regardless of treatment regimen undertaken. Overall, those with advanced prostate cancer at time of diagnosis remains essentially incurable, and do poorly after androgen withdrawal therapy developing progressive disease that is resistant to further hormone manipulation. For these patients with castration-resistent prostate cancer (CRPC), and particularly patients with metastatic disease, options till few years ago have been limited. However, as newer agents become available, higher rate of biochemical and clinical response are being achieved, providing a new hope for the management of these patients [2].

CRPC is defined as patients with serum castration levels of testosterone (< 50 ng/dL or < 1.7 nmol/L), PSA and/or clinical progression to castration, and progression despite anti-androgen withdrawal for at least 4-6 weeks. PSA progression is defined as three consecutive rises of PSA, 1 week apart, resulting in two 25% increases over the nadir, with a PSA level > 2 ng/dL above the nadir. Clinical progression includes progression of bone lesions (two or more lesions on bone scan) or soft tissue progression using Respond Evaluation Criteria In Solid Tumors (RECIST) criteria [3].

Although patients with CRPC have, by definition, castrate levels of circulating testosterone, most tumors continue to remain dependent on androgen and on signaling from the androgen receptor (AR). This may occur through constitutive activation of the AR (gene amplification, alternative splicing, AR-activating gene mutations), intratumoral production of androgen, promiscuity of the AR (and binding of other hormones), activation of downstream targets by dysregulation of transcription factors (eg, binding of the frequently rearranged and overexpressed ETS oncogenic factors to androgen-regulated promoters), and alternative yet unidentified mechanisms [1, 2].

CRPC status includes patient cohorts with significantly different median survival times and different sensitivity to second hormonal manipulations. However, the vast majority of patients eventually develop progressive disease that is resistant to further hormone manipulation. We now know that although this group of patients progress to androgen deprivation, they might still be hormone-sensitive. Until 2004, cytotoxic chemotherapy was considered to be relatively ineffective in men with CRPC. In 2004, 2 landmark trials, TAX 327 and Southwest Oncology Group (SWOG) 99-16, showed for the first time a survival benefit in men with metastatic HRPC. Specifically, docetaxel-based chemotherapy demonstrated a median improvement in survival of 2.5 months as compared with mitoxantrone and prednisone in metastatic HRPC [4, 5]. Regimens that include docetaxel, have demonstrated higher rates of objective and biochemical PSA response, as well as longer survival durations. In contrast, metastatic CRPC has become a more complicated disease to be properly treated. Since then, newer treatments in this stage of the disease have been approved optimizing survival and quality of life.

## 2. Mechanisms involved in the development and progression of the disease

To understand prostatic growth in diseased states, it is important to understand the hormonal influences at play in normal prostate development and function. Testosterone is the primary circulating androgen in men. Within the prostate, testosterone is converted to a more potent androgen dihydrotestosterone (DHT) by the action of intracellular 5α-reductase enzymes [6]. Circulating DHT levels are low (1 : 10) when compared with testosterone, whereas in the prostate, this ratio is reversed, making DHT the primary prostatic androgen [7].

Dihydrotestosterone is essential for the development of the prostate gland. Inside the prostate, both testosterone and DHT bind to the androgen receptor (AR), stimulating the AR signalling axis that promotes cell-cycle regulation, cell survival and lipogenesis [8]. Although both the androgens are capable of binding AR, DHT has a stronger affinity than testosterone and a slower dissociation rate [9, 10]. DHT is also more potent at stimulating prostatic growth than testosterone [9]. These combined effects of DHT enhance the androgen signalling pathway in tissues where 5α-reductase enzymes are highly expressed [10].

Depending on the developmental stage of the individual, DHT signalling could promote the differentiation of the male external genitalia (gestation) or the maturation of the prostate gland (puberty) [7]. Throughout adulthood, DHT androgen signalling acts as a regulator of homoeostasis, maintaining the prostate epithelium by balancing cell proliferation and cell death [8]. Unlike testosterone, DHT does not exhibit an age-related decline in serum concentration. Some studies have shown a steady decline of testosterone every decade in healthy men [11, 12], whereas the levels of DHT either decline slightly or remain unchanged [13, 14]. It has been suggested that DHT levels remain constant in ageing individuals because the pathway of conversion from testosterone is saturated at low levels of testosterone. Morgentaler and Traish present a critical revision of the traditional view of T and PC [15]. They use a saturation model that is consistent with regression of cancer when T is reduced to castrate levels but lacks observed growth when serum T is increased. The saturation model starts from the observation that PCa growth is sensitive to variation in serum T concentrations at or below the castrate range and is insensitive to T variation above this concentration. Considering the actual interest in using T replacement therapies in men, a new definition of the relationship between T and PCa is of considerable importance. Evidence supports the hypothesis that T administration in hypogonadal men without PCa does not increase the risk for PCa growth if T levels are normalised [16-18].

Compelling evidence that implicates DHT as the primary prostatic androgen comes from the discovery of the Dominican pseudohermaphrodites or Guevedoce. This population has a deficiency in 5α-reductase and therefore their DHT levels are markedly lower, whereas their testosterone levels remain normal [19]. The prostate of these affected men is non-palpable and the prostate volume is one-tenth that of normal age-matched controls. Administration of DHT in these individuals results in prostate enlargement, strongly implicating DHT as a necessary component of prostate growth and development [20].

Androgen receptor signaling remains active even with castrate levels of serum testosterone, contrary to the previous notion that disease progression after gonadal ablation necessarily implied androgen-independent escape mechanisms. This is supproted by studies, which report high intratumoral androgens, continued AR signaling [21], and overexpression of enzymes key to androgen síntesis, which suggests that CRPC may synthesize androgens de novo [22, 23]. Until recently, available strategies that target the AR, such as antiandrogens, ketoconazole, estrogens or glucocorticoids, result in modest benefit. New drugs such as abiraterone, or MDV 3100 have shown a much more supression activity of the AR by different pathways.

The key components of DHT production are the 5α reductase enzymes. There are two well-characterised isoforms, type 1 and type 2 [24, 25]. Type 1 is present throughout all stages of life and is primarily localised in extraprostatic tissues including the non-genital skin, liver and certain brain regions. Although type 1 expression was originally thought to be absent from the prostate gland, certain studies have found type 1 within the prostatic tissue predominantly localised to the secretory luminal epithelium [26]. The type 2 5α-reductase iso-form is prevalent in the prostatic tissue as well as the genital skin, seminal vesicle and epididymis. Although this isoform is present through all stages of prostate development, it has a single wave of expression in the skin and scalp that begins at birth and ends at ages 2–3 years [26]. Type 2 5α-reductase is deficient in the Guevedoce and therefore these individu-als do not generate enough DHT to promote normal development of the prostate gland and the man's external genitalia [20].

## 3. Natural history of prostate cancer

Although the natural history of prostate cancer (PCa) has not been fully elucidated, it is thought to arise from damaged prostate epithelium and progressively develop over many decades [27]. Prostate disease is heterogeneous and multifocal, further complicating the un-derstanding of its progression. Based on autopsy studies, about one-third of men over the age of 50 years display histological evidence of PCa. However, a majority of these cases re-main clinically insignificant, underscoring the variability in PCa and the protracted nature of this disease [3, 28].

The likelihood of disease progression of PCa is difficult to predict. Detection of cancer from a biopsy can result in a localised diagnosis; however, upon a prostatectomy, it may be re-vealed that the disease had grown outside the margins of the gland or even had metastas-ised. Conversely, certain men diagnosed with PCa may live out their natural lives without suffering any morbidity or mortality from the disease.Therefore, it becomes imperative to determine whether or not a particular lesion will stay localised or spread beyond the con-fines of the gland [3]. The usually slow progression of prostate cancer allows delaying or avoiding definitive treatment (active surveillance) in selected patients if some prerequisites are fulfilled. The younger a candidate is for active surveillance, the more strict the tumour-related criteria that should be used [29].

Research has revealed insights into the likely progression of prostate tumours. It has been shown that certain high-grade tumours proceed on a more aggressive course than low-grade, well-differentiated tumours and therefore should be managed accordingly [30]. The Gleason score is one of the most powerful prognostic factors in prostate cancer [31]. In elder-ly patients with clinically localised, conservatively managed prostate cancer, the probability to survive the disease for at least 10 years ranges from 77% to 98% when the Gleason score is 7 or less, whereas this rate is only 33–75% in patients with a Gleason score of 8–10 [32]. The prolonged nature of PCa progression highlights the opportunities for clinical therapeutic in-terventions that could reduce the risk of disease development and slow it or treat the exist-ing disease. Through the Cancer and Leukimia Group B (CALGB) cooperative study group, Halabi and colleagues performed a polled analysis combining data from 6 trials and more than 1100 patients with CRPC accured from 1991 to 2001 [33], and created a prognostic mod-el for risk stratification of metastatic CRPC patients. The observed median survival dura-tions (in months) were 7.5 (95% confidence interval [CI] 6.2–10.9], 13.4 (95% CI 9.7–26.3],

18.9 (95% CI 16.2–26.3], and 27.2 (95% CI 21.9–42.8] for the first, second, third, and fourth risk groups, respectively. The factors involved in this model can be broadly divided into clinical variables that reflect the condition of the host (eg, performance status, anemia, fatigue), the tumor burden (eg, sites of metastatic disease, PSA level, alkaline phosphatase level), or the biologic aggressiveness of the cancer itself (eg, lactate dehydrogenase [LDH] levels, Gleason sum).

The clinical course of metastatic castration-resistant prostate cancer has changed considerably, primarily because of factors such as earlier diagnosis, stage migration and changes in clinical practice patterns. Earlier initiation of androgen-deprivation therapy and the increased use of diagnostic imaging have contributed to earlier detection of metastatic disease in androgen-deprived patients. Furthermore, new treatments have further extended the time to the terminal phase of the disease, estimating the duration of the course of metastatic castration-resistant prostate cancer measured from the first documented metastasis (in the castrate state) until death may now extend beyond 5 years.

## 4. Mechanisms and targets in CRPC

The key for the development of new drugs and to optimize androgenic suppression in advanced stages of CRPC is the identification and characterization of molecular targets and mechanisms that lead to tumor growth. Disease progression involves the development of cellular adaptive pathways of survival in an androgen-depleted environment [34]. Experimental evidence assigns an important role to the continuous activation of the androgenic receptors (ARs) in tumor growth, as well as alternative independent routes [35]. In general, resistance mechanisms can be divided into 6 groups.

- *Increased Expression of Enzymes Involved in Steroidogenesis.* Studies have suggested that, in CRPC patients, even castrate serum levels of androgen are still sufficient for AR activation and able to maintain cancer cells survival. Indeed, the intratumoral levels of testosterone in CRPC patients are equal of those found in noncastrate patients [36]. The source of these androgens is thought to be derived from the synthesis of androgens directly in prostate cancer cells due to an upregulation of the enzymes and activation of the routes necessary for the synthesis of androgens such as testosterone and dihydrotestosterone [34, 37, 38]. Also bone metastases contain intact enzyme pathways for conversion of adrenal androgens to testosterone and dihydrotestosterone [36]. Montgomery and colleagues showed that there was marked reversal of the DHT : testosterone ratio in the metastatic tumor. These tumor cells express significantly lower levels of SRD5A2, which catalyses the conversion of testosterone to DHT, and higher levels of UGT2B15 and UGT2B17, which mediate the irreversible glucuronidation of DHT metabolites. Marked up regulation of CYP19A1, which mediates the aromatization of testosterone to estradiol, was also observed in the metastases samples [34, 36-38].

- *Increased Expression of AR.* The overexpression of AR have been involved in the progression of prostate cancer [34]. The activated AR pathways observed in these CRPC patients has been postulated as a result of genetic phenomena that promotes increased sensitivity of AR. DNA amplifications are responsible for AR overexpression and for its activation in presence of low levels of ligand (androgens) [34, 38].

- *AR Gene Mutations and Altered Ligand Specificity.* While the androgens are the main factors of tumor growth and AR signaling, the presence of AR mutations leads to its activation by nonandrogenic steroid molecules and antiandrogens [34]. The majority AR mutations are point mutations in the AR ligand-binding domain, and initially this was considered relevant to explain why 10–30% of patients receiving antiandrogens treatment experience paradoxical PSA drop on cessation of treatment [35]. However the AR mutations could occur in other regions such as the amino terminus or the DNA binding domain that confer oncogenic properties to the AR [37]. At the present, the role of AR mutations in the anti-androgen withdrawal phenomena is called into questioned and a new explanation is offered since the discovery of alternative splicing of the AR. In fact, in recent reports [39, 40], it was shown that splice variants of AR with deletion of exons 5, 6, and 7 could result in AR capable to translocate to the nucleus without ligand binding.

- *Downstream Signaling Receptor for Androgens.* One of the most important mechanisms in the development of castration resistance is the activation of different signal transduction pathways in CRPC cells. They could enhance the activity of the AR or its coactivators in the presence of low levels or even in the absence of androgen. These include other receptors such as epithelial growth factors, insulin growth factors, and tyrosine-kinase receptor [40].

- *Bypass Pathways.* The induction of bypass pathways independent of AR, is an important mechanism of castration resistance, that can overcame apoptosis induced by androgen-deprivation therapy. One such example of this is the up-regulation of antiapoptotic proteins, including the protein Bcl-2 gene [34, 40].

- *Stem Cells.* Prostatic cancer stem cells are rare and undifferentiated cells that do not express AR on their surface, being independent of androgens to survive [34]. Currently it is thought that these cells can be responsible for maintaining tumor growth and development, because they are able to survive under androgen-deprivation therapy. The identification of these cells is possible based on the expression of surface protein ($\alpha1\beta1$ integrin and CD133), which could allow new targets therapies [34].

# 5. New therapeutics settings in the treatment of castration resistant prostate cancer

Being able to predict which patients will develop metastasis and death with rising PSA levels after treatment with androgen ablation is essential for deciding therpeutic interventions and gauging prognosis. The major biologic processes under therpeutic investigation in prostate cancer involve growth and survival, chemotherapy and hormone therapy resistance, extragonadal androgen production, modulation of the androgen receptor, angiogenesis, the bone interface, immune surveillance and escape, epigenetic regulation and stem cell renewal. A better understanding of this mechanisms responsible for prostate cancer growth and metastatic spread has allowed for the development of a wide array of new therapies.

The growth of prostate cancer is originally androgen dependent and metastatic tumors are generally treated with androgen ablation therapy, with or without antiandrogen supplementation [41, 42, 43]. However, resistance to hormonal therapy occurs within 12–18 months (remissions last on average 2-3 years, progression occurs even under castration [37, 44, 45], referred to as hormone-refractory or CRPC [41]. Resistance to hormones (in patients with metastatic disease) is probably shorter than 2-3 years, using PSA. Until recently, patients with castration-resistant prostate cancer had limited treatment options after docetaxel chemotherapy. However, in 2010, new options emerged [46]. The three nonhormonal systemic approaches that have been found to prolong survival are docetaxel as first line [4] chemotherapy, cabazitaxel as second-line cytotoxic chemotherapy [46, 47] and a vaccine named sipuleucel-T [48]. A new hormonal manipulation with abiraterone acetate [45] also showed to prolong survival in CRPC.

The current palliative treatment options for patients with CRPC can be divided in different groups such as secondary hormonal therapies, chemotherapy agents, vaccine-based immune therapy, bisphosphonates, radiotherapy and novel targets.

## 5.1. Antiandrogen therapies

Drugs that reduce circulating levels of androgens or that competitively inhibit the action of androgens remain central to the treatment of prostate cancer. The surgical or medical castration with orchiectomy or gonadotropin-releasing hormone (GnRH) agonists, respectively, suppresses testicular testosterone generation. However, the duration of response to castration is short [12–33 months) and, in almost all patients, is followed by the emergence of a castration-resistant phenotype [34]. The combination with antiandrogens to achieve the maximum androgen blockade (MAB) did not prove to prolong survival and 30% of the patients have a drop in PSA after discontinuing antiandrogens [3, 43]. For patients whose disease progresses after a MAB, antiandrogen can be discontinued [49], or can be switched to an alternative antiandrogen as showed in several reports [3, 43]. High-dose [150 mg daily) bicalutamide as second-line hormonal therapy resulted in ≥50% PSA reduction in 20%–45% of patients [12, 34].

- **Oral Glucocorticoids** (10 mg/day) can result in temporary PSA responses for 25% of the patients, presumably due to adrenal androgen suppression [34, 50].

- **Diethylstilboestrol** (DES), a synthetic estrogen, as well as the other estrogens, suppresses the hypothalamic-pituitary-gonadal axis and it reduces ≥50% the total PSA in 26% to 66% of patients with CRPC. However, the important thromboembolic toxicity limited is use [50,51].

- **Ketoconazol** is an antifungal agent that can be given to CRPC patients after antiandrogen withdrawal because it inhibits cytochrome P-450 enzyme-mediated steroidogenesis in testes and adrenal glands and when given at high-dose (1200 mg/day) or low dose (600 mg/day) it resulted in ≥50% PSA reduction in 27% to 63% and 27 to 46%, of patients, respectively [49]. However, the narrow therapeutic window of ketoconazole + hydrocortisone versus hydrocortisone alone must be kept in mind due to secondary effects of ketoconazole.

- **Abiraterone acetate**, a prodrug of abiraterone, is a potent and highly selective inhibitor of androgen biosynthesis that blocks cytochrome P450 c17 (CYP17] a critical enzyme in androgen synthesis in the testes, adrenals and in the tumor itself [52]. This enzyme catalyzes two sequential reactions: the conversion of pregnenolone and progesterone to their 17-α-hydroxy derivates and the subsequent formation of dehydroepiandrosterone (DHEA) and androstenedione, respectively. These two androgens are precursors of testosterone. As a result, plasma testosterone levels are significantly lower than those achieved with conventional hormone therapies; in addition, a reduction in intratumoral levels of androgens is obtained. The COU-AA-301, a phase III trial in post-docetaxel refractory CRPC, resulted in a significant improvement in overall survival in the abiraterone group [53]. Furthermore there is a second randomized phase III trial (COU-AA-302) targeting men with docetaxel and ketoconazole-naïve CRPC showing positive results in the interim analysis in the Abiraterone group, achieving a delay in disease progression and fairly long expected survival. For this reason the study was recently unblinded before completion at the recommendation of the Independent Data Monitoring Committee.

- **MDV3100** (Enzalutamide) is an androgen-receptor antagonist that blocks androgens from binding to the androgen receptor and prevents nuclear translocation and co-activator recruitment of the ligand-receptor complex. It also induces tumour cell apoptosis, and has no agonist activity. MDV 3100 was found clinically active for metastatic castration-resistant prostate cancer patients in ongoing phase I and II trials. The AFFIRM trial (a phase III trial) compared MDV3100 versus placebo in patients with docetaxel-refractory CRPC [34, 54]. The trial will determine the effectiveness of enzalutamide in patients who have previously failed chemotherapy treatment with docetaxel. In November 2011, this trial was halted after an interim analysis revealed that patients given the drug lived for approximately 5 months longer than those taking placebo, estimating a median survival of 18.4 months for men treated with MDV3100, compared with 13.6 months for men treated with placebo. This translates into a 37% reduction in the risk for death with MDV3100 (hazard ratio, 0.631]. As a result, the trial's Independent Data Monitoring Committee recommended that AFFIRM should be stopped earlier and that men who were receiving placebo should be offered MDV3100. The recommendation was based on the fact that the study's prespecified interim efficacy stopping criteria were successfully met. The committee also examined the safety profile to date and determined that MDV3100 demonstrated a risk/benefit ratio that was favorable enough to stop the study. It is expected to file for FDA approval sometime in 2012. There is another phase III trial, known as PREVAIL, that is investigating the effectiveness of enzalutamide with patients who have not yet received chemotherapy [55].

- **Orteronel** (TAK-700]. Is an androgen synthesis inhibitor. It selectively inhibits the enzyme CYP17A1 which is expressed in testicular, adrenal, and prostatic tumor tissues. It is a very promising drug, but we still have to wait for results of two phase III clinical trials currently recruiting participants in CRPC patients and high risk patients [56].

## 5.2. Chemotherapy

**Cabazitaxel** is a new tubulin-binding taxane that has shown to be as potent as docetaxel in cell lines, and is the first chemotherapy shown to improve survival in patients with docetaxel-refractory metastatic castration resistant prostatic cancer. Moreover, it has demonstrated antitumor activity in models resistant to docetaxel due to its poor affinity for the ATP-dependent drug efflux pump, a member of the multidrug resistance protein family [57]. The TROPIC trial, a phase III trial in post-docetaxel refractory CRPC, compared cabazitaxel plus prednisone versus mitoxantrone plus prednisolone, in patients with docetaxel-refractory prostate cancer concluding in a significant improvement in overall survival in the cabazitaxel group.

**Epothilones**, namely, ixabepilone and patupilone, have shown significant activity in men with CRPC [58, 59]. These molecules were evaluated in second-line chemotherapy in two phase II trials after progression with prior taxane [60, 61]. Phase III trials with ixabepilone are in development and two phase II trial of patupilone are completed [59].

**Eribulin mesylate** (E7389] is a synthetic analog of the marine macrolide halichondrin B, which acts as a novel microtubule modulator with a distinct mechanism of action (different from taxanes) [60]. An open-label, multicenter, single-arm, phase II study was conducted in patients with CRPC stratified by prior taxane therapy [62]. Primary efficacy endpoint was PSA response rate defined as two consecutive ≥50% decreases in PSA levels from baseline. The secondary endpoints were duration of PSA response rate and objective response rate by RECIST criteria. One hundred and eight patients were available for analyses. Of these 50 were taxane pretreated. Eribulin showed activity in patients with metastatic CRPR, especially in those with taxane naïve disease. Side effects, mainly hematological toxicity (grade 3 and 4 leucopenia and neutropenia), fatigue, and peripheral neuropathy were manageable [62].

**Satraplatin** (JM-216] is an oral third-generation platinum compound evaluated in the SPARC trial, a phase III trial, in combination with prednisone in second-line therapy after docetaxel [34, 51]. In this trial, satraplatin plus prednisone resulted in significant improvement in PFS (11.1 weeks versus 9.7 weeks) but there were no improvement in median overall survival compared with prednisone alone (61.3 weeks versus 61.4 weeks).

Other chemotherapy treatments, studied in CRPC are Mitoxantrone with two pivotal studies in the late 90's that could not demonstrate to be superior to palliative corticosteroid therapy. Encourarging results with alternative treatments, including Vinorelbine, a semi-synthetic vinca alkaloid, and oral cyclophosphamide, have being obtained in prospective clinical phase II trials. However the lack of representative randomized phase III trials and unknown long-term efficacy are the major problems associatied with all these studies [63, 64, 65].

## 5.3. Vaccines-based immunotherapy

**Sipuleucel-T** is an active cellular immunotherapy consisting of autologous peripheral-blood mononuclear cells, including antigen-presenting cells (APCs), which have been activated ex vivo with a recombinant fusion protein known as PA2024, composed of prostatic acid phosphatase (PAP) linked to granulocyte-macrophage colony-stimulating factor (GM-CSF). In the first two randomized trials, sipuleucel-T, the primary endpoint was not accomplished since these studies did not show a significant effect on the time to disease progression comparing with placebo. Despite this, the hazard ratios were in favor of sipuleucel-T [66, 67]. The IMPACT trial, a phase III trial in CPRC asyntomatic patients, resulted in a longer median survival time in the Sipuleucel-T group, with limited toxicity. Approved by the Food and Drugs Administration (FDA), currently Sipuleucel-T is not approved to been used in Europe [68].

**GVAX** (CGI940/CG8711] is a cellular vaccine composed of two allogeneic prostate cancer cell lines (LNCaP and PC-3] that is genetically modified to secrete GM-CSF [69]. This vaccine showed clinical benefit with limited toxicity in phase I and II trials [70, 71]. However, the two phase III trials (VITAL-1 and VITAL-2] evaluated GVAX against docetaxel plus prednisone in naïve CRPC and both were closed prematurely [70]. The VITAL-1 study was closed when the unplanned futility analysis revealed a <30% chance of meeting its predefined primary endpoint of OS improvement and the VITAL-2 terminated when an interim analysis revealed more deaths in the GVAX arm than in the control [71].

**PROSTVAC-VF** is a cancer vaccine consisting of a recombinant vaccinia vector as a priming immunization with subsequent multiple booster vaccinations, using a recombinant fowlpox vector. This agent presented in the context of 3 costimulatory molecules (ICAM-1, BLA-7, and LFA-3] which, when taken together, demonstrate an increase in strength of the target immunologic response [48]. This vaccine was evaluated in phase I and II trials. The phase I trial showed PSA stabilization in 40% of patients and limited toxicity and, in the phase II study, patients in the PROSTVAC-VF arm achieved an 8.5-month improvement in median OS [25.1 months versus 16.6 months) and a 44% reduction in the death rate (Hazard ratio 0.56], [72]. Phase III trial are being planned and other vaccines are under current development [73].

### 5.4. Bone-targeted treatments

**Zoledronic Acid.** Metastatic prostate cancer has an affinity to spread to the bone. Bone metastases occur in up to 90% of patients with HRPC. These metastases can lead to significant morbidity, including severe pain, fractures, and spinal cord compression tumors in the bone may cause pain, compression, or pathologic fratures, known as skeletal related events (SRE's). Because of the frequent involvement of vertebrae by metastatic prostate cancer, the incidene of cord compression is of particular concern. Zoledronic acid has been shown to prevent or delay skeletal complications in men with bone metastases, as well as to palliate bone pain [74, 75]. At an average followup of 24 months, there was a significant reduction in the frequency of skeletal related events (SREs) in men receiving zoledronic acid compared to placebo [38 versus 49 percent), and the median time to develop an SRE was significantly longer with zoledronic acid [488 versus 321 days) [76]. Biphosphonates may also have a role in preventing osteopenia that frequently accompanies the use of androgen-deprivation therapy [77, 78]

**Denosumab.** Is a human monoclonal antibody directed against RANKL that inhibits osteoclast-mediated bone destruction. In a phase III study [79]. Denosumab showed to be better than zoledronic acid for the prevention of skeletal-related events. Although is not yet available in Europe, it is expected to be approved soon.

### 5.5. External beam radiotherapy and radioisotope drugs

Focal external beam radiation therapy (RT) is a palliative treatment possibility that should be considered for men with CRPC and bone pain that is limited to one or a few sites. Several clinical trials as well as a systematic review of the literature suggest that single treatments with fractionation schedules provide palliation with cost effectiveness and patient convenience [80].

**Hemibody** RT could also be considered in selected patients with symptomatic disease limited to one side of the diaphragm, in order to rapid pain relief, when multiple bone metastases are present [81]. However, this technique has frequently been replaced by the administration of radioisotope pharmaceuticals which may be associated with less toxicity and are more appropriated for patients with multiple painful lesions [82]. In order for these patients to be treated with radioisotopes the presence of uptake on bone scan due to metastatic disease at sites that correlate with pain is necessary. These radioisotopes are used in men with advanced prostate cancer with osteoblastic bone metastasis. These patients are often characterized by a high ratio of bone to soft tissue metastases. Multiple radioisotopes have been used but the most extensive data are with 89-strontium (89Sr), Radium-223 and 153-samarium [153Sm]. Several clinical trials provide the rational for the use of this approach in carefully selected patients [83, 84, 85].

**Lexidronam** (Samarium 153]. Is a complex of a radioisotope of the lanthanide element samarium with the chelator EDTMP. Particularly useful in patients with CRPC and multiple painful bone metastases, who have relapsed following initial course of hormonal or cytotoxic chemotherapy, and in patients with progressive or recurrent symptoms at the treated sites. The goal in this stage of the disease is to maintain quality of life while managing the symptoms of the progressing cancer. Extensive data support the use of Samarium SM 153 in this group of patients [8, 9].

**Alpharadin** (Radium-223]. Alpharadin uses alpha radiation from radium-223 decay to kill cancer cells. Radium-223 naturally self-targets to bone metastases by virtue of its properties as a calcium-mimic. Alpha radiation has a very short range of 2-10 cells (when compared to current radiation therapy which is based on beta or gamma radiation), and therefore causes less damage to surrounding healthy tissues (particularly bone marrow). Radium-223 has a half life of 11.4 days, making it ideal for targeted cancer treatment. Furthermore, any Alpharadin that is not taken up by the bone metastases is rapidly cleared to the gut and excreted. In the phase III ALSYMPCA trial [86], Alpharadin succesfully met the primary endpoint of overall survival. When compared with placebo, Radium-223 was associated with improved overall survival (median 14.0 versus 11.2 months; HR, 0.69. A recent phase III trial envoluving Alpharadin, showed a significant improvement in the median overall survival in chemo-naïve patients as well as in those treated previously with docetaxel.

## 5.6. Antiangiogenic strategies

**Bevacizumab**. Tumor angiogenesis is likely to be an important biologic component of pros-tate cancer growth and progression. An elevated levels of the potent angiogenic molecule vascular endothelial growth factor (VEGF) have been shown to correlate with advanced clinical stage and survival. Microvessel density in clinically localized prostate cancer is an independent prognostic for progression and survival [87, 88]. Antiangiogenic agents using monoclonal antibodies to VEGF, such as bevacizumab (Avastin®) have been studied in prostate cancer. Although single-agent studies have failed to demonstrate significant results, a phase II trial conducted by the CALGB added bevacizumab to docetaxel and estramustine in men with HRPC; 79% of patients had a greater than 50% decline in PSA level, median time to progression of 9.7 months, and overall median survival of 21 months [89]. On the basis of these promising results, a randomized, double-blind, placebo-controlled, phase III trial has been designed comparing docetaxel 75 mg/m² every 3 weeks with prednisone 10 mg orally daily with either bevacizumab 15 mg/kg IV or placebo every 3 weeks (CALGB 90401]. The primary endpoint for this trial is overall survival, and secondary endpoints in-clude progression-free survival, PSA reduction, and grade 3 toxicities. This trial opened in April 2005 and is actively accruing.

**Thalidomide**. Is a synthetic glutamic acid derivative. Thalidomide was noted to have anti-inflammatory, immunomodulatory and antiangiogenic effects. alone or in combination with docetaxel were studied in phase II trials with promising results. Microvessel density (MVD) has been reported to be higher in prostate cancer tissue than in adjacent hyperplastic or be-nign tissue [90]. Preclinical evidence also suggests that angiogenesis may play a key role in the development of aggressive prostate cancer lesion [91]. Clinical studies have observed a correlation between increased angiogenesis in primary tumor specimens and the future de-velopment of metastatic disease. The apparent importance of angiogenesis in the evolution of prostate cancer provides a rationale for the investigation of antiangiogenesis agents in CRPC. A phase II trial of thalidomide resulted in a > 40% fall in PSA levels in 27% of pa-tients and improvement in clinical symptoms in all responding patients. PSA declines often resulted in striking reductions in measurable disease on positron emission tomographic scan. Thalidomide plus docetaxel versus docetaxel monotherapy, in a phase II trial in pa-tients with metastatic CRPC, showed a ≥50% PSA decrease (53% versus 37%) and improve-ment in median overall survival (28.9 months versus 14.7 months) for patients in the thalidomide group [92, 93].

The combination of docetaxel, thalidomide, bevacizumab, and prednisolone was also evalu-ated in a phase II trial with a ≥50% PSA reduction in 89.6% of patients. The median time to progression was 18.3 months and the median overall survival was 28.2 months [93]. More studies are needed before prescribing angiogenesis inhibitors outside clinical trials.

## 5.7. Other targets

**Dasatinib**. Is a small molecular kinase inhibitor of Src family kinases (SFK), being studied for prostate cancer because Src signaling is involved in androgen-induced proliferation. In a phase II trial in chemotherapy-naïve patients with metastatic CRPC, dasatinib [100 mg orally twice daily) showed lack of progression in 43% of patients at week 12 and in 19% in patients at week 24. It also revealed a decrease in the markers of bone metabolism (N-telopeptide and bone alkaline phosphatase) A randomized phase III trial with dasatinib plus docetaxel is ongoing [94].

**Ipilimumab.** Blockade of the T-cell inhibitory receptor CTL-associated antigen-4 (CTLA-4] augments and prolongs T-cell responses and is a strategy to elicit antitumor immunity [95]. Ipilimumab, an anti-CTLA-4 antibody, was tested in order to potentiate endogenous antitumor immunity to prostate cancer through combination immunotherapy with CTLA-4 blockade and GM-CSF [96]. The results showed that this combination immunotherapy can induce the expansion not only of activated effector CD8 T cells *in vivo* but also of T cells that are specific for known tumor-associated antigens from endogenous immune repertoire.

In a pilot trial of CTLA-4 blockade with ipilimumab patients with CRPC were given a single dose of 3 mg/kg [95]. Results showed that this approach was safe and did not result in significant clinical autoimmunity. PSA modulating effects presented need further investigation in order to be fully understood. Two phase III trials are now recruiting patients in order to compare ipilimumab with placebo [96]. One trial [97] will evaluate this approach in patients with metastatic disease, with at least one bone metastasis, prior treatment with docetaxel, and castrate levels of serum testosterone. The other trial [98] will include patients with metastatic castration-resistant prostate cancer who are asymptomatic or minimally symptomatic and who have not received prior chemotherapy or immunotherapy.

Atrasentan. The Endothelins (ETs) constitute a family of three 21-amino-acid peptides (ET-1, ET-2, and ET-3] that are synthesized as propeptides and are transformed to their active forms by sequential endopeptidase and ET-converting enzyme-mediated cleavage [99]. ETs are regulators of cell proliferation, vasomotor tone, and angiogenesis. The ETs bind to two receptors, endothelin-A (ET-A) and endothelin-B (ET-B), and play an important role in angiogenesis, proliferation, escape from apoptosis, invasion, tumor growth, new bone formation, and bone metastasis [73, 74]. ET and their receptors have emerged as a potential targets in CRPC [99]. Efficacy and safety of ET-A receptor blockade—atrasentan (ABT-627]—have been evaluated in a double-blind, randomized, placebo-controlled, phase II trial [99], Two hundred and eighty-eight asymptomatic patients were randomized to one of three study groups: placebo, 2.5 mg atrasentan, 10 mg atrasentan. Primary endpoint was time to progression. Secondary end points were time to PSA progression, bone scan changes, and changes in bone and tumor markers. Target therapy with atrasentan was well tolerated and results showed a potential to delay progression of CRPC.

Based on these results other phase III studies also evaluated atrasentan. In one of these studies [100], atrasentan did not reduce the risk of disease progression relative to placebo. However exploratory analyses showed that alkaline phosphatase and PSA levels were significantly lower in the treatment arm [90]. Another phase III study (SWOG S0421) tested atrasentan combined with docetaxel/prednisone in metastatic CRPC as a first-line therapy [100]. SWOG trial S0421 closed earlier based on interim finding that atrasentan added to docetaxel and prednisone did not confer additional survival benefit to patients with hormone-refractory prostate cancer. The Data and Safety Monitoring Committee has determined that patients in phase III S0421 receiving atrasentan in addition to a standard chemotherapy regimen for advanced prostate cancer did not have longer survival or longer progression-free survival.

**Zibotentan** (ZD 4054]. Is another ET-A receptor antagonist, which showed evidence of activity in a randomized phase II trial in men with castrate-resistant prostate cancer and bone metastases [101]. Following these results two phase III trials [102, 103] were conducted. ENTHUSE M0 was discontinued following the results of an early efficacy review by the Independent Data Monitoring Committee. The company has concluded that zibotentan was unlikely to meet its primary efficacy endpoints progression free survival and overall survival. Results from ENTHUSE M1C are still awaited.

**Tyrosine kinase inhibitors** (TKIs) are important new class of target therapy that interfere with specific cell signaling pathways and thus allow target specific therapy for selected malignancies. Sorafenib and sunitinib have been tested in prostate cancer in phase I and II trials.

**Sorafenib**. In the first stage of a phase II trial with sorafenib [104] 22 metastatic CRPC were enrolled. Most of the patients [59%) had received prior therapy with docetaxel or mitoxantrone. Sorafenib therapy failed to show >50% PSA reduction [51]. A second stage of the trial was conducted with 24 more patients [105]. Of the 24 patients, 21 had previous chemotherapy with docetaxel. All patients had bone metastases, either alone (in 11] or with soft-tissue disease (in 13]. At a median potential followup of 27.2 months, the median progression-free survival was 3.7 months and the median overall survival was 18.0 months. For the whole trial of 46 patients the median survival was 18.3 months. The authors concluded that sorafenib has moderate activity as a second-line treatment for metastatic castration-resistant prostate cancer in this trial population [106].

Another phase II study [98] included 57 chemotherapy naïve CRPC patients. Fifty-five patients were evaluable. Two of these patients had >50% PSA reduction and 15 patients had stable disease. Analysis of the results from a third phase II trial suggests that sorafenib therapy could affect PSA production or secretion regardless of its antitumor activity [107].

**Sunitinib**. A phase I/II trial of sunitinib in combination with docetaxel and prednisone showed a PSA response in 56% of patients, a median time to PSA progression of 42.1 weeks, and a partial response of measurable disease in 39% patients [108]. Sunitinib was also tested in CRPC naïve and docetaxel refractory patients in other phase II trials [106, 107]. A phase III trial comparing sunitinib plus prednisone versus prednisone alone, in patients with docetaxel refractory metastatic CRPC, is ongoing. Overall survival is the primary endpoint of this study [109].

**Cabozantinib**. Is an inhibitor of MET and VEGFR2 [90]. Both the MET and VEGF-type 2 receptor signaling pathways appear to play important roles in the function of osteoblasts and osteoclasts. MET signaling promotes tumor growth, invasion, and metastasis. Results from cabozantinib trial were presented at ASCO Meeting, 2011. The authors concluded that cabozantinib showed clinical activity regardless of prior docetaxel in metastatic CRPC patients, particularly in patients with bone disease, in addition to improvements in hemoglobin and tumor regression.

There are also other potential targets, such as IGF-1R signaling, vitamin D receptor, PTEN, and phosphoinositide 3-kinase signaling; those are quite promising and could lead us to new treatment options [3, 34]. New mechanisms, drugs, and clinically relevant molecular targets show survival advantage and are new options available for patients after traditional chemotherapy. As ongoing studies using all the mentioned agents continue to evolve, our understanding of how and where these agents fit into the treatment paradigm for patients with CRPC will become clearer. Improvements in progression-free survival and OS rates, observed with novel agents, in metastatic prostate cancer have led to a shift in treatment paradigm. The challenge will be to position the current established and expected novel treatments in the new landscape of metastatic prostate cancer and to determine at what point and time in the disease course they can best be administered. It is clear, however, that our knowledge of the biologic mechanisms involved iin teh progression of metastaic castration-resistant prostate cancer has reached a level at which the discovery of more effective targeted approaches will probably futher improve outcomes.

## Author details

Miguel Álvarez Múgica[1], Jesús M. Fernández Gómez[2,3], Antonio Jalón Monzón[2], Erasmo Miguelez García[1] and Francisco Valle González[1]

1 Urology Department, Hospital Valle Nalón, Spain

2 Urology Department, HUCA, Spain

3 University of Oviedo, Spain

## References

[1] American Cancer Society. http://www.cancer.org (accessed September 2010).

[2] Dolfsson J, Oksanen H, Salo JO, Steineck G. Localized prostate cancer and 30 years of follow-up in a population-based setting. Prostate Cancer Prostatic Dis2000; 3: 37-42.

[3] Scardino PT. The Gordon Wilson Lecture. Natural history and treatment of early stage prostate cancer. Trans Am Clin Climatol Assoc 2000; 111: 201–41.

[4] Tannock IA, de Wit R, Berry WR, Horti J, Pluzanska A, Chi KN, Oudard S, Théodore C, James N, Turesson I, Rosenthal MA, Eisenberger MA. Docetaxel plus Prednisone or Mitoxantrone plus Prednisone for Advanced Prostate Cancer. N Engl J Med 2004; 351: 1502-12.

[5] Petrylak DP, Tangen CM, Hussain MHA, et al. Docetaxel and estramustine compared with mitoxantrone and prednisone for advanced refractory prostate cancer. N Engl J Med 2004; 351: 1513–20.

[6]  Zhu YS, Sun GH. 5α-reductase isozymes in the prostate. J Med Sci 2005; 25: 1–12.

[7]  Marks LS. 5α-reductase: history and clinical importance. Rev Urol 2004; 6(suppl 9): 11–21.

[8]  Dutt SS, Gao AC. Molecular mechanisms of castration-resistant prostate cancer progression. Fut Oncol 2009; 5: 1403-13.

[9]  Pereira de Jésus-Tran K, Côté PL, Cantin L, Blanchet J, Labrie F, Breton R. Comparison of crystal structures of human androgen receptor ligand-binding domain complexed with various agonists reveals molecular determinants responsible for binding affinity. Protein Sci 2006; 15: 987–99.

[10]  Askew EB, Gampe RT Jr, Stanley TB, Faggart JL, Wilson EM. Modulation of androgen receptor activation function 2 by testosterone and dihydrotestosterone. J Biol Chem 2007; 282: 25801–16.

[11]  Morley JE, Kaiser FE, Perry HM III et al. Longitudinal changes in testosterone, luteinizing hormone, and follicle-stimulating hormone in healthy older men. Metabolism 1997; 46: 410-3.

[12]  Harman SM, Metter EJ, Tobin JD, Pearson J, Blackman MR. Longitudinal effects of aging on serum total and free testosterone levels in healthy men. Baltimore Longitudinal Study of Aging. J Clin Endocrinol Metab 2001; 86: 724–31.

[13]  Gray A, Feldman HA, McKinlay JB, Longcope C. Age, disease, and changing sex hormone levels in middle-aged men: results of the Massachusetts Male Aging Study. J Clin Endocrinol Metab 1991; 73: 1016–25.

[14]  Pirke KM, Doerr P. Age related changes in free plasma testosterone, dihydrotestosterone and oestradiol. Acta Endocrinol (Copenh) 1975; 80: 171–8.

[15]  Morgentaler A, Traish AM. Shifting the paradigm of testosterone and prostate cancer: the saturation model and the limits of androgen-dependent growth. Eur Urol 2009; 55: 310–21.

[16]  Morgentaler A, Rhoden EL. Prevalence of prostate cancer among hypogonadal men with prostate-specific antigen levels of 4.0 ng/ml or less. Urology 2006; 68: 1263–7.

[17]  Lane BR, Stephenson AJ, Magi-Galluzzi C, Lakin MM, Klein EA. Low testosterone and risk of biochemical recurrence and poorly differentiated prostate cancer at radical prostatectomy. Urology 2008; 72: 1240–5.

[18]  Sofikerim M, Eskicorapci S, Oruc O, Ozen H. Hormonal predictors of prostate cancer. Urol Int 2007; 79: 13–8.

[19]  Imperato-McGinley J, Guerrero L, Gautier T, Peterson RE. Steroid 5α-reductase deficiency in man: an inherited form of male pseudohermaphroditism. Science 1974; 186: 1213–5.

[20]  Imperato-McGinley J, Zhu YS. Androgens and male physiology the syndrome of 5α-reductase-2 deficiency. Mol Cell Endocrinol 2002; 198: 51–9.

[21]  Titus MA, Schell MJ, Lih FB, et al. Testosterone and dihydrotestosterone tissue levels in recurrent prostate cancer. Clin Cancer Res 2005; 11: 4653-7.

[22]  Stanbrough M, Bubley GJ, Ross K, et al. Increased expresión of genes converting adrenal androgens to testosterone in androgen-independent prostate cancer. Cancer Res 206; 66: 2815-25.

[23]  Holzbeierlein J, Lal P, La Tulippe E, et al. Gene expresión analysis of human prostate carcinoma Turing hormonal therapy identifies androgen-responsive genes and mechanisms of therapy resistance. Am J Pathol 204; 164: 217-27.

[24]  Andersson S, Russell DW. Structural and biochemical properties of cloned and expressed human and rat steroid 5α-reductases. Proc Natl Acad Sci USA 1990; 87: 3640–4.

[25]  Jenkins EP, Andersson S, Imperato-McGinley J, Wilson JD, Russell DW. Genetic and pharmacological evidence for more than one human steroid 5α-reductase. J Clin Invest 1992; 89: 293–300.

[26]  Wright AS, Thomas LN, Douglas RC, Lazier CB, Rittmaster RS. Relative potency of testosterone and dihydrotestosterone in preventing atrophy and apoptosis in the prostate of the castrated rat. J Clin Invest 1996; 98: 2558–63.

[27]  Rittmaster RS. 5α-reductase inhibitors in benign prostatic hyperplasia and prostate cancer risk reduction. Best Pract Res Clin Endocrinol Metab 2008; 22: 389–402.

[28]  Gudmundsson J, Sulem P, Steinthorsdottir V et al. Two variants on chromosome 17 confer prostate cancer risk, and the one in TCF2 protects against type 2 diabetes. Nat Genet 2007; 39: 977–83.

[29]  Klotz L. Active surveillance for prostate cancer: a review. Curr Urol Rep 2010; 11: 165–71.

[30]  Chodak GW, Thisted RA, Gerber GS et al. Results of conservative management of clinically localized prostate cancer. N Engl J Med 1994; 330: 242–8.

[31]  Epstein JI. An update of the Gleason grading system. J Urol 2010; 183: 433–40.

[32]  Lu-Yao GL, Albertson PC, Moore DF et al. Outcomes of localized prostate cancer following conservative management. JAMA 2009; 302: 1202–9.

[33]  Halabi S, Small E, Kantoff P, et al. Prognostic model for predicting survival in men with hormone-refractory metastatic prostate cancer. J Clin Oncol 2003; 21: 1232-7.

[34]  Attard G, Sarker D, Reid A, Molife R, Parker C, De Bono JS. Improving the outcome of patients with castration-resistant prostate cancer through rational drug development. Br J Cancer 206; 95 (7): 767-74.

[35]  Cooperberg MR, Lubeck DP, Meng MV, Mehta SS, Carroll PR. The changing face of low-risk prostate cancer: trenes in clinical presentation and primary management. J Clin Oncol 2004; 22: 2141-9.

[36]  Harris WP, Mostaghel EA, P. S. Nelson, and B. Montgomery, "Androgen deprivation therapy: progress in understanding mechanisms of resistance and optimizing androgen depletion," Nature Clinical Practice Urology 2009; 6 (2): 76–85.

[37]  Attar RM, Takimoto CH, Gottardis MM. Castration-resistant prostate cancer: locking up the molecular escape routes Clinical Cancer Research 2009: 15 (10); 3251–5.

[38]  Serafini AN, Houston SJ, Resche I, et al. Palliation of pain associated with metastático bone cancer using samarium-153 lexidronam: a double-blind placebo-controlled clinical trial. J Clin Oncol 1998; 16: 1574-81.

[39]  Sun S, Sprenger CT, Vessella RL. Castration resistance in human prostate cancer is conferred by a frequently occurring androgen receptor splice variant. J Clin Invest 2010; 120: 2715-30.

[40]  Watson PA, Chen YF, Balbas M. Constitutively active androgen receptor splice variants expressed in castration-resistant prostate cancer require full-length androgen receptor. Proceedings of the National Academy of Sciences of the United States of America 2010; 107: 16759–65.

[41]  Marques RB, Dits NF, Erkens-Schulze S, Weerden WM, Jenster G. Bypass mechanisms of the androgen receptor pathway in therapy-resistant prostate cancer cell models. PLoS ONE 2010; 5: 13500-5.

[42]  Crawford ED, Eisenberger MA, McLeod DG. A controlled trial of leuprolide with and without flutamide in prostatic carcinoma. N Eng J Med 1989; 321: 419-24.

[43]  Eisenberger MA, Blumenstein BA, Crawford ED. Bilateral orchiectomy with or without flutamide for metastatic prostate cancer. N Eng J Med 1998; 339: 1036-42.

[44]  Harris WP, Mostaghel EA, Nelson PA, Montgomery B. Androgen deprivation therapy: progress in understanding mechanisms of resistance and optimizing androgen depletion. Nature Clin Prac Urol 2009; 6: 76-85.

[45]  Ang JA, Olmos D, De Bono JS. CYP17 blockade by abiraterone: further evidence for frequent continued hormone-dependence in castration-resistant prostate cancer. Br J Cancer 2009; 100: 671-5.

[46]  Paller CJ, Antonarakis ES. Cabazitaxel: a novel second-line treatment for metastatic castration-resistant prostate cancer. Drug Design, Develop Ther 2011; 5: 117-24.

[47]  Pal SK, Twardowski P, Sartor O. Critical appraisal of cabazitaxel in the management of advanced prostate cancer. Clin Interv Aging 2010; 5: 395-402.

[48]  Sonpave G, Slawin KM, Spencer DM, Levitt JM. Emerging vaccine therapy approaches for prostate cancer. Rew Urol 2010; 12: 25-34.

[49]  Small EJ, Halabi S, Dawson NA. Antiandrogen withdrawal alone or in combination with ketoconazole in androgen-independent prostate cancer patients: a phase III trial (CALGB 9583). J Clin Oncol 2004; 22 (6): 1025-33.

[50]  Berthold DR, Sternberg CN, TannockIF. Management of advanced prostate cancer after first-line chemotherapy. J Clin Oncol 2005; 23: 8247-52.

[51]  Kim SJ, Kim SM. Current treatment strategies for castration-resistant prostate cancer. Korean J Urol 2011; 52: 157-65.

[52]  O'Donell A, Judson I, Dowsett M, et al. Hormonal impact of the 17 alpha-hydrosy-lase/C(17,20)-lyase inhibitor abiraterone acetate (CB7630) in patients with prostate cancer. Br J Cancer 2004; 90: 2317-25.

[53]  de Bono JS, Logothetis CJ, Molina A, et al. Abiraterone and increased survival in metastatic prostate cancer. New Engl J Med 2011; 364: 1995-2005.

[54]  Safety and Efficacy Study of MDV3100 in Patients With Castration-Resistant Prostate Cancer Who Have Been Previously Treated With Docetaxel-based Chemotherapy (AFFIRM).

[55]  ClinicalTrials.gov, United States National Institutes of Health. Retrieved 2011-11-06. "A Safety and Efficacy Study of Oral MDV3100 in Chemotherapy-Naive Patients With Progressive Metastatic Prostate Cancer (PREVAIL)". "NCT01212991".

[56]  Kaku T, Hitaka T, Ojida A, Matsunaga N, Adachi M, Tanaka T, Hara T, Yamaoka M, Kusaka M, Okuda T, Asahi S, Furuya S, Tasaka A. Discovery of orteronel (TAK-700), a naphthylmethylimidazole derivative, as a highly selective 17,20-lyase inhibitor with potential utility in the treatment of prostate cancer. Bioorg Med Chem. 2011; 19(21): 6383-99.

[57]  Pouessel D, Oudard S, Gravis G, Priou F, Shen L, Culine S. Cabazitaxel for metastatic castration-resistant prostate cancer progressing after docetaxel treatment: the TROP-IC study in France. Bull Cancer 2012; 99: 731-741.

[58]  Galsky MD, Small EJ, Oh WK. Multi-institutional randomized phase II trial of the epothilone B analog ixabepilone (BMS-247550) with or without estramustine phosphate in patients with progressive castrate metastatic prostate cancer. J Clin Oncol 2005; 23 (7): 1439-46.

[59]  Chi KN, Beardsley EK, Venner PM. A phase II study of patupilone in patients with metastatic hormone refractory prostate cancer (HRPC) who have progressed after docetaxel. J Clin Oncol 2008; 26 (15): 5166-71.

[60]  Beardsley EK, Saad F, Eigl B. A phase II study of patupilone in patients (patients) with metastatic castration-resistant prostate cancer (CRPC) who have progressed after docetaxel. J Clin Oncol 2009; 27: 5319.

[61]  Rosenberg JE, Weinberg VK, Kelly WK. Activity of second-line chemotherapy in do-cetaxel-refractory hormone-refractory prostate cancer patients: randomized phase 2 study of ixabepilone or mitoxantrone and prednisone. Cancer 2007; 110: 556–63.

[62]  Bono JS, Maroto P, Calvo E. Phase II study of eribulin mesylate (E7389) in patients (pts) with metastatic castration-resistant prostate cancer (CRPC) stratified by prior taxane therapy. Ann Oncol 2011; 1: 380-5.

[63]  De Bono JS, Oudard S, Ozguroglu M. Prednisone plus cabazitaxel or mitoxantrone for metastatic castration-resistant prostate cancer progressing after docetaxel treat-ment: a randomised open-label trial. Lancet 2010; 376: 1147-54.

[64]  Park SI, Liao J, Berry JE, Li X, Koh AJ, Michalski ME, Eber MR, Soki FN, Sadler D, Sud S, Tisdelle S, Daignault SD, Nemeth JA, Snyder LA, Wronski TJ, Pienta KJ, McCauley LK. Cyclophosphamide creates a receptive microenvironment for prostate cancer skeletal metastasis. Cancer Res 2012; 72(10): 2522-32.

[65]  Grenader T, Goldberg A. Reinduction of hormone sensitivity to goserelin following chemotherapy with vinorelbine in castration-resistant prostate cancer. Scientific World Journal 2010; 10: 1814-7.

[66]  Small EJ, Schellhammer PF, Higano CS. Placebo-controlled phase III trial of immuno-logic therapy with Sipuleucel-T (APC8015) in patients with metastatic, asymptomatic hormone refractory prostate cancer. J Clin Oncol 2006; 24: 3089-94.

[67]  Higano CS, Schellhammer PF, Small EJ. Integrated data from 2 randomized, double-blind, placebo-controlled, phase 3 trials of active cellular immunotherapy with sipu-leucel-T in advanced prostate cancer. Cancer 2009; 115: 3670-9.

[68]  Kantoff PW, Higano CS, Shore ND. Sipuleucel-T immunotherapy for castration-re-sistant prostate cancer. New Eng J Med 2010: 363: 411–2.

[69]  Small EJ, Sacks N, Nemunaitis J. Granulocyte macrophage colony-stimulating factor-secreting allogeneic cellular immunotherapy for hormone-refractory prostate cancer. Clin Canc Res 2007; 13: 3883-91.

[70]  Hussain M, Smith MR, Sweeney C. Cabozantinib (XL184) in metastatic castration-re-sistant prostate cancer (mCRPC): results from a phase II randomized discontinuation trial. J Clin Oncol 2011; 29: 4516-9. 71. Cha E, Fong L. Therapeutic vaccines for pros-tate cancer. Current Opinion Mol Ther 2010; 12 (1): 77-85.

[71]  Cha E, Fong L. Therapuetic vaccines for prostate cancer. Current Opinion Mol Ther 2010; 12 (1): 77-85.

[72]  Kantoff PW, Schuetz TJ, Blumenstein BA. Overall survival analysis of a phase II randomized controlled trial of a Poxviral-based PSA-targeted immunotherapy in metastatic castration-resistant prostate cancer. J Clin Oncol 2010; 28 (7): 1099-105.

[73]  Carducci MA, Jimeno A. Targeting bone metastasis in prostate cancer with endothe-lin receptor antagonists. Clin Canc Res 2006; 12: 6296-300.

[74]  Saad F, Gleason DM, Murray R. A randomized, placebo-controlled trial of zoledronic acid in patients with hormone-refractory metastatic prostate carcinoma. J Nat Canc Inst 2002; 94: 1458-68.

[75]  Weinfurt KP, Anstrom KJ, Castel LD, Schulman KA, Saad F. Effect of zoledronic acid on pain associated with bone metastasis in patients with prostate cancer. Ann Oncol 2006; 17 (6): 986-9.

[76]  Saad F, Gleason DM, Murray R. Long-term efficacy of zoledronic acid for the prevention of skeletal complications in patients with metastatic hormone-refractory prostate cancer. J Nat Canc Inst 2004; 96: 879-82.

[77]  Diamond TH, Winters J, Smith A. The antiosteoporotic efficacy of intravenous pamidronate in men with prostate carcinoma receiving combined androgen blockade: a double blind, randomized, placebo-controlled crossover study. Cancer 2001; 92 (6): 1444-50.

[78]  Smith MR, Eastham J, Gleason DM, Shasha D, Tchekmedyian S, Zinner N. Randomized controlled trial of zoledronic acid to prevent bone loss in men receiving androgen deprivation therapy for nonmetastatic prostate cancer. J Urol 2003; 169 (6): 2008-12.

[79]  Cavalli L, Brandi ML. Targeted approaches in the treatment of osteoporosis: differential mechanism of action of denosumab and clinical utility. Ther Clin Risk Manag 2012; 8: 253-6.

[80]  Chow E, Harris K, Fan G, Tsao M, Sze WM. Palliative radiotherapy trials for bone metastases: a systematic review. J Clin Oncol 2007; 25 (11): 1423-36.

[81]  Salazar OM, Sandhu T, Da Motta NW. Fractionated half-body irradiation (HBI) for the rapid palliation of widespread, symptomatic, metastatic bone disease: a randomized Phase III trial of the International Atomic Energy Agency (IAEA). Int J Rad Oncol Biol Physic 2001; 50 (3): 765-75.

[82]  Dearnaley DP, Bayly RJ, A'Hern RP, Gadd J, Zivanovic MM, Lewington VJ. Palliation of bone metastases in prostate cancer. Hemibody irradiation or strontium-89?. Clin Oncol 1992; 4 (2): 101-7.

[83]  Lewington VJ, McEwan AJ, Ackery DM. A prospective, randomised double-blind crossover study to examine the efficacy of strontium-89 in pain palliation in patients with advanced prostate cancer metastatic to bone. Eur J Canc 1991; 27 (8): 954-8.

[84]  Buchali K, Correns HJ, Schuerer M, Schnorr D, Lips H, Sydow K. Results of a double blind study of 89-strontium therapy of skeletal metastases of prostatic carcinoma. Eur J Nuc Med 1988; 14 (7): 349-51.

[85]  Sartor O, Reid RH, Hoskin PJ. Samarium-153-lexidronam complex for treatment of painful bone metastases in hormone-refractory prostate cancer. Urology 2004; 63 (5): 940-5.

[86] Cheetham PJ, Petrylak DP. Alpha particles as radiopharmaceuticals in the treatment of bone metastases: mechanism of action of radium-223 chloride (Alpharadin) and radiation protection. Oncology 2012; 26(4): 330-7.

[87] Kelly WK, Halabi S, Carducci M, George D, Mahoney JF, Stadler WM, Morris M, Kantoff P, Monk JP, Kaplan E, Vogelzang NJ, Small EJ. Randomized, double-blind, placebo-controlled phase III trial comparing docetaxel and prednisone with or without bevacizumab in men with metastatic castration-resistant prostate cancer: CALGB 90401. J Clin Oncol. 2012; 30(13): 1534-40.

[88] Redding MB, Surati M. Emerging treatments for castrate-resistant prostate cancer. J Pharm Pract. 2011; 24(4): 366-73.

[89] Weisshardt P, Trarbach T, Dürig J, Paul A, Reis H, Tilki D, Miroschnik I, Ergün S, Klein D. Tumor vessel stabilization and remodeling by anti-angiogenic therapy with bevacizumab. Histochem Cell Biol. 2012; 137(3): 391-401.

[90] Meng LJ, Wang J, Fan WF, Pu XL, Liu FY, Yang M. Evaluation of oral chemotherapy with capecitabine and cyclophosphamide plus thalidomide and prednisone in prostate cancer patients. J Cancer Res Clin Oncol 2012; 138 (2): 333-9.

[91] Emerging novel therapies for advanced prostate cancer. Osanto S, Van Poppel H. Ther Adv Urol 2012; 4 (1): 3-12.

[92] Dahut WL, Gulley JL, Arlen PM. Randomized phase II trial of docetaxel plus thalidomide in androgen-independent prostate cancer. J Clin Oncol 2004; 22 (13): 2532-9.

[93] Ning YM, Gulley JL, Arlen PM. Phase II trial of bevacizumab, thalidomide, docetaxel, and prednisone in patients with metastatic castration-resistant prostate cancer. J Clin Oncol 2010; 28 (12): 2070-6.

[94] National Institutes of Health Clinical Trials database, http://clinicaltrials.gov/.

[95] Small EJ, Tchekmedyian NS, Rini BI, Fong L, Lowy I, Allison JP. A pilot trial of CTLA-4 blockade with human anti-CTLA-4 in patients with hormone-refractory prostate cancer. Clin Canc Res 2007; 13 (6): 1810-5.

[96] Fong L, Kwek SS, O'Brien S. Potentiating endogenous antitumor immunity to prostate cancer through combination immunotherapy with CTLA4 blockade and GM-CSF. Cancer Res 2009; 69 (2): 609-15.

[97] NCT00861614 A Randomized, Double-Blind, Phase 3 Trial Comparing Ipilumumab vs. Placebo Following Radiotherapy in Subjects With Castration Resistant Prostate Cancer That Have Received Prior Treatment With Docetaxel.

[98] NCT01057810 Randomized, Double-Blind, Phase 3 Trial to Compare the Efficacy of Ipilumumab vs Placebo in Asymptomatic or Minimally Symptomatic Patients With Metastatic Chemotherapy-Naïve Castration Resistant Prostate Cancer.

[99] Carducci MA, Padley RJ, Breul J. Effect of endothelin-A receptor blockade with atra-sentan on tumor progression in men with hormone-refractory prostate cancer: a randomized, phase II, placebo-controlled trial. J Clin Oncol 2003; 21 (4): 679-89.

[100] Phase III Study of Docetaxel and Atrasentan Versus Docetaxel and Placebo for Pa-tients With Advanced Hormone Refractory Prostate Cancer National Institutes of Health. Clinical Trials 2011, http://clinicaltrials.gov/.

[101] James ND, Caty A, Payne H. Final safety and efficacy analysis of the specific endo-thelin A receptor antagonist zibotentan (ZD4054) in patients with metastatic castra-tion-resistant prostate cancer and bone metastases who were pain-free or mildly symptomatic for pain: a double-blind, placebo-controlled, randomized Phase II trial. Br J Urol Int 2010; 106 (7): 966-73.

[102] A Phase III Trial of ZD4054 (Zibotentan) (Endothelin A Antagonist) in Non-metastat-ic Hormone Resistant Prostate Cancer (ENTHUSE M0) NCT00626548.

[103] A Phase III Trial of ZD4054 (Zibotentan) (Endothelin A Antagonist) and Docetaxel in Metastatic Hormone Resistant Prostate Cancer (ENTHUSE M1C) NCT00617669.

[104] Dahut WL, Scripture C, Posadas E. A phase II clinical trial of sorafenib in androgen-independent prostate cancer. Clin Canc Res 2008; 14 (1): 209-14.

[105] Aragon-Ching JB, Jain L, Gulley JL. Final analysis of a phase II trial using sorafenib for metastaticcastration-resistant prostate cancer. Br J Urol Int 2009; 103: 1636-40.

[106] Steinbild S, Mross K, Frost A. A clinical phase II study with sorafenib in patients with progressive hormone-refractory prostate cancer: a study of the CESAR Central Euro-pean Society for Anticancer Drug Research-EWIV. Br J Cancer 2007; 97 (11): 1480-5.

[107] Chi KN, Ellard SL, Hotte SJ. A phase II study of sorafenib in patients with chemo-naive castration-resistant prostate cancer. Ann Oncol 2008; 19 (4): 746-51.

[108] Zurita AJ, Liu G, Hutson T. Sunitinib in combination with docetaxel and prdnisone in patients (pts) with metastatic hormone-refrectory prostate cancer (mHRPC). J Clin Oncol 2009; 27 (15): 5166-71.

[109] Sonpavde G, Periman PO, Bernold D. Sunitinib malate for metastatic castration-re-sistant prostate cancer following docetaxel-based chemotherapy. Ann Oncol 2010; 21 (2): 319-24.

# Chapter 13

# Intermittent Androgen Suppression Therapy for Prostate Cancer Patients: An Update

Gerhard Hamilton and Gerhard Theyer

Additional information is available at the end of the chapter

## 1. Introduction

Prostate cancer is the leading cause of cancer and the second leading cause of cancer-related deaths among men in the Western world [1]. For early stage prostate cancer treatment with surgery and radiation is often curative; however, about 10–20% of men with prostate cancer present with metastatic disease at diagnosis, while 20–30% of patients diagnosed with localized disease will eventually develop metastases [2]. Primary tumor involvement outside the prostatic capsule or relapse following radical prostatectomy results generally in incurability [3,4]. Androgen suppression (AS) is the mainstay of initial therapy in these patients, and orchidectomy or use of LHRH analogs and steroidal or nonsteroidal antiandrogens consistently results in a 90–95% reduction in circulating testosterone levels [5]. However, nearly all patients that respond initially will develop progressive disease, termed castration-resistant prostate cancer (CRPC), after a median duration of 18–24 months. Although CRPC may respond to secondary hormonal manipulations (including antiandrogens, estrogens and ketoconazole) this benefit is usually short-lived.

Although continuous androgen suppression [CAS] therapy has been a cornerstone of the management of prostate cancer for more than 50 years, controversy remains regarding its optimum application. Generally, AS is performed as continuous treatment, resulting in apoptotic regression of the tumor cells in a high percentage of cases. The side-effects of CAS are well described and include anaemia, osteoporosis, impotence, cognitive functional effects, gynaecomastia, muscle atrophy, depression, dyslipidaemia and generalized lethargy [5]. Following failure of the antiandrogenic therapy, chemotherapy is used as secondary treatment. However, responses to cytotoxic therapy are low and only recently several studies revealed a possible benefit of incorporating chemotherapeutic agents in treatment regimen for prostate cancer [6]. In the last years new agents were approved by the U.S. Food and Drug Administration (FDA), comprising an immunotherapeutic product (sipuleucel-T), the novel taxane, cabazitaxel, which showed a survival advantage over mitoxantrone in docetaxel-pretreated patients and an androgen synthesis inhibitor, abiraterone acetate, which was also reported to improve survival when evaluated against placebo in docetaxel-pretreated patients [3,7].

In order to reduce side effects of the CAS and to prolong the duration of the hormone-responsive state of prostate cancers intermittent androgen suppression (IAS) was introduced as new clinical concept [8]. Stopping CAS has the hypothetical advantage of reducing the selection pressure which favors the clones that have initiated molecular adaptations to achieve androgen-independent growth. If there is a population of androgen-dependent clones left then these will proliferate and repopulate the gland, and androgen dependence will resume. Experimental animal models involving androgen-dependent xenografts supported the hypothesis that during limited regrowth in the antiandrogenic treatment cessation periods tumorigenic cells are residing in an androgen-responsive state. The concept of IAS was experimentally developed using the androgen-dependent Shionogi mouse mammary tumor, investigating regular phases of growth, regression and recurrence of xenograft tumors during serial transplantation [9]. For the androgen-dependent Shionogi carcinoma regular cycles of treatment cessations and castration-induced regressions were successfully repeated four times before tumor growth became androgen-independent during the fifth cycle [10]. The average duration of one cycle was 30 days and progression to androgen-insensitivity was observed after 150 days. Serial determinations of the proportion of stem cells in the Shionogi tumor revealed a constant part during the first three cycles, but a 15-fold increase between the third and fourth cycles [11]. Therefore, it was concluded that independent of intermittent or continuous androgen withdrawal, conversion to hormone-insensitivity occurs when the tumor has accumulated one-third to one-half of the total stem cell compartment with androgen-independent cells. The next step included the switch to a human prostate cancer xenograft model using the LNCaP androgen-dependent prostate cancer cell line, where serum PSA levels correlated well with tumor volume and decreased rapidly following castration, followed by appearance of androgen-independency after 3-4 weeks [12]. IAS therapy prolonged time to androgen-independent PSA production threefold, from an average of 26 days in the CAS group to 77 days in the IAS group. It was concluded that IAS in the LNCaP model delayed the onset of androgen-independent PSA gene regulation markedly, most likely due to androgen-induced differentiation and/or downregulation of androgen-suppressed gene expression. In summary, the animal experimental data indicated that androgen-dependent tumor xenografts can be subjected to several cycles of androgen withdrawal/replacement and revealed prolonged hormone-dependency compared to CAS.

Since induction of androgen independence may occur early after treatment initiation, cessation of antiandrogen therapy prior to this switch is expected to maintain the apoptotic potential of the tumor cells and keep them sensitive to retreatment. Serial serum PSA determinations are used to decide on AS, treatment cessation and reinitiation of therapy [13]. Generally, IAS consists of an initial androgen suppression period of up to nine months combining LHRH antagonists and antiandrogens, which is followed by treatment cessation until a certain PSA threshold is reached, then AS is reinitiated for the same time period as the initial suppression phase (Figure 1) In initial pilot trials regrowing tumors of patients undergoing IAS were consistently reported to be sensitive to several cycles of androgen withdrawal [14,15]

## Intermittent Androgen Suppression (IAS)

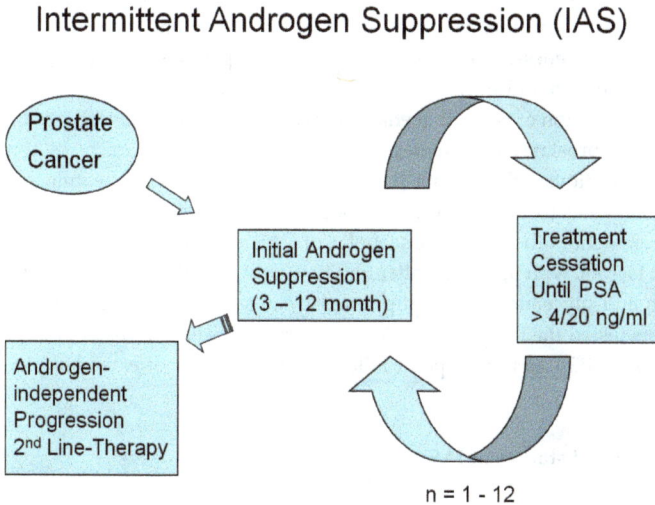

Figure 1. Schematic presentation of IAS. Patients undergo an initial phase of AS. If successful, AS is paused until progression to 4 (localized disease) or 10-20 (metastatic disease) ng/ml PSA. Then AS is resumed and cycles repeated until progression to androgen-independent disease that is treated with diverse regimens second-line.

Therefore, the primary goal of IAS was the prolongation of the hormone-sensitivity of the tumors, which in turn was expected to result in increased survival eventually. Furthermore, IAS was expected to reduce the side effects of CAS, comprising reduced sexual activity, cardiovascular problems, metabolic consequences and osteoporosis among others. Based on the available evidence, IAS nowadays represents a valid treatment option for patients with non-metastatic prostate cancer, including those with locally advanced disease, either with or without lymph node involvement, and those who biochemically relapsed following apparently curative treatment. IAS has been researched since the mid-1980s in a number of clinical phase II and III trials in an effort to prolong hormone-dependency and reduce adverse effects and costs of CAS [16]. With preclinical evidence suggesting a potential benefit for IAS in terms of time to androgen independence, with phase II and phase III studies producing optimistic results, and with the potential for decreased costs and complications IAS has now become a popular modality of therapy worldwide. Quite recently, according to results of a Phase III trial presented in a plenary session at the 2012 ASCO Annual Meeting, IAS was shown to be less effective than CAS for a subgroup of patients with hormone-sensitive metastatic prostate cancer, questioning the use of IAS as standard therapy for these patients [17].

# 2. Clinical evaluation of intermittent androgen suppression

## 2.1. Introduction

Maximal androgen ablation through combination therapy increases treatment-related side effects and expenses and fails to prolong time to progression to androgen-independence and, furthermore, preliminary evidence indicates that a low androgen milieu is associated with tumor aggressiveness. Transition to androgen-independence is a complex process and involves both selection and outgrowth of preexisting androgen-resistant clones, as well as adaptative upregulation of genes that enable cancer cells to survive and grow after CAS [18]. CAS in men with prostate cancer increases the risk of osteoporotic fractures, type 2 diabetes and, possibly, cardiovascular events [19]. The benefits of CAS in treating non-metastatic prostate cancer need to be carefully weighed against the risks of CAS-induced adverse events. Management of the metabolic sequelae of CAS includes optimal reduction of cardio-vascular risk factors, with particular attention to weight, blood pressure, lipid profile, smoking cessation and glycemic control. Supported by preclinical and first clinical IAS results, several centers tested the feasibility of IAS in non-randomized groups of prostate cancer patients with serum PSA as trigger point followed by a number of extended phase II and III trials [16,20]

## 2.2. Clinical phase II studies of IAS

### 2.2.1. Comparison of therapeutic efficacies of IAS and CAS

Following apparently successful pilot studies, a number of phase II IAS trials were conducted (Table 1) [16]. Since the end points of most phase II studies were safety and feasibility of IAS, survival data were not reported in general. Out of the 19 studies reviewed by Abrahamsson only five involved more than 100 patients (102, 103, 146, 250 and 566 patients, respectively) and the other smaller studies employed a mean number of 52 patients [16]. Although patients with advanced, metastatic prostate cancer were included in several studies, most patients treated in phase II IAS trials had localized disease or biochemical progression following prostatectomy/radiation therapy. The number of IAS cycles given ranged from 1 to 12, with an average of 2–3 per patient, and the length of time off therapy generally decreased or remained stable with each succeeding cycle. Most of the studies reported off-treatment periods of approximately 50% of the duration of the IAS cycles, dependent on the tumor stage of the respective prostate cancer patients [16]. A metaanalysis by Shaw et al. involving ten phase II trials reported a median number of two cycles per patient and a median time off-therapy of 15.4 months [21]. Time on treatment also varied but was usually in the region of 6–9 months [16]. The proportion of men in whom serum testosterone normalized was generally high following the first cycle (70–90%) but tended to decrease during subsequent cycles [16]. Factors influencing time to delay in testosterone normalization may include advanced age, low baseline testosterone levels, and duration of AS. Testosterone recovery to baseline values was achieved in 79% during the first and in 65% during the second IAS cycle, respectively [22]. No significant difference was observed up to 1000 days between IAS and CAS with regard to time to androgen-independent tumor progression.

| Authors | # | Endpoint(s) | Tumor stage | Androgen suppression |
|---|---|---|---|---|
| Calais da Silva et al. [13] | 626 | Time to subjective or objective progression | Locally advanced or metastatic | GnRH agonist + cyproterone acetate |
| De Leval et al. [36] | 68 | Time to androgen-independence | Locally advanced, metastatic or recurrent | Goserelin + flutamide |
| Miller et al. [37] | 335 | Time to clinical or biochemical progression | Locally advanced or D1/D2 | Goserelin + bicalutamide |
| Mottet et al. [38] | 173 | Overall survival | Metastatic PCa (D2) | Leuprorelin + flutamide |
| TULP [39,40] | 290 | Time to clinical progression or PSA escape | Advanced or locally advanced | Buserelin depot + nilutamide |
| Tunn et al [22] | 184 | Clinical or PSA progression | PSA relapse after radical prostatectomy | Leuprorelin + cyproterone acetate |
| Verhagen et al. [35] | 366 | QoL | Metastatic | Cyproterone acetate |
| Klotz et al.[34] | 1386 | Survival | PSA recurrence after radical Radiotherapy | All types of AS |
| Salonen et al. [41,42] | 554 | Progression/Survival | Advanced or locally advanced | Goserelin + cyproterone acetate |
| Hussain et al. [17] | 1345 | Survival | Advanced (D2) | Goserelin + bicalutamide |

**Table 1.** Overview of the published phase II IAS trials

In a study by Bruchovsky et al. men who quickly recovered serum testosterone levels experienced a more rapid rise in PSA levels and a shorter time off therapy [23]. Generally, low levels (2–16%) of progression to hormone-refractory prostate cancer have been reported [16,22]. In a review by Zhu et al. there were 16 trials that compared IAS with CAS with a total of 3264 patients (1624 with IAS and 1640 with CAS) [24]. Pooled effects indicated no significant difference between IAS and CAS groups in terms of death and progression rate (hazard ratio HR=0.99, 95% CI 0.80-1.23, and HR=1.03, 95% CI 0.84-1.26 respectively). Calculated results indicated that quality of live (QoL) on sexual activity was significantly higher in the IAS group (HR=0.24, 95% Cl 0.17-0.33, p<0.00001). Moreover, IAS could effectively reduce side effects associated with AS. Thus, the therapeutic efficacy was not significantly different between the IAS and CAS groups. However, IAS could effectively preserve the QoL (in particular sexual life) and reduce the side effects.

### 2.2.2. Comparison of the side effects/QoL of IAS and CAS

Because it became increasingly clear that the time to androgen-independence seems not to be prolonged by IAS, trials focussed on the impact of the intermittent therapy on side effects of AS and QoL. Malone et al estimated that approximately 50% of patients recovered from anaemia during off-therapy periods and that the weight gain normally associated with CAS was prevented [25]. Bouchot et al reported hot flushes in most cases during the on-therapy period, which showed significant improvement during treatment cessation periods and pain significantly improved during on-therapy periods with no new pain occurring once therapy was withdrawn [26]. Goldenberg et al. observed that all patients tolerated therapy well and responded in a positive physical and psychological manner to the cycling approach [27]. The attenuation of spine and hip bone mineral density (BMD) decline after 3-year IAS compared with those reported for CAS appears to be due to testosterone-driven BMD recovery in the cessation period [28]. Failure of testosterone recovery was associated with worse final BMD. Patients experienced the greatest average change in BMD during early treatment periods of IAS with a smaller average change thereafter and fractures were rare [29]. During the first off-treatment period (median duration 37.4 weeks), BMD recovery at the spine was significant; however, subsequent periods had heterogeneous changes of BMD without significant average changes. By reducing the potential risk for adverse bone complications, intermittent therapy may become an important consideration when the therapeutic ratio is narrow [30]. We examined the effect of IAS on bone metabolism by determinations of CrossLaps levels, a biochemical marker of collagen degradation, in blood samples of prostate cancer patients. Measurements of the CrossLaps concentration in patients under IAS revealed that treatment cessation phases rapidly reversed increased bone degradation, which was associated with the AS phases, in good agreement with the clinical observations of reduced loss of BMD in IAS [31]. Since pretreatment concentrations of CrossLaps were restored within several months of treatment cessation and mean duration of the off-treatment periods ranged from 8–16 months in our patients, this protective effect of IAS is expected to be effective for several treatment cycles. Additionally, procollagen I N-terminal peptide (PINP), a parameter of bone synthesis was increased during off-treatment phases in IAS [32].

Improvement of sexual activity was highlighted in several studies and concerned approximately half of the patients [16]. Sato et al reported significant worsening of potency and physical well-being during AS and significant improvements in potency, lack of energy, social/family well-being, and ability to enjoy life during off-therapy periods [33]. In a study by Spry et al. QoL scores also deteriorated during androgen suppression, but had generally achieved baseline levels by the end of the off-treatment period [28]. In summary, IAS showed benefits in the treatment of prostate cancer with respect to QoL in the majority of trials.

### 2.2.3. IAS phase II studies – conclusion

In phase II studies there has been considerable variation in the particular approaches in regard to medication, duration of AS phases, target PSA nadir and selection of the PSA value for restarting therapy. At that time preliminary results of the the ongoing randomized controlled trials have generated evidence that the use of IAS in patients with advanced or locally advanced disease was at least as safe as CAS [16,24]. In conclusion, phase II studies of IAS demonstrated that several cycles of IAS were feasible, the duration of response was not worse than historical controls of CAS and well-being was better during treatment cessation periods. Patients with localized disease fared superior under IAS compared to patient with extended disease. The need for randomized phase III trials was stressed in order to get firm data on progression-free and overall survival (OS) as well as time to androgen insensitivity for IAS and CAS, respectively.

## 2.3. Clinical phase III studies of IAS

Nowadays a number of phase III trials have been completed comparing IAS with CAS [16]. Of the ten reported trials, two included patients with relapse after radical prostatectomy or radiation therapy, all others studied locally advanced and metastatic disease [22,34]. The number of patients in these trials varied from 68 to 1386, but only four involved >500 patients; the average age of patients was around 70 years. Full details of trial design are not available for all studies, several reports are available only in abstract form [16]. The treatment regimen in all but one of the trials consisted of a LHRH agonist and an antiandrogen. The exception was Verhagen et al., in which antiandrogen monotherapy (cyproterone acetate/CPA) was the sole regimen studied [35]. Although there was generally consistency in the PSA levels designated for AS discontinuation (0.1/4 ng/ml or 20% of the initial PSA value), the criteria for resuming treatment were less uniform, with 4 ng/ml for biochemical relapses and 10 or 20 ng/ml 20 ng/ml for locally advanced or metastatic disease, respectively. The low PSA nadir and reinitiation values used by Tunn et al. and Klotz et al. are due to the fact that the study involved patients who had relapsed after radical prostatectomy [22,34]. End points in these studies also varied to some degree: whereas the majority had time to progression as the primary end point, three assigned survival and one focussed on QoL outcomes [35]. Average follow-up times in these studies have all been >2 yr, with a maximum of 12 years cited by Calais da Silva et al. [13].

### 2.3.1. South European uroncological trial [13]

Patients with locally advanced or metastatic with histologically confirmed prostate adenocarcinoma, cT3–cT4 M0, cT3–cT4 M1, PSA >4 ng/ml, were recruited for this study and end point was time to subjective or objective progression. All registered patients had an initial 3-months induction treatment with CPA (200 mg daily for two weeks) followed by monthly depot injections of a LHRH analog plus 200 mg of CPA daily. Patients (n = 626) whose PSA level decreased to <4 ng/ml or by at least 80% of the initial level by the end of the induction were randomized. Time to any progression was slightly longer in the continuous arm, with an HR of progression of 0.81. Both metastatic status and PSA level were independent predictors of progression, with M1 and PSA level > 4 ng/ml associated with a greater hazard of progressing. In the intermittent and continuous arm there was no significant difference in OS (p = 0.84) and the HR was 0.99 for CAS compared with IAS. The greater number of cancer deaths in the IAS treatment group was balanced by a greater number of cardiovascular deaths under CAS. Both PSA level and metastatic status at randomization were independently associated with survival. A significant interaction of metastatic status with treatment was almost reached (p = 0.07). Among M0 patients, the HR for continuous therapy compared with intermittent therapy was 0.86 (95% CI: 0.65–1.14), favouring continuous; among M1 patients, the HR was 1.26 (95% CI: 0.90–1.78), favouring intermittent. It was concluded that IAS should be considered for use in routine practice because it is associated with no reduction in survival, no clinically meaningful impairment in QoL, better sexual activity, and considerable economic benefit to the individual and the community. Since this study used only three months of therapy before stopping treatment in the intermittent arm, without impairing survival, there are significant savings for a patient receiving IAS for one year relative to CAS.

### 2.3.2. Study by De Leval et al. [36]

In this trial, a total of 68 evaluable patients with hormone-naive advanced or relapsing prostate cancer were randomized to receive AS (goserelin and flutamide) according to a continuous (n = 33) or intermittent (n = 35) regimen. The outcome variable was time to androgen-independence and mean follow-up was 30.8 months. The estimated 3-year progression rate was significantly lower in the IAS group (7.0%) than in the CAS group (38.9%). It was concluded that IAS treatment may maintain the androgen-dependent state of advanced human prostate cancer, as assessed by PSA measurements, at least as long as CAS treatment. This study may be regarded as underpowered to assess the full impact of IAS and the authors recommended further studies with longer follow-up times and larger patient cohorts to determine the comparative impacts of CAS and IAS with certainty.

### 2.3.3. Study by Miller et al. [37]

This randomized study compared AS with goserelin + bicalutamide in CAS with IAS. The primary endpoint was time to clinical and/or biochemical progression of the disease and secondary endpoints were survival time, QoL and side effects. Patients had histologically confirmed adenocarcinoma of the prostate in clinical stage T1-4N1-3M0 or T1-4N0-3M1 (D1 or D2). After an induction phase of six months with AS, 335 patients whose PSA decreased under 4 ng/ml or 90% from baseline were randomized. About two-thirds of the patients of both the intermittent and the continuous therapy arm (65% versus 66%, ITT population) experienced a clinical and/or biochemical disease progression. The median time to progression was longer for patients randomised to IAS (16.6 months) compared with patients randomized to CAS (11.5 months; difference not significant). The median time to death from any cause was 51.4 months in the intermittent arm compared and 53.8 months in the continuous therapy arm (p = 0.658). There were no differences in the incidence of patients with any safety parameter. Patients' self-assessment of their overall health and of their sexual activity appeared to be favourable in the IAS therapy arm. It was concluded that IAS in D1 and D2 prostate cancer patients seems to be safe and superior in respect to QoL.

### 2.3.4. TAP22 investigators group trial [38]

This study aimed at comparing CAS to IAS with AS consisting of leuproreline and flutamide in patients with newly diagnosed metastatic prostate cancer with bone metastases (stage D2). All patients had a positive bone or CT scan and a PSA > 20 ng/ml. After a 6 months induction period with AS, they were randomized into two groups if the PSA was < 4 ng/ml. CAS was continued after randomization and in the IAS group treatment was discontinued until PSA > 10 ng/ml or clinical progression. AS was then resumed for

3 months periods until the PSA became < 4 ng/ml and then treatment was then stopped again until the next progression for a new cycle. 341 patients were selected and received a 6 months induction AS period, and 173 were randomized: 83 to CAS and 86 to IAS. Patients were off-treatment approximately 50% of the first cycle, without decline in succeeding cycles and most had testosterone recovery. A progression occurred in 127 patients (73.4%). The overall QoL did not differ significantly between both arms. Median OS was 52 months for CAS and 42.2 months for IAS (p=0.74) and the median progression-free survial was 15 months for CAS and 20.7 months for IAS (p=0.73). This randomized trial comparing CAS to IAS in metastatic prostate cancer patients suggests that IAS may be as safe as CAS in D2 prostate cancer patients.

### 2.3.5. Therapy Upgrading Life in Prostate cancer (TULP) study [39,40]

Eligible patients (n = 290) had histologically proven advanced prostate cancer with positive lymph nodes or distant metastases (T2-4N1-3M0 or T2-4NxM1). They received AS with buserelin and nilutamide for 6 months. Patients who had a normalisation of PSA (< 4 ng/ml) after the course, were randomized between IAS (n=97) or CAS (n=96). Median time to clinical progression or PSA escape was 18.0 months in the IAS arm and 24.1 months in the CAS arm. In particular, the 2-year risk of progression for baseline PSA < 50 ng/ml, 50 to <500 ng/ml, and ≥500 ng/ml was 25%, 55%, and 76% (P = 0.03) in CAS, and 38%, 64%, and 85% (p = 0.006) in IAS, respectively. There was no clinically significant difference in QoL scores between patients. Metastatic prostate cancer patients with high baseline PSA, pain, and high PSA nadir, after a 6-months induction course, have a poor prognosis with hormonal therapy. Overall, in this study patients on IAS seem to do worse than CAS patients. Also, patients receiving IAS with low PSA nadir had significantly higher progression rates than CAS patients. In IAS testosterone recovery during the off-treatment phase was incomplete, explaining the missing benefit for QoL, even though more side effects occurred during CAS. Therefore, it was concluded from this study that IAS constitutes not a good treatment option for most metastatic prostate cancer patients.

### 2.3.6. European trial EC507 [22]

In this multicentre European prospective randomized phase III trial EC507, testosterone serum concentrations under AS were analyzed in prostate cancer patients with PSA progression after radical prostatectomy. Patients were randomized to either CAS or IAS therapy using a 3-months depot with leuprorelin acetate as microcapsule formulation. In 109 patients testosterone recovery to baseline values was achieved in 79% during the first and in 65% during the second IAS cycle, respectively. Median time to testosterone normalization was 100 days in the first and 115 days in the second cycle, respectively. There also appeared to be a QoL benefit during off-treatment intervals owing to the recovery of serum testosterone levels. No significant difference was observed up to 1000 days between IAS and CAS with regard to time to androgen-independent progression. This was the first prospective study of leuprolide, demonstrating normalization of testosterone levels in the off-treatment period in patients undergoing IAS.

### 2.3.7. Study by Verhagen et al. [35]

This randomized trial compared efficacy and QoL of IAS and CAS treatment by CPA of asymptomatic patients with prostate cancer metastatic to the bone. A total of 366 patients with metastatic prostate cancer received 3 to 6 months CPA (100 mg daily) depending on their PSA response. Patients with a good or moderate response were randomized to continuous or intermittent treatment. Intermittent hormonal therapy of metastatic prostate cancer by CPA has advantages in important QoL domains. However, cognitive function scores appeared reduced in the intermittent group.

### 2.3.8. NCIC CTG PR.7/SWOG PR.7/CTSU JPR.7/UK trial [34]

This Intergroup randomized phase III trial compared IAS vs. CAS to test for non-inferiority of IAS with respect to OS. Patients had rising PSA > 3.0 ng/ml >1 year post radical radiotherapy (RRT), either initial or salvage, for localized prostate cancer. Stratification factors were time since RRT (>1-3 vs >3 years), initial PSA (<15 vs >15), prior radical prostatectomy and prior AS. IAS was delivered for 8 months in each cycle with restart when PSA reached >10 ng/ml off-treatment. Primary endpoint was OS, secondary endpoints included time to hormone refractory state, QoL, duration of treatment/non-treatment intervals, time to testosterone and potency recovery. The trial was halted after a planned interim analysis demonstrated that a prespecified stopping boundary for non-inferiority was crossed. 1,386 patients were randomized to IAS (690) or CAS (696) arms. IAS patients completed a median of 2 x 8 months cycles (range: 1-9) and median follow-up was 6.9 years. 524 deaths were observed (268 on IAS vs. 256 on CAS). Median OS was 8.8 vs. 9.1 years on IAS and CAS arms, respectively (HR 1.02, 95%CI 0.86-1.21; p for non-inferiority [HR IAS vs CAS ≥ 1.25] = 0.009). The IAS arm had more disease related (122 vs. 97) and fewer unrelated (134 vs. 146) deaths. Time to androgen insensitivity was statistically significantly improved on the IAS arm (HR 0.80, 95%CI 0.67-0.98; p = 0.024). IAS patients had reduced hot flashes, but otherwise there was no evidence of differences in adverse events, including myocardial events or osteoporotic fractures. Thus, in men with PSA recurrence after RRT IAS was non-inferior to CAS with respect to OS.

### 2.3.9. SWOG 9346 intergroup trial [17]

The largest trial comparing IAS and CAS in metastatic patients was reported by Hussain et al. [17]. Between 1995 and 2008, the study enrolled 3040 men with newly diagnosed metastatic disease and PSA levels ≥ 5 ng/mL. The study population was preselected for hormone sensitivity and when PSA level fell to ≤ 4 ng/mL, patients were randomized to either IAS (n = 770) stopping treatment at that point until a rise in PSA level was observed (an increase to 20 ng/mL, or for those with baseline value < 20 ng/mL, when PSA returned to baseline) or CAS (n = 765). Hormone therapy consisted of goserelin and bicalutamide for 7 months, which was in use in 1995 when the study was launched. At randomization, patients were stratified according to performance status, extent of disease, and prior exposure to hormone therapy.

At a median follow-up of 9.2 years, median overall survival was 5.1 years with IAS and 5.8 years with CAS, an absolute difference of slightly more than 6 months favoring CAS in the entire study population. The study design specified that survival with IAS would be non-inferior to CAS if the upper 95% confidence bound for the HR did not reach or include 1.2. This specification would rule out with high confidence the possibility of a 20% or greater increase in the relative risk of death with IAS. The difference between the two treatments resulted in a HR of 1.09 in favor of CAS, but the upper boundary of the 95% confidence interval was 1.24, so the conclusion was that the two treatments could not be called equivalent and survival with IAS therapy was regarded inferior to IAS by these authors. For this study, survival in both arms was much better than the expected 3-year median OS. In all examined subgroups, CAS was slightly better than IAS, with exception of extensive disease, where IAS achieved comparable survival (5 years on IAS vs 4.4 years on CAS). In this subgroup analysis, patients with minimal disease had a median overall survival of 5.2 years in the IAS group vs. 7.1 years with CAS, suggesting that the loss of almost two years of life in the intermittent group could not be ruled out. In this study "minimal disease" was defined as disease that had not spread beyond the lymph nodes or the bones of the spine or pelvis and "extensive disease" as disease that had spread beyond the spine pelvis, and lymph nodes or to the lungs or liver.

Trial participants also compared QoL measures across the two study arms during the first 15 months following patient randomization, including measures of sexual function (impotence and libido), physical and emotional function, and energy level. They found improved sexual function in men who received IAS as compared to those on continuous therapy.

### 2.3.10. FinnProstate study VII [41,42]

The FinnProstate study VII enrolled 852 men with locally advanced or metastatic prostate cancer to receive AS for 24 weeks [41]. Study inclusion criteria were M1 disease at any PSA, M0 disease at PSA 60 ng/ml or greater, or T3-4 M0 prostate cancer at PSA 20 ng/ml or greater, or previously surgically or radiotherapy treated localized prostate cancer and PSA recurrence of 20 ng/ml or greater. Patients in whom PSA decreased to less than 10 ng/ml, or by 50% or more if less than 20 ng/ml at baseline, were randomized to IAS or CAS. In the intermittent therapy arm AS was withdrawn and resumed again for at least 24 weeks based mainly on PSA decrease and increase. Of the 852 men, 554 patients were randomized and observed for a median follow-up of 65.0 months. Of these patients 71% died, including 68% in the intermittent and 74% in the continuous arm (p = 0.12). There were 248 prostate cancer deaths, comprised of 43% under IAS and 47% under CAS (p = 0.29). Median times to progression were 34.5 and 30.2 months in the intermittent and continuous arms, respectively. Median times to death (all cause) were 45.2 and 45.7 months, to prostate cancer death 45.2 and 44.3 months, and to treatment failure 29.9 and 30.5 months, respectively. Therefore, according to this trial, IAS is a feasible, efficient and safe method to treat advanced prostate cancer compared with CAS. However, the prevalence of adverse events was not significantly lower with IAS [42].

### 2.3.11. Phase III studies - Summary

In general, the phase III trials comparing IAS with CAS involved a varying number of patients, prostate cancer tumor stages ranging from biochemical relapse to metastatic and recurring disease and widely differing durations of initial AS as well as differing PSA values for the start of treatment cessations and reinitiations. Therefore, conclusions to be drawn are restricted to specific tumor stages and treatment schemes.

### 2.3.11.1. IAS – phase III – impact on survival

The Miller randomized trial of IAS versus continuous CAS in 335 patients with advanced (lymph node-positive or metastatic) prostate cancer demonstrated equivalent survival [37]. Patients in the intermittent arm were off-treatment >40% of the time. It is important to note that testosterone recovery after discontinuation of the LHRH agonist is often delayed and may depend on treatment duration, age, baseline testosterone, and ethnicity [22,43]. In the TULP trial of IAS versus CAS for advanced prostate cancer, 193 patients were randomized and, after a mean follow-up of 34 months, no difference in survival was observed [40]. The larger de Silva trial randomized 312 men to CAS and 314 men to IAS [13]. With a median follow-up of 51 months from randomization, there were fewer cancer deaths (84 vs. 106), more cardiovascular deaths (52 vs 41), and an equivalent number of total deaths (169 vs. 170) in the continuous versus intermittent arms respectively. Median time off AS was 52 weeks for patients in the intermittent arm [13]. It should be noted that the randomization criteria for all of these trials are a PSA decline of 80–90%, or to <4ng/ml, on initial AS.

In the study by Miller et al. about two thirds of patients receiving either IAS or CAS experienced clinical and/or biochemical progression, with no significant differences between groups with respect to median time to tumour progression or median time to death [37]. Similarly, Mottet et al. reported no significant difference between patients receiving IAS and CAS with respect to median overall survival (OS; 1265 vs 1560 days) and median progression-free survival (PFS) (620 vs 452 days) [38]. Tunn et al. also reported equivalency between IAS and CAS with respect to PFS (91.7 vs 93.6%) and median time to progression (1.86 vs 2.36 yr), although estimated mean PFS was longer in the IAS group compared with the CAS group (1234 vs 1010 days) [22]. In the TULP study, median time to progression was longer in the CAS arm (24.1 vs 18 months; significance not stated); more recent data from this study show no difference in OS between groups (mean follow-up of 66 months) [39,40]. The Intergroup randomized phase III trial demonstrated non-inferiority of IAS with respect to OS and time to hormone refractory state for patients with biochemical relapses after radical radiotherapy [34]. Similarly, the FinnProstate Study VII, found no significant differences in time to progression and OS, concluding that IAS is an efficient method to treat advanced prostate cancer compared with CAS [41].

However, differences in OS between CAS and IAS have been reported in two studies. De Leval et al. reported that the estimated risk of 3-year progression in CAS patients was significantly higher than in the IAS group (38.9% vs. 7%; p = 0.0052) [36]. In patients with a Gleason score >6, 3-year progression rates were significantly higher in CAS than in IAS patients (p = 0.018) but not in patients with lower Gleason scores. Compared with CAS, the IAS group had better results with respect to the number of deaths from hormone-refractory disease (4 vs. 2), number of patients with disease progression (10 vs. 3), and mean time to progression (21 vs. 28 months) (level of significance not stated for any outcome). In patients without bone metastases at initiation, risk of progression was significantly higher in CAS than IAS patients (p < 0.001). The largest trial comparing IAS to CAS is the SWOG 9346 intergroup trial, which included metastatic prostate cancer patients [17]. At a median follow-up of 9.2 years, the median overall survival was six months longer with CAS in the entire study population. This was caused by a comparable survival in extensive disease and an inferior survival in response to IAS in patients with minimal metastatic disease. The results of these two studies point to an inferior clinical results of IAS in metastatic prostate cancer.

*2.3.11.2. IAS – phase III – impact on QoL*

Early results from the study by Calais da Silva et al. showed no clinically meaningful differences between groups in virtually all QoL parameters and no evidence that IAS carries a significantly higher risk of death [13]. Mottet et al. also reported no significant difference in QoL outcomes in patients receiving either IAS or CAS [38]. However, updated results from a larger cohort of the Calais da Silva study (maximum follow-up of 7 years; median: 2 years) suggest a better tolerability profile for IAS versus CAS, with up to three times as many patients in the CAS arm reporting side effects compared with IAS patients (hot flushes: 23% vs. 7%; gynaecomastia: 33% vs. 10%; headaches: 12% vs. 5%; all p < 0.0001) [44]. Levels of sexual activity also increased in the IAS group compared with the CAS group, reported in 28 vs. 10% of patients after 15 months. Similarly, Miller et al. reported that patients' self-assessment of their overall health and sexual activity appeared to favour IAS; however, no differences in incidence of adverse events or other safety parameters were noted in this study [37]. Further evidence of QoL advantages comes from Verhagen et al. who note that EORTC scores on physical and emotional function were significantly better in the IAS group than in the CAS group. Role and social function were equivalent between groups, although cognitive function was surprisingly reduced in the IAS group, but not in the CAS group [35]. AS-related side effects were reported in most patients by de Leval et al., most of which resolved in the IA group on discontinuation of therapy [36]. In the TULP study, 26 preliminary withdrawals were reported due to adverse events, 20 in the CAS group and 6 in the IAS group [39,40]. The FinnProstate Study VII reported no significant difference in the prevalence of adverse with IAS [42]. Improved sexual function in men who received IAS as compared to CAS was confirmed in the SWOG 9346 intergroup trial [17].

*2.3.11.3. IAS – phase III trials – Conclusion*

Following pilot and phase II clinical trials comparing IAS to CAS, results of phase III studies were awaited eagerly to get a definite judgement of these different regimens of AS. The clinical results, time to progression and OS, seem to be comparable between IAS and CAS for prostate cancer patients with biochemical relapses and localized disease. With the exception of two studies, namely trials performed by the South European Uroncological Group and the SWOG 9346 intergroup, IAS was not inferior to CAS in respect to progression of disease and OS in metastatic prostate cancer. In the two dissenting studies, patients with limited metastatic disease seem to have an impaired OS under IAS. However, the statement that IAS is possibly inferior to CAS and not standard therapy of all prostate cancer patients is an oversimplification [17]. Improvements in QoL parameters were confirmed by most studies, depending on testosterone recovery and extent of disease.

| NCI Trial # | Treatment | End point/Study subject | Start | Status |
| --- | --- | --- | --- | --- |
| NCT00283803 | Exisulind | Duration of off-treatment period | 2006 | Unknown |
| NCT00686036 | Zactima ( 18 mo) | Duration of off-treatment period | 2008 | Terminated |
| NCT00553878 | Dutasteride | Duration of off-treatment period | 2007 | Ongoing |
| NCT00668642 | Dutasteride | Androgen-Response Gene Expression | 2008 | Recruiting |
| NCT00801242 | Degarelix (1 mo) | Duration of off-treatment period | 2008 | Ongoing |
| NCT00928434 | Degarelix IAS | Duration of off-treatment period /QoL | 2009 | Ongoing |
| NCT01512472 | Degarelix (4 vs 10 mo) | Duration of off-treatment period | 2011 | Recruiting |
| NCT00002651 | IAS vs. CAS | Survival/QoL Prostate cancer D2 | 1999 | Recruiting |
| NCT00223665 | IAS | Progression/QoL Localized Prostate Cancer | 2005 | Recruiting |
| NCT00378690 | ELIGARD | Survival/QoL Metastatic Prostate Cancer | 2006 | Ongoing |

**Table 2.** Overview of the IAS trials currently under investigation

### 2.4. IAS trials currently under investigation

Table 2. lists the trials comprising IAS treatment of prostate cancer patients registered in the United States National Institute of Health (NIH) clinical studies site. With exception of a few further trials comparing IAS to CAS in metastatic cancer patients, several drugs are investigated for their potential to prolong the off-treatment phase of IAS. Exisulind (Aptosyn or sulindac sulfone) may be useful as a treatment for men with advanced prostate cancer, achieving disease stabilization. This drug increases the rate of programmed cell death in cancer cells without damaging normal tissue by interfering with cyclic GMP phosphodiesterase in abnormally growing precancerous and cancerous cells [45]. Zactima (vandetanib) is an oral inhibitor of vascular endothelial growth factor receptor 2 (VEGFR-2), epidermal growth factor receptor (EGFR) and Ret tyrosine kinases involved in tumor growth, progression and angiogenesis [46]. Although, as single agent, no significant antitumor activity has been observed for Zactima in small cell lung cancer, advanced ovarian, colorectal, breast, prostate cancer and multiple myeloma. Further drugs target the androgen-stimulated growth by exploiting distinct mechanism or new formulations. Dutasteride is a non-selective inhibitor of steroid 5α-reductase, an enzyme responsible for conversion of testosterone to a more potent androgen dihydrotestosterone (DHT) approved for clinical use in treatment of benign prostate hyperplasia (BPH) and currently tested in clinical trials for prevention and treatment of prostate cancer [47]. Degarelix is a GnRH antagonist, that was found to be at least as effective as leuprolide in the ability to suppress serum testosterone to < or =0.5 ng/mL for up to 1 year in prostate cancer patients in different doses and in depot form [48]. Finally, Eligard constitutes a new leuprorelin acetate formulation that appears to achieve a testosterone suppression of 20 ng/dL in 98% of patients, while maintaining a side effect profile comparable to other products in its class [49]. It remains to be investigated, whether this use of drugs targeting androgen-independent mechanisms or improving AS can prolong the duration of the off-treatment periods of IAS and, possibly, contribute to extended survival compared to CAS.

## 3. Discussion

In many patients with prostate cancer, androgen deprivation therapy is administered over prolonged periods of time. The benefits of long-term AS in patients with advanced disease are well established, nevertheless, because this therapy has potential long-term side effects strategies should be applied that manage or prevent long-term complications [50]. One such strategy is IAS, in which patients receive regular cycles of AS, the duration of which is usually determined by PSA levels [51]. Canadian prostate cancer researchers have led the field of androgen withdrawal therapy for many years, from Nobel prize winner (Halifax born) Charles Huggins in 1940 to Nicholas Bruchovsky's Vancouver team's preclinical and clinical work on intermittent therapy in the early 1990s [52]. The basic premise of IAS is that periods (or cycles) on androgen deprivation for cancer control are followed by periods off therapy for testosterone recovery and improvements in quality of life parameters (such as libido, sexual function, energy, cognition and sense of masculinity). Preclinical studies suggest that the reintroduction of testosterone into the cellular milieu during the off-treatment period keeps the remaining cancer cells androgen-dependent, allowing for the next successful round of AS and delaying progression to hormone-resistant prostate cancer [51]. Accumulating data indicate that this approach improves the tolerability of AS and patients' QoL, without compromising clinical outcomes.

Consequently, the latest European Association of Urology guidelines state that IAS should no longer be considered investigational. Furthermore, given the adverse effects of CAS, there may be beneficial effects and potential cost savings in time off therapy with intermittent treatment, particularly if suppressive effects on prostate cancer are equivalent to CAS [53,54]. Seruga and Tannock, reviewing >1000 randomised patients, concluded that compelling data indicate that IAS should be regarded as standard therapy [54]. Likewise, Spendlove and Crawford put forward a strong argument that IAS has now demonstrated that it is no less effective than CAS and that it clearly reduces the impact of the side effects of hormone therapy on patient QoL [55]. Although current evidence suggests that IAS may be reasonable for some patients with hormone-sensitive prostate cancer, there are still questions about patient selection, timing, and methodology of IAS [56].

Results of the IAS phase III trials were expected to finally give some answers in regard to the clinical applicability and feasibility of this novel form of AS in prostate cancer patients. Phase II trials pointed to a non-inferiority of IAS as compared to CAS and improved tolerability of AS; however, these findings were only partially confirmed in phase III studies. According to the part of these trials involving patients with biochemical progression and confined disease, IAS can be regarded as non-inferior to CAS and superior in respect to QoL. For metastatic prostate cancer patients the situation seems to be different: whereas in patients with extended disease the intermittent and continuous form of AS were equivalent in respect to disease progression and OS, patients with limited metastatic disease fare worse, according to preliminary data stemming from the South European Uroncological Group trial and to definitive data from the SWOG 9346 intergroup trial [13,17]. The latter study could not exclude the loss of two years in OS in patients in which the disease that had not spread beyond the lymph nodes or the bones of the spine or pelvis. The results of Hussain et al. did not apply to men without metastases, who constitute a much larger group getting hormonal therapy. For those men IAS remain a reasonable option and even men with metastatic cancer might still opt for IAS to give their years more live instead of giving their live more years. It should be noted that the metastatic prostate cancer patients in this study had an unusual mean OS and AS consisted of a 7 months course, that may be short of the minimum of 8 months requested by Bruchovsky et al. for full downstaging [57].

The question that needs to be discussed is the selection of the prostate cancer patients who will get an optimal benefit from IAS instead of CAS. Men with local or biochemical failures after radiotherapy would benefit from IAS because they are treatment-free for longer periods of time and so are less likely to develop hormone-refractory disease [58]. De la Taille et al. identified patients >70 years of age with localised prostate cancer, a Gleason score of < 7, and a first off-therapy period of >1 year as the best candidates for IAS [59]. Grossfeld et al. recommend investigation of IAS in patients with clinically localised cancer who are not appropriate for definitive local treatment, but have significant risk of tumour progression, patients who refuse all local treatment options despite risk of progression, and those who have failed prior local therapy [60]. Poor candidates for IAS have been described as those with initial bulky tumors, with numerous lymph nodes or bone metastases, PSA doubling time <9 months, and initial serum PSA >100 ng/ml or severe pain [61]. Gleave et al. suggest that patients who fail to achieve a PSA nadir of <4 ng/ml after 6 months of therapy and most men with TxNxM1 disease should not be offered IAS, whereas those with TxN1-3M0 who are sexually active, compliant, or intolerant of AS side effects make good candidates, as long as they are informed of its investigational status [62]. Patients most likely to benefit are those with locally advanced prostate cancer with or without lymph node metastases but without any evidence of bone metastases. Also, those patients with biochemical failure following radiologic or surgical therapy for prostate cancer, those who cannot tolerate side effects of CAS, and those who wish to remain sexually active would appear to be good candidates. However, treatment should be restricted to those who can comply with close follow-up. Clearly, IAS is impossible in a significant fraction of men who do not respond to an initial course of AS.

Although the American Urological Association has not yet included IAS in its treatment guidelines for prostate cancer, the European Association of Urology acknowledged that IAS is at present widely offered to patients with prostate cancer in various clinical settings and states that its status should no longer be regarded as investigational [63,64]. This is in contrast to the American Society of Clinical Oncology practice guidelines, which state that there are currently insufficient data to support the use of IAS outside of clinical trials [65]. The 2008 UK National Institute for Health and Clinical Excellence (NICE) recommends that IAS be offered as a first-line hormonal therapy option to men with newly diagnosed or relapsing metastatic cancer, provided they are aware of its unproven status [66]. They also note that results from uncontrolled studies have shown satisfactory outcomes and that IAS will probably be more cost effective than CAS, despite the need for close monitoring. Irrespective of official guideline recommendations, IAS is a treatment option used worldwide by both urologists and oncologists outside of clinical trials. Based on available evidence and general clinical opinion, IAS is a valid treatment option in non-metastatic prostate cancer cases, that is, patients with locally advanced disease with or without lymph node involvement and those experiencing relapse following curative treatment. These patients have a higher chance of survival than those with more advanced disease, making QoL a key consideration.

Since the introduction of PSA screening in the late 1980s, more prostate cancers have been detected, and at an earlier stage that are low grade and slow growing and will not need aggressive therapy [67,68]. With this long natural history and a median survival without treatment that often approaches at least 15 to 20 years many patients will die rather with than of prostate cancer. Approximately one-third of patients who undergo radical prostatectomy will develop a detectable PSA level within 10 years [69]. Management of PSA recurrence is controversial, as prostate cancer may take an indolent course, or it may develop aggressively into metastatic disease. Prostate cancer is over-treated at present but a short course of AS might identify those patients for whom the outcome would be good with IAS by identifying those with a good PSA response. Multivariate models show the power of the initial PSA level and PSA nadir, and type of treatment and the PSA threshold for restarting treatment, in predicting outcome [21]. In those patients who rapidly achieve a good PSA nadir it is safe to shorten treatment to < 4 months. In the presence of evidence of metastasis, treatment must be protracted to ≥ 8 months. Restarting treatment when the PSA level approaches 15 ng/mL is associated with improved survival in patients with metastases, indicating the need for a more aggressive treatment strategy in these patients. Maximum androgen blockade or LHRH analog should be the standard for patients treated with IAS. The duration of biochemical remission after a period of IAS is a durable early indicator of how rapidly progression and death will occur, and will make a useful endpoint in future trials. The initial PSA level and PSA nadir allow the identification of patients with prostate cancer in whom it might be possible to avoid radical therapy.

Twenty years ago it was expected that the IAS regimen would be associated with extended survival, mainly through postponing the castration-resistant status [70]. The expected associated benefits were a decrease in the adverse effects of castration, such as hot flushes, decreased libido and erection, bone and muscle problems, depression, and metabolic syndrome (Table 3). Regarding the expected QoL and adverse effects benefits, few prospective data from randomized trials are available comparing IAS to CAS treatment. The report from Salonen et al. shows some benefit in QoL for activity limitation, physical capacity, and sexual functioning [41,42]. Surprisingly, no difference was observed in drug-induced adverse effects, such as hot flushes or night sweats. This lack of a clear sexual benefit is disappointing and a little different from what is observed in other trials, especially the South European Urooncological Group or the Miller trial [13,37]. The different questionnaires might partly explain this difference, as might the different treatment modalities, such as varied duration of treatment cycles and combined treatments or monotherapy. It was also hoped that IAS would decrease the treatment adverse effects; this decrease, at best, has been marginally obtained as the claimed QoL benefit. The thresholds, which were different from trial to trial, were only empirically chosen. The lower the PSA level after the AS induction period, the longer the survival. Therefore, the threshold of 4 ng/ml to stop the treatment in most metastatic trials might be too high and the threshold of 20 ng/ml to resume treatment might also be too high; however, it allows a longer off-treatment period, although not long enough to lead to a clear large QoL benefit [70]. Mottet concludes that apart from treatment cost, IAS does not hold to its promises and should probably be considered with caution in the most advanced situations, even in patients with a clear PSA response.

Initial goals of IAS

- Prolongation of androgen dependence and survival
- Therapy working in most stages of prostate cancer
- Reduction of the side effects of CAS
- Reduction of adverse events associated with CAS
- Reduction of the costs of prostate cancer treatment
-

Current status of IAS

- Survival under IAS not inferior to CAS?
- Prolongation of androgen-dependence of tumor not confirmed
- Most suitable for relapse after prostatectomy/radiation therapy
- Reduction of side effects of AS in most studies?
- Improved quality of life during off treatment dependent on testosterone recovery
- No consistent and optimal scheme for the implementation of IAS?
- Reduced costs of IAS compared to CAS

**Table 3.** Summary of the achievements and shortcomings of IAS

These findings for IAS are far from what was initially expected, and the presented SWOG 9346 trial added even more questions regarding IAS [17]. It has long been said that IAS does not appear to be inferior to CAS. Those results were obtained from under-powered trials or large trials including heterogeneous patients, such as the FinnProstate Study VII [41] or even the large, recently presented SWOG JPR7 [17] trial in postradiotherapy relapsing patients. None of the trials even suggested increased overall or specific survival. IAS was expected to postpone androgen independence; this finding, however, as well as an increase in OS has never been obtained in any trial. Thus, the marked elongation of hormone-dependency in the Shionogi mouse model could not be materialized in patients, which may be most likely due to increased cycle length of several months in humans compared to one month these animals, allowing for better adaptation to hormone deprivation. Furthermore, the Shionogi study was done on androgen-dependent mouse mammary carcinoma. This animal model may be insufficient to explain homeostasis of human stem cells and their progenies in relation to human prostate cancer. Miki et al. reported that human prostate cancer stem cells had no androgen receptors or PSA [71]. Guzmán-Ramírez and coworkers presented a similar protein expression pattern of prostate cancer stem cells [72]. There is a high probability that human prostate cancer stem cells are really androgen-independent. Another possibility is that two populations of stem cells exist within human prostate cancer and that the first population is androgen-sensitive and the second is androgen-independent. Our knowledge of prostate cancer stem cells is still too immature to support the rational approach for IAS therapy. Furthermore, Pfeiffer and Schalken reported difficulties in finding stem cells within established prostate cell lines in vitro, reflecting their limited use in such research [73].

In the world of medicine it has been estimated that it takes an average of 17 years for practice changing evidence to reach the bedside [52]. The first phase II study of IAS was published in 1995 and after 17 years it was advised to accept that multiple randomized controlled trials have supported its use as a non-inferior option to CAS in defined populations and to reintroduce suitable men with prostate cancer intermittently to the pleasure of their androgens [52]. High-risk patients seem to be poor candidates for any type of androgen suppression. In summary, it can be concluded from the trials that IAS is neither inferior nor superior to CAS with respect to clinical end points, namely the time period until hormone-resistance as well as cancer-specific survival, but offers significant advantages in terms of adverse effects, quality of life and costs. The off-treatment periods particularly offer the possibility to apply drugs, such as finasteride, or chemotherapeutics in order to delay disease progression [74]. However, the clinical lack of prolongation of the hormone-sensitive state of prostate cancers by IAS raises doubts about the underlying hypothesis of keeping the prostate cancer cell in an androgen responsive state by cycling between AS and off-treatment periods. Fundamental tumor biology studies in patients would be needed to clarify this issue. Otherwise IAS may be regarded as treatment regimen aiming simple for AS reduction to a level that does not permit efficient tumor growth and simultaneously lowers the side effects of AS. Patients that respond well to a first cycle of AS may go on off-treatment for years [75]. Clearly, IAS is not standard therapy for all prostate cancer patients, but a valid and favourable regimen for a significant part of selected patients.

## Acknowledgment

We thank all the patients and staff involved in our IAS trial.

## Author details

Gerhard Hamilton[1] and Gerhard Theyer[2]

*Address all correspondence to: gerhard.hamilton@toc.lbg.ac.at

1 Ludwig Boltzmann Cluster of Translational Oncology, Vienna, Austria

2 LKH Kittsee, Burgenland, Austria

## References

[1] Siegel R, Naishadham D, Jemal A. Cancer statistics. CA Cancer J. Clin.2012; 62, 10–29.

[2] Fitzpatrick JM, Schulman C, Zlotta AR, Schroeder FH. Prostate cancer: a serious dis-ease suitable for prevention. BJU Int 2009;103, 864-870.

[3] Felici A, Pino MS, Carlini P. A Changing Landscape in Castration-Resistant Prostate Cancer Treatment.Front Endocrinol (Lausanne). 2012;3:85.

[4] Lassi K. and Dawson NA. Emerging therapies in castrate-resistant prostate can-cer.CurrOpinOncol 2009;21, 260-265.

[5] Kollmeier, M.A. and Zelefsky, M.J. What is the role of androgen deprivation therapy in the treatment of locally advanced prostate cancer? Nat ClinPractUrol 2008;5, 584-585.

[6] Chang, S.S., and Kibel, A.S. The role of systemic cytotoxic therapy for prostate can-cer. BJU Int 2009;103, 8-17.

[7] Madan, R.A., Pal, S.K., Sartor, O. &Dahut, W.L. Overcoming chemotherapy resist-ance in prostate cancer. Clin Cancer Res 2011;17(12), 3892-3902.

[8] Bruchovsky, N., Goldenberg, S.L., Rennie, P.S. &Gleave M. Theoretical considera-tions and initial clinical results of intermittent hormone treatment of patients with advanced prostatic carcinoma. Urologe-A 1995;34, 389-392.

[9] Bruchovsky, N., Rennie, P.S., Coldman, A.J., Goldenberg, S.L., To, M. & Lawson D. Effects of androgen withdrawal on the stem cell composition of the Shionogi carcino-ma. Cancer Res 1990;50(8), 2275-2282.

[10]  Akakura, K., Bruchovsky, N., Goldenberg, S.L., Rennie, P.S., Buckley, A.R. & Sullivan L.D.Effects of intermittent androgen suppression on androgen-dependent tumors. Apoptosis and serum prostate-specific antigen. Cancer 1993;71(9), 2782-2790.

[11]  Rennie, P.S., Bruchovsky, N. &Coldman, A.J. Loss of androgen dependence is associated with an increase in tumorigenic stem cells and resistance to cell-death genes. J Steroid BiochemMolBiol 1990;37(6), 843-847.

[12]  Gleave, M., Santo, N., Rennie, P.S., Goldenberg, S.L., Bruchovsky, N. & Sullivan, L.D. Hormone release and intermittent hormonal therapy in the LNCaP model of human prostate cancer. ProgUrol 1996;6(3), 375-385.

[13]  Calais da Silva, F.E., Bono, A.V., Whelan, P., Brausi, M., Marques Queimadelos, A., Martin J.A., Kirkali, Z., Calais da Silva, F.M. & Robertson C. Intermittent androgen deprivation for locally advanced and metastatic prostate cancer: results from a randomised phase 3 study of the South European Uroncological Group. EurUrol 2009;55(6), 1269-1277.

[14]  Bruchovsky, N., Snoek, R., Rennie, P.S. Akakura, K., Goldenberg, L.S. &Gleave M. Control of tumor progression by maintenance of apoptosis. Prostate 1996;6S, 13-21.

[15]  Theyer, G. and Hamilton G. Current status of intermittent androgen suppression in the treatment of prostate cancer. Urology 1998;53, 353-359.

[16]  Abrahamsson P.A. Potential Benefits of Intermittent Androgen Suppression Therapy in the Treatment of Prostate Cancer.EurUrol 2010;57(1), 49-59.

[17]  Hussain M, Tangen CM, Higano CS, et al. Intermittent (IAD) versus continuous androgen deprivation (CAD) in hormone sensitive metastatic prostate cancer (HSM1PC) patients: results of S9346 (INT- 0162), an international phase III trial. J ClinOncol 2012;30(Suppl), abstract LBA 4.

[18]  Corona, G., Baldi, E. & Maggi, M. Androgen regulation of prostate cancer: Where are we now? J Endocrinol Invest 2011;34(3), 232-243.

[19]  Grossmann, M., Hamilton, E.J., Gilfillan, C., Bolton, D., Joon, D.L. &Zajac, J.D. Bone and metabolic health in patients with non-metastatic prostate cancer who are receiving androgen deprivation therapy. Med J Aust 2011;194(6), 301-306.

[20]  Buchan NC, Goldenberg SL. Intermittent androgen suppression for prostate cancer. Nat Rev Urol. 2010;7(10):552-560.

[21]  Shaw GL, Wilson P, Cuzick J, Prowse DM, Goldenberg SL, Spry NA, Oliver T. International study into the use of intermittent hormone therapy in the treatment of carcinoma of the prostate: a meta-analysis of 1446 patients. BJU Int. 2007;99(5):1056-1065.

[22]  Tunn UW, Canepa G, Kochanowsky A, Kienle E. Testosterone recovery in the off-treat ment time in prostate cancer patients undergoing intermittent androgen deprivation therapy. Prostate Cancer Prostatic Dis. 2012, in press.

[23] Bruchovsky N, Klotz L, Crook J, Phillips N, Abersbach J, Goldenberg SL.Quality of life, morbidity, and mortality results of a prospective phase II study of intermittent androgen suppression for men with evidence of prostate-specific antigen relapse after radiation therapy for locally advanced prostate cancer. ClinGenitourin Cancer. 2008;6(1):46-52.

[24] Zhu J, Wang Y, Xu S, Sun Z. Intermittent androgen blockade or continuous androgen blockade in advanced prostate cancer: a meta-analysis of efficacy, quality of life and side effects. J BUON. 2012;17(2):350-356.

[25] Malone S, Perry G, Segal R, Dahrouge S, Crook J. Long-term side effects of intermittent androgen suppression therapy in prostate cancer: results of a phase II study. BJU Int 2005;96:514–20.

[26] Bouchot O, Lenormand L, Karam G, et al. Intermittent androgen suppression in the treatment of metastatic prostate cancer. EurUrol 2000;38:543–9.

[27] Goldenberg SL, Gleave ME, Taylor D, Bruchovsky N. Clinical experience with intermittent androgen suppression in prostate cancer: Minimum of 3 years' follow-up. MolUrol 1999;3:287–292.

[28] Spry NA, Kristjanson L, Hooton B, et al. Adverse effects to quality of life arising from treatment can recover with intermittent androgen suppression in men with prostate cancer. Eur J Cancer 2006;42: 1083–1092.

[29] Yu EY, Kuo KF, Gulati R, Chen S, Gambol TE, Hall SP, Jiang PY, Pitzel P, HiganoCS.Long-term dynamics of bone mineral density during intermittent androgen deprivation for men with nonmetastatic, hormone-sensitive prostate cancer. J ClinOncol. 2012;30(15):1864-1870.

[30] Spry NA, Galvão DA, Davies R, La Bianca S, Joseph D, Davidson A, Prince R. Long-term effects of intermittent androgen suppression on testosterone recovery and bone mineral density: results of a 33-month observational study. BJU Int. 2009;104(6): 806-12.

[31] Theyer G, Holub S, Olszewski U, Hamilton G (2010) Measurement of bone turnover in prostate cancer patients receiving intermittent androgen suppression therapy. OA Journal of Urology 2010;2: 155-159.

[32] Hamilton G, Olszewski-Hamilton U, Theyer G. Type I collagen synthesis marker procollagen I N-terminal peptide (PINP) in prostate cancer patients undergoing intermittent androgen suppression. Cancers 2011;3: 3601-3609.

[33] Ng E, Woo HH, Turner S, Leong E, Jackson M, Spry N. The influence of testosterone suppression and recovery on sexual function in men with prostate cancer: observations from a prospective study in men undergoing intermittent androgen suppression. J Urol. 2012;187(6):2162-2166.

[34] L. Klotz, C. J. O'Callaghan, K. Ding, D. P. Dearnaley, C. S. Higano, E. M. Horwitz, S. Malone, S. L. Goldenberg, M. K. Gospodarowicz, J. M. Crook. A phase III random-

ized trial comparing intermittent versus continuous androgen suppression for patients with PSA progression after radical therapy: NCIC CTG PR.7/SWOG PR.7/CTSU JPR.7/UK Intercontinental Trial CRUKE/01/013. J ClinOncol 29: 2011 (suppl 7; abstr 3).

[35] Verhagen, P.C.M.S.1, Wissenburg, L.D.1, Wildhagen, M.F.1, Bolle, W.A.B.M.1, Verkerk, A.M.1, Schroder, F.H.1, Bangma, C.H.1, Mickisch, G.H.2 Quality of life effects of intermittent and continuous hormonal therapy by cyproterone acetate (CPA) for metastatic prostate cancercancer [abstract 541]. Presented at: 23rd Annual Congress of the European Association of Urology; March 26–29, 2008; Milan, Italy.

[36] de Leval J, Boca P, Yousef E, Nicolas H, Jeukenne M, Seidel L, Bouffioux C, Coppens L, Bonnet P, Andrianne R, Wlatregny D. Intermittent versus continuous total androgen blockade in the treatment of patients with advanced hormone-naive prostate cancer: results of a prospective randomized multicenter trial. Clin Prostate Cancer. 2002;1(3):163-171.

[37] Miller K, Steiner U, Lingnau A, et al. Randomised prospective study of intermittent versus continuous androgen suppression in advanced prostate cancer [abstract 5105]. Presented at: American Society of Clinical Oncology; June 1–5, 2007; Chicago, IL, USA.

[38] Mottet N, Van Damme J, Loulidi S, Russel C, Leitenberger A, Wolff JM, the TAP22 Investigators Group. Intermittent hormonal therapy in the treatment of metastatic prostate cancer: a randomized trial. BJU Int. In press.

[39] Langenhuijsen JF, Schasfoort EMC, Heathcote P, et al. Intermittent androgen suppression in patients with advanced prostate cancer: an update of the TULP survival data [abstract 538]. Presented at: 23rd Annual Congress of the European Association of Urology; March 26–29, 2008; Milan, Italy.

[40] Langenhuijsen JF, Badhauser D, Schaaf B, Kiemeney LA, Witjes JA, Mulders PF. Continuous vs. intermittent androgen deprivation therapy for metastatic prostate cancer.UrolOncol. 2011, in press.

[41] Salonen AJ, Taari K, Ala-Opas M, Viitanen J, Lundstedt S, Tammela TL; FinnProstate Group. The FinnProstate Study VII: Intermittent Versus Continuous Androgen Deprivation in Patients with Advanced Prostate Cancer. J Urol. 2012;187(6):2074-2081.

[42] Salonen AJ, Taari K, Ala-Opas M, Viitanen J, Lundstedt S, Tammela TL; the FinnProstate Group. Advanced Prostate Cancer Treated with Intermittent or Continuous Androgen Deprivation in the RandomisedFinnProstate Study VII: Quality of Life and Adverse Effects. Eur Urol. 2012, in press.

[43] Gulley JL, Figg WD, Steinberg SM, et al. A prospective analysis of the time to normalization of serum androgens following 6 months of androgen deprivation therapy in patients on a randomized phase III clinical trial using limited hormonal therapy. J Urol 2005;173:1567–1571.

[44] Calais da Silva FE, Goncales F, Santos A, et al. Evaluation of quality of life, side effects and duration of therapy in a phase 3 study of intermittent monotherapy versus continuous androgen deprivation [abstract 540]. Presented at: 23rd Annual Congress of the European Association of Urology; March 26–29, 2008; Milan, Italy.

[45] Webster WS, Leibovich BC. Exisulind in the treatment of prostate cancer.Expert Rev Anticancer Ther. 2005;5(6):9579-62.

[46] Morabito A, Piccirillo MC, Costanzo R, Sandomenico C, Carillio G, Daniele G, Giordano P, Bryce J, Carotenuto P, La Rocca A, Di Maio M, Normanno N, Rocco G, Perrone F. Vandetanib: An overview of its clinical development in NSCLC and other tumors. Drugs Today (Barc). 2010;46(9):683-698.

[47] Schmidt LJ, Tindall DJ. Steroid 5 α-reductase inhibitors targeting BPH and prostate cancer. J Steroid BiochemMol Biol. 2011;125(1-2):32-38.

[48] Steinberg M. Degarelix: a gonadotropin-releasing hormone antagonist for the management of prostate cancer. ClinTher. 2009;31Pt 2:2312-2331.

[49] Berges R, Bello U. Effect of a new leuprorelin formulation on testosterone levels in patients with advanced prostate cancer. CurrMed Res Opin. 2006;22(4):649-655.

[50] Schulman C, Irani J, Aapro M. Improving the management of patients with prostate cancer receiving long-term androgen deprivation therapy.BJU Int.2012;109Suppl 6:13-21.

[51] Hamilton G, Olszewski-Hamilton U., Theyer G. Intermittent Androgen Suppression Therapy for Prostate Cancer Patients: A Choice for Improved Quality of Life? Prostate Cancer - Diagnostic and Therapeutic Advances, 2011;18;363-378.

[52] Ischia J, S., Goldenberg L. Intermittent Androgen Suppression—Ready for Prime Time? J Urol, 2012;187(6), 1956–1957.

[53] Seruga B, Tannock F. Intermittent androgen blockade should be regarded as standard therapy in prostate cancer. Nat ClinPractOncol 2008;5:574–576.

[54] Sharifi N, Gulley JL, Dahut WL. Continuous ADT versus intermittent ADT.An update on androgen deprivation therapy for prostate cancer.EndocrRelat Cancer. 2010;17(4):R305-315.

[55] Spendlove J, Crawford D. Intermittent Versus Continuous Androgen Deprivation Therapy. AUA News,2012;16(5), 13-14.

[56] Keizman D, Carducci MA Intermittent androgen deprivation--questions remain. Nat Rev Urol. 2009;6(8):412-414.

[57] Gleave, M.E, Goldenberg, S.L., Jones, E.C., Bruchovsky N. & Sullivan L.D. Maximal biochemical and pathological downstaging requires eight months of neoadjuvant hormonal therapy prior to radical prostatectomy. J Urol 1996;155, 213-219.

[58] Crook JM, Szumacher E, Malone S, Huan S, Segal R. Intermittent androgen suppression in the management of prostate cancer. Urology 1999;53:530–534.

[59] de la Taille A, Zerbib M, Conquy S, et al. Intermittent androgen suppression in patients with prostate cancer. BJU Int 2003;91:18–22.

[60] Goldenberg SL, Gleave ME, Taylor D, Bruchovsky N. Clinical experience with intermittent androgen suppression in prostate cancer: Minimum of 3 years' follow-up. MolUrol 1999;3:287–292.

[61] Grossfeld GD, Small EJ, Carroll PR. Intermittent androgen deprivation for clinically localized prostate cancer: initial experience. Urology 1998;51:137–44.

[62] Gleave M, Klotz L, Taneja SS. The continued debate: intermittent vs.continuous hormonal ablation for metastatic prostate cancer. UrolOncol 2009;27:81–86.

[63] American Urological Association. Guideline for the management of clinically localized prostate cancer: 2007 update. Linthicum, MD: American Urological Association; 2007.

[64] Heidenreich A, Aus G, Bolla M, et al. Guidelines on prostate cancer. European Association of Urology 2007;1–114.

[65] Loblaw DA, Virgo KS, Nam R, et al. Initial hormonal management of androgen- sensitive metastatic, recurrent, or progressive prostate cancer: 2006 update of an American Society of Clinical Oncology practice guideline. J ClinOncol 2007;25:1596–1605.

[66] National Institute for Health and Clinical Excellence. Prostate cancer: diagnosis and treatment. February 2008. http://www.nice.org.uk/CGO58. Accessed on 3 July 2008.

[67] Gjertson CK, Albertsen PC. Use and assessment of PSA in prostate cancer. Med Clin North Am. 2011;95(1):191-200.

[68] Carroll PR. Early stage prostate cancer – do we have a problem with overdetection, overtreatment or both? J Urol 2005; 173:1061–1062.

[69] Tzou K, Tan WW, Buskirk S. Treatment of men with rising prostate-specific antigen levels following radical prostatectomy. Expert Rev Anticancer Ther. 2011;11(1): 125-136.

[70] Mottet N. Intermittent Androgen Deprivation Therapy in Prostate Cancer: Is Everything So Clear?Eur Urol. 2012 in press.

[71] Miki J. Investigations of prostate epithelial stem cells and prostate cancer stem cells. Int J Urol. 2010;17(2):139-147.

[72] Guzmán-Ramírez N, Völler M, Wetterwald A, Germann M, Cross NA, Rentsch CA, Schalken J, Thalmann GN, Cecchini MG. In vitro propagation and characterization of neoplastic stem/progenitor-like cells from human prostate cancer tissue.Prostate. 2009;69(15):1683-1693.

[73]  M.J. Pfeiffer, J.A. Schalken. Stem cell characteristics in prostate cancer cell lines. Eur-Urol, 2010;57:246–255.

[74]  Locke, J.A. &Bruchovsky, N. Prostate cancer: finasteride extends PSA doubling time during intermittent hormone therapy.Can J Urol 2010;7(3), 5162-5169.

[75]  Theyer, G., Ulsperger, E., Baumgartner, G., Raderer, M. & Hamilton, G. Prolonged response to a single androgen suppression phase in a subpopulation of prostate cancer patients. Ann Oncol 2000;11, 877-881.

# Permissions

The contributors of this book come from diverse backgrounds, making this book a truly international effort. This book will bring forth new frontiers with its revolutionizing research information and detailed analysis of the nascent developments around the world.

We would like to thank Gerhard Hamilton, PhD, for lending his expertise to make the book truly unique. He has played a crucial role in the development of this book. Without his invaluable contribution this book wouldn't have been possible. He has made vital efforts to compile up to date information on the varied aspects of this subject to make this book a valuable addition to the collection of many professionals and students.

This book was conceptualized with the vision of imparting up-to-date information and advanced data in this field. To ensure the same, a matchless editorial board was set up. Every individual on the board went through rigorous rounds of assessment to prove their worth. After which they invested a large part of their time researching and compiling the most relevant data for our readers. Conferences and sessions were held from time to time between the editorial board and the contributing authors to present the data in the most comprehensible form. The editorial team has worked tirelessly to provide valuable and valid information to help people across the globe.

Every chapter published in this book has been scrutinized by our experts. Their significance has been extensively debated. The topics covered herein carry significant findings which will fuel the growth of the discipline. They may even be implemented as practical applications or may be referred to as a beginning point for another development. Chapters in this book were first published by InTech; hereby published with permission under the Creative Commons Attribution License or equivalent.

The editorial board has been involved in producing this book since its inception. They have spent rigorous hours researching and exploring the diverse topics which have resulted in the successful publishing of this book. They have passed on their knowledge of decades through this book. To expedite this challenging task, the publisher supported the team at every step. A small team of assistant editors was also appointed to further simplify the editing procedure and attain best results for the readers.

Our editorial team has been hand-picked from every corner of the world. Their multi-ethnicity adds dynamic inputs to the discussions which result in innovative outcomes. These outcomes are then further discussed with the researchers and contributors who give their valuable feedback and opinion regarding the same. The feedback is then collaborated with the researches and they are edited in a comprehensive manner to aid the understanding of the subject.

Apart from the editorial board, the designing team has also invested a significant amount of their time in understanding the subject and creating the most relevant covers. They scrutinized every image to scout for the most suitable representation of the subject and create an appropriate cover for the book.

The publishing team has been involved in this book since its early stages. They were actively engaged in every process, be it collecting the data, connecting with the contributors or procuring relevant information. The team has been an ardent support to the editorial, designing and production team. Their endless efforts to recruit the best for this project, has resulted in the accomplishment of this book. They are a veteran in the field of academics and their pool of knowledge is as vast as their experience in printing. Their expertise and guidance has proved useful at every step. Their uncompromising quality standards have made this book an exceptional effort. Their encouragement from time to time has been an inspiration for everyone.

The publisher and the editorial board hope that this book will prove to be a valuable piece of knowledge for researchers, students, practitioners and scholars across the globe.

# List of Contributors

**Martin Dörr, Anne Schlesinger-Raab and Jutta Engel**
Munich Cancer Registry (MCR), Clinic Großhadern / IBE, Ludwig-Maximilians-University (LMU), Germany

**Ugo Rovigatti**
University of Pisa Medical School, Pisa, Italy

**Mario Bernardo Filho**
Coordenadoria de Pesquisa, Instituto Nacional de Câncer and Departamento de Biofísica e Biometria, Instituto de Biologia Roberto Alcântara Gomes, Universidade do Estado do Rio de Janeiro, Rio de Janeiro, RJ, Brasil

**Mauro Luis Barbosa Júnior**
Departamento de Medicina de Integral Familiar e Comunitária, Hospital Universitário Pedro Ernesto, Universidade do Estado do Rio de Janeiro, Rio de Janeiro, RJ, Brasil

**Luke A Robles, Shihning Chou and Amanda Griffiths**
Institute of Work, Health & Organisation, The University of Nottingham, Nottingham, UK

**Owen J Cole**
Department of Urology, The Medical Specialist Group, Guernsey

**Akhlil Hamid**
Department of Urology and University of Western Australia, Royal Perth Hospital, Western Australia

**Kavita Vedhara**
Division of Primary Care, The University of Nottingham, Nottingham, UK

**Shinji Kariya**
Department of Diagnostic Radiology and Radiation Oncology, Kochi Medical School, Kohasu, Oko-town, Kochi, Japan

**Zachary Klaassen, Kelvin A. Moses, Rabii Madi and Martha K. Terris**
Department of Surgery, Section of Urology, Georgia Health Sciences University, Augusta, Georgia

**Ray S. King**
Department of Surgery, Georgia Health Sciences University, Augusta, Georgia

Pedro J. Prada
Department of Radiation Oncology, Hospital Universitario Marques de Valdecilla, Santander, Spain

Tine Hajdinjak
Center UROL Maribor, Slovenia
Medical Faculty, University of Maribor, Maribor, Slovenia
Division of Urology, Department of Surgery, General Hospital Murska Sobota, Slovenia

Glenn Tisman
Whittier Cancer Research Building, Whittier, CA, USA

Sarah M. Rudman and Peter G. Harper
Dept of Oncology, Guys & St Thomas' NHS Foundation Trust, Great Maze Pond, London, SE1 9RT, UK

Christopher J. Sweeney
Lank Center for Genitourinary Oncology, Dana Farber Cancer Institute, 450 Brookline Ave, Boston, MA, USA

Jorge A. R. Salvador
Laboratório de Química Farmacêutica, Faculdade de Farmácia, Universidade de Coimbra, Pólo das Ciências da Saúde, Azinhaga de Santa Comba, Coimbra, Portugal
Centro de Neurociências e Biologia Celular, Universidade de Coimbra, Coimbra, Portugal

Vânia M. Moreira
Division of Pharmaceutical Chemistry, Faculty of Pharmacy, Viikinkaari, University of Helsinki, Helsinki, Finland

Samuel M. Silvestre
Health Sciences Research Centre, Faculdade de Ciências da Saúde, Universidade da Beira Interior, Covilhã, Portugal

Miguel Álvarez Múgica, Erasmo Miguelez García and Francisco Valle González
Urology Department, Hospital Valle Nalón, Spain

Jesús M. Fernández Gómez and Antonio Jalón Monzón
Urology Department, HUCA, Spain

Jesús M. Fernández Gómez
University of Oviedo, Spain

Gerhard Hamilton
Ludwig Boltzmann Cluster of Translational Oncology, Vienna, Austria

Gerhard Theyer
LKH Kittsee, Burgenland, Austria